Prakash's

Atlas of Primary Hip Arthroplasty

N o sponsorship or benefits have been received from any commercial organization or company for production of this book.

This book does not advocate or propagate any particular brand, design or company or their total hip joints or brand of bone cement. That choice is left to the reader.

All my income from the sale of this book would be used for pure and applied research into the normal and abnormal joints, and for performing surgeries on economically underprivileged patients.

L Prakash

Books by Same Author

Orthopaedic Books

Prakash's

Atlas of Primary Hip Arthroplasty

The Book is accompanied by 6 Disks with the following contents

A. Operative DVDs

5 DVDs describing various procedures

B. Audiobook

1 Audio CD containing the whole audiobook. Each chapter as a separate to act.

L Prakash

MS (Orth), MCh (Orth) (Liverpool)

Institute for Special Orthopaedics
Chennai, Tamil Nadu

CBS

CBS Publishers & Distributors Pvt Ltd

New Delhi • Bengaluru • Chennai • Kochi • Kolkata • Mumbai
Hyderabad • Nagpur • Patna • Pune • Vijayawada

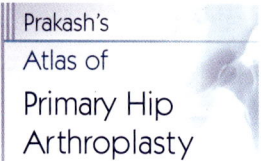

Prakash's
Atlas of
Primary Hip
Arthroplasty

ISBN: 978-93-86217-74-5

Copyright © Author and Publisher

First Edition: 2017

Published by Satish Kumar Jain and produced by Varun Jain for

CBS Publishers & Distributors Pvt Ltd

4819/XI Prahlad Street, 24 Ansari Road, Daryaganj, New Delhi 110 002, India.
Ph: 23289259, 23266861, 23266867 Website: www.cbspd.com
Fax: 011-23243014   e-mail: delhi@cbspd.com; cbspubs@airtelmail.in.
Corporate Office: 204 FIE, Industrial Area, Patparganj, Delhi 110 092

Ph: 4934 4934   Fax: 4934 4935   e-mail: publishing@cbspd.com; publicity@cbspd.com

Branches

- **Bengaluru:** Seema House 2975, 17th Cross, K.R. Road,
  Banasankari 2nd Stage, Bengaluru 560 070, Karnataka
  Ph: +91-80-26771678/79   Fax: +91-80-26771680   e-mail: bangalore@cbspd.com
- **Chennai:** 7, Subbaraya Street, Shenoy Nagar, Chennai 600 030, Tamil Nadu
  Ph: +91-44-26680620, 26681266   Fax: +91-44-42032115   e-mail: chennai@cbspd.com
- **Kochi:** Ashana House, No. 39/1904, AM Thomas Road, Valanjambalam,
  Ernakulam 682 016, Kochi, Kerala
  Ph: +91-484-4059061-65   Fax: +91-484-4059065   e-mail: kochi@cbspd.com
- **Kolkata:** 6/B, Ground Floor, Rameswar Shaw Road, Kolkata-700 014, West Bengal
  Ph: +91-33-22891126, 22891127, 22891128   e-mail: kolkata@cbspd.com
- **Mumbai:** 83-C, Dr E Moses Road, Worli, Mumbai-400018, Maharashtra
  Ph: +91-22-24902340/41   Fax: +91-22-24902342   e-mail: mumbai@cbspd.com

Representatives

- **Hyderabad** 0-9885175004 • **Nagpur** 0-9021734563 • **Patna** 0-9334159340
- **Pune** 0-9623451994 • **Vijayawada** 0-9000660880

Printed at Rashtriya Printers, Dilshad Garden, Delhi, India

About this Atlas

This is an illustrated book teaching the technique of primary hip arthroplasty. Independent of the design or method of fixation used, the long-term success of a hip replacement depends on three points.

1. Accurate placement of the acetabular component.
2. Precise balance of the hip abductor mechanism and a correct limb length achievement.
3. Perfect preparation of bone surfaces for an excellent bone/implant interface.
4. Correct cementation with a perfect bone-cement-implant bond in a cemented hip.
5. Best and precise fit between implants and bone in cementless hips.

This is a 50% *pictures* and 50% *text* Atlas, and I hope the reader enjoys reading it at least as much as I enjoyed writing it!

L Prakash

Foreword

Dr L Prakash has been my close friend for the last thirty years. He was one of the early arthroplasty surgeons in this country, who was manufacturing cementless hips and ceramic heads way back in 1991.

I have always felt that Prakash has been extremely lucky to be at the right place at the right time. He saw hip replacements evolve, and saw history being made. His unending passion for arthroplasty took him to every surgeon of repute and he has worked under the legends in joint replacement, including Mullar, Ring, Freeman, Goodfelow, Monk, Wroblowski, Young, Taylor, and many others, each of whom bears a joint in their name. He has donned many a hat, as a surgeon, industrialist, implant manufacturer, and then an author, artist, sculptor, designer, inventor, scientist and teacher. His current avatar as a medical illustrator and author is most welcome, because he has begun filling important gaps in medical literature. Orthopaedic books are usually written in a dull stiff language, making it difficult for non native English speakers to understand them fully.

Using a simple language and short sentences, Prakash has written this book in his own narrative style.

The accompanying DVDs are shot really well from correct angles. The narration and text are perfect. The book is abundant in illustrations and short in words, explaining everything with great clarity.

The book would be of great use to any surgeon involved with arthroplasty and is a must-read for every young resident hoping to specialize in this exciting field. Written with great passion, full of personal anecdotes, this book reads like a story book, but is more informative than most textbooks on primary hip arthroplasty.

He has devoted an entire section on hemiarthroplasties, something I have never seen in most arthroplasty books. Sprinkled with personal advice and many tricks and tips one does not find in the literature, this atlas is a pleasure to read and savour.

It is a pleasure to write the Foreword to this book.

Mayilvahanan Natarajan

Former Vice Chancellor
MGR Medical University

Former President
Indian Orthopaedic Association

Acknowledgments

My parents Mr TS Lakshmanane and Radha Lakshman, I owe my existence to them.

Dr TS Ramaswamy and Dr Pramila Ramaswamy, who made my life worth living, and because of whom I am now a medical teacher and scientist.

Dr Mayil, my best friend, and more importantly my foul weather friend.

TG Seshadri, my medical assistant, who learnt photography, designed a sterilizable camera sleeve, and who scrubbed up in every case, to take the brilliant closeup photos and the excellent videos in this book.

Jagga, my biomedical engineer, Puliarasi my orthopaedic nurse, and Babu my Man Friday, who help me to stretch my day beyond twenty-four hours.

Mr LR Ashok, my editor, who has rendered the book flawless as far as the language and grammar are concerned. My patients who placed their trust in me from the time I began implanting locally forged and machined implants twenty-five years ago.

L Prakash

Contents

1

Anatomy of The Hip Joint

THE HIP JOINT

Bony Landmarks and Surface Anatomy

The following bony landmarks are easily identifiable:
1. Symphysis Pubis
2. Anteriosuperior iliac spine and Iliac crest
3. Posteriosuperior iliac spine
4. Greater Trochanter
5. Ischial tuberosity
6. Pubic tubercle

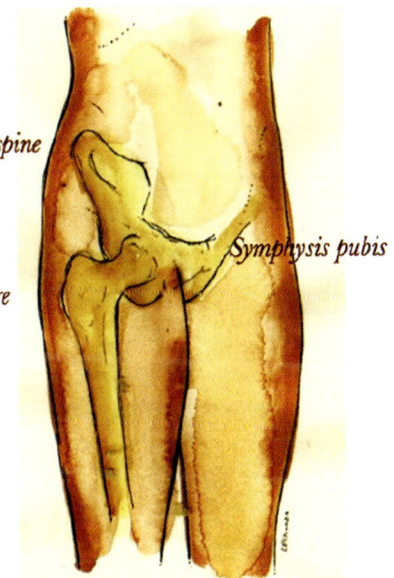

Surface landmarks of the hip joint

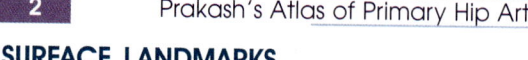

SURFACE LANDMARKS

It is important to have a thorough idea of the entire surface landmarks; as all of these will be the reference points whilst the surgery is in progress. The anterosuperior iliac spine, is the most prominent anterior part of the pelvis and, is the principal reference for limb length measurement, for pelvic orientation and for a reference point for cup placement.

The Iliac crest follows this lateral to posterior and; the second prominence of the crest lying posteriorly is the posterosuperior Iliac spine. From the midpoint of these two crests if one runs down a finger, the next prominent part is the flare of the greater trochanter and; this is the midpoint of most skin incisions for the lateral and posterior approaches to the hip joint.

The trochanteric flare can be identified and located with ease, as one rotates the limb whilst the palm is kept on the upper lateral part of the thigh when the mobile flare lump is obvious.

The anterior part of the head of the femur is palpable at the inguinal region with the femoral artery pulsations being a landmark and reference.

Both knee joint levels are identified by locating the joint line by knee movements, and Medial and Lateral Malleoli are other reference points to measure limb length, or the rotational and axial positioning of the femoral component.

Vital Structures Around the Hip

The surgeon has to be very careful of six arteries, four nerves, two veins and two cutaneous nerves; which are the important structures around the hip.

These are

Arteries: Femoral artery, medial circumflex artery, lateral circumflex artery, obturator, superior gluteal and inferior gluteal arteries.

Nerves: Sciatic, femoral, superior gluteal and obturator are the deep nerves, while lateral and posterior cutaneous nerves are superficial.

Veins: Femoral and long saphenous are the larger veins.

The three drawings below show the anterior, posterior and sectional anatomy of the hip.

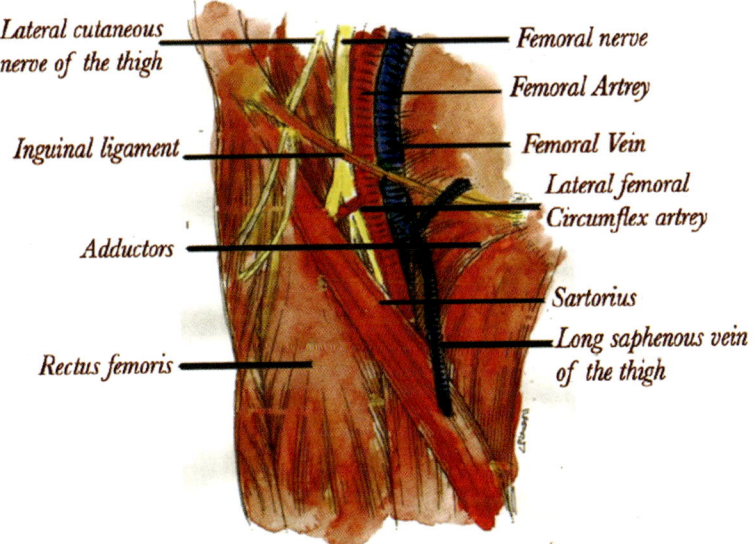

Lateral cutaneous nerve of the thigh

Inguinal ligament

Adductors

Rectus femoris

Femoral nerve

Femoral Artrey

Femoral Vein

Lateral femoral Circumflex artrey

Sartorius

Long saphenous vein of the thigh

Structures on the anterior side

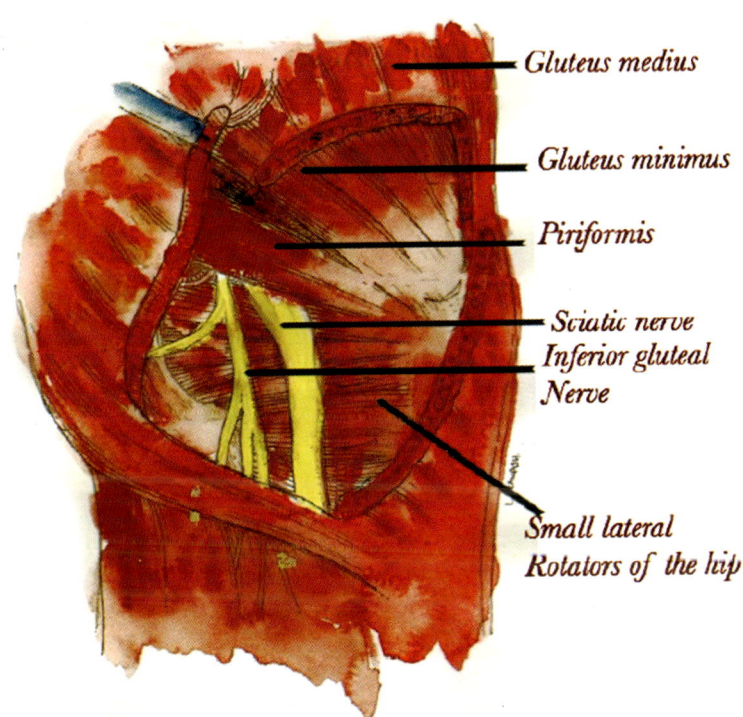

Gluteus medius

Gluteus minimus

Piriformis

Sciatic nerve

Inferior gluteal Nerve

Small lateral Rotators of the hip

Structures posteriorly

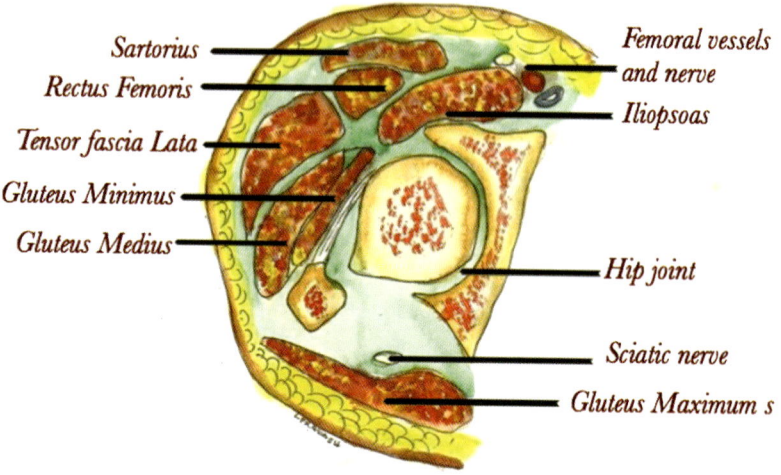

Anatomical planes for hip approach

The line between the pubic tubercle to the anteriosuperior iliac spine is the groin crease. Over its midpoint lie the femoral neurovascular structures.

The sciatic nerve lies at the midpoint of a line between greater trochanter and ischial tuberosity.

The femoral and superior gluteal nerves are under risk with anterior approaches, while the sciatic nerve should be identified and protected in posterior approaches.

Likewise obturator nerve is at risk with medial approaches.

THE RELATIONS OF THE HIP JOINT

As opposed to an anatomist, the surgeon has to understand the circumferential centrifugal anatomy of the joint in a three dimensional perspective. Starting from the inside (with the acetabulum and the head of the femur, as the central point), as one goes outside; one has to have a fair idea of the structures he will encounter. As there are many approaches to the hip joint, the Surgeon should at least have an absolute familiarity to the structures he will encounter, as he approaches it from the incision he wants to use.

All around the joint is the fibrous capsule which is a strong and dense structure. It is attached to the margin of the acetabulum 5 mm beyond the acetabular labrum in front, to the outer margin of the labrum, and to the transverse acetabular ligament and the edge of the obturator foramen.

On the femoral side it is attached in front to the trochanteric line, above to the base of the neck, behind to the neck above the trochanteric crest, and below to the lower part of the neck closer to the lesser trochanter. This sleeve like structure can be imagined enveloping the neck arising from the baso trochanteric area and going up to the acetabular margins.

The capsule is surrounded by muscles on all sides. *Anteriorly,* lie the lateral fibres of the pectineus and the femoral vein. Lateral to pectineus, the tendon of the psoas major, with the Iliacus on its lateral side runs downwards across the front of the capsule. At this level the femoral artery is on the psoas tendon and the femoral nerve lies deeply in the groove behind the tendon and the Iliacus.

More laterally, the straight head of Rectus Femoris crosses the joint and the deep layer of the iliotibial band blends with the fibrous capsule.

Superiorly, the reflected head of the Rectus Femoris and Gluteus Minimus are present with the latter being closely adherent to it.

Inferiorly, the lateral fibres of pectineus lie on the capsule as they incline backwards and more posteriorly, the obturator externus crosses obliquely to reach the posterior aspect of the joint.

Posteriorly, the lower part of the capsule is covered with the tendon of the obturator externus, which separates it from the quadratus Femoris and is accompanied by the ascending branch of the medial circumflex femoral artery. Above that are the tendon of obturator internus and the two gamelli which lie between the joint and the sciatic nerve.

The uppermost part of the posterior aspect of the articular capsule is crossed by the piriformis.

THE ANATOMY OF THE HIP AS PERTINENT TO ARTHROPLASTY

Hip joint is the largest ball and socket of the body. The acetabular part; formed by all the three components of the pelvis, articulates with the femoral head. In the undiseased, this is probably one of the stablest joints. A deep cup and an almost spherical head lead to a mechanical stability which is augmented with the presence of ligamentum teres which binds the two components.

FEMUR

There are three points of importance as regards the upper femur. The anteversion, the neck shaft angle and the relation of the femoral medulla with reference to the greater and lesser trochanters.

ANTEVERSION

The anteversion is the angle at which the head faces in the coronal plane with reference to the long axis of the bone. For simple explanation, we could look the femur end on from the top and compare the axis of the deviation of the femoral head in relation with the lesser trochanter; and this will be the anteversion.

Thus if the patient lies supine and the femoral condyles lie parallel to the bed, the head will be lifted towards the ceiling to about 9 degrees to 16 degrees -which is the normal anteversion.

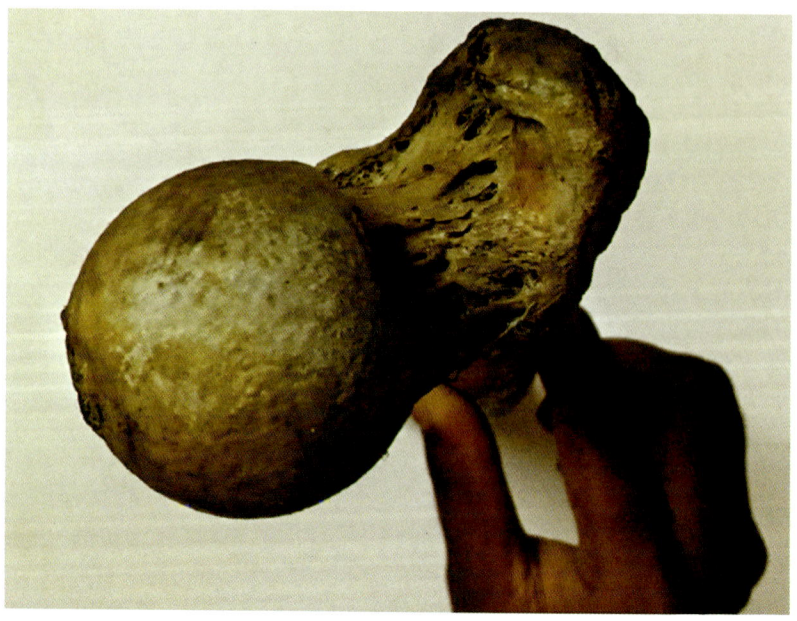

If the head were to face the ceiling the head would be markedly anteverted. On the contrary, if it were to get closer to the bed or even go further posteriorly it would move on from anteversion to neutral and thence to retroversion.

At the cost of repetition

Anteversion is the extent to which the femoral head deviates from the axis of the shaft.

When one replaces the upper end of femur this aspect of anatomy becomes quite important, because if the head faces too much posteriorly when the toes point towards the roof, a large amount of the femoral head will be uncovered in the back and a little internal rotation will cause the hip to dislocate.

In a neutral position only a small portion of head remains uncovered, and a full coverage is achieved in 15 degrees of anteversion. This is because of the position of acetabulum in relation to the long axis of the body. Any further facing of the head greater than this 15 degrees causes an opening anteriorly and this would result in excess of anteversion causing anterior instability.

THE NECK SHAFT ANGLE

Whilst the anteversion is the orientation of the head to the shaft in coronal plane, the neck shaft angle is the orientation in the sagittal plane.

This can be seen easily in the AP radiograph and by simply drawing a line through the long axis of the femoral shaft and that of the head and neck one can deduce the angle. With an average of 133 degrees, verticality an increase of the angle is called Valgus and bringing it closer to a right angle is called Varus.

A pre operative assessment of the existing anatomical Valgus is very important because in the manmade implants the neck is straight, whereas in anatomical specimens and the patient, there are slight deviations and curvature which allow for stability and a uniform distribution of forces across the joints.

When the head is vertical the upper part of the femoral head remains uncovered with the leg in neutral position and this uncovering increases as the limb is adducted. With abduction

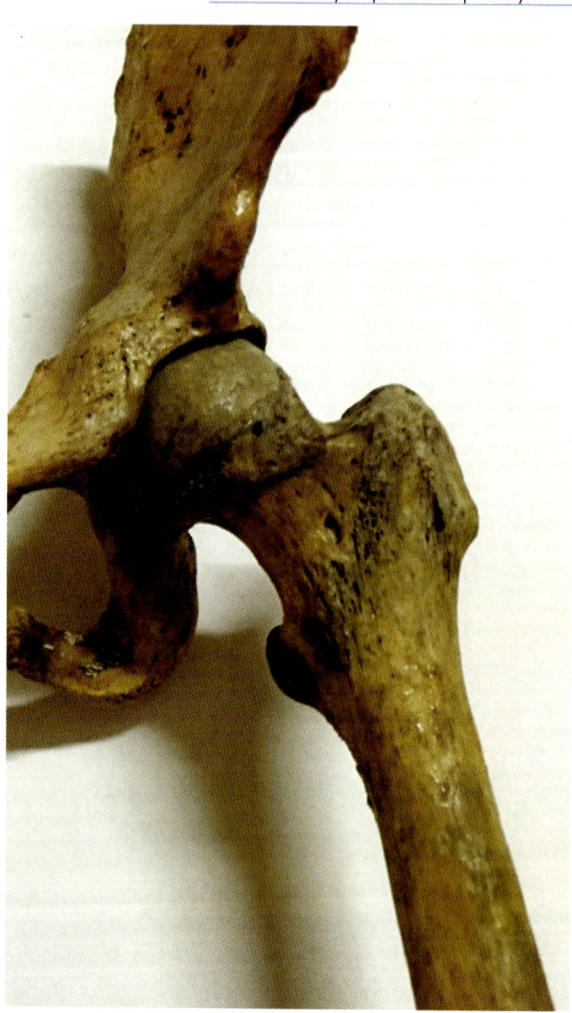

the coverage increases. Likewise if the head is horizontal or in varus; in neutral there is an inferior uncovering which reduces with adduction but increases with abduction of the limb. In an ideal situation with the limb in neutral position with reference to abduction and adduction, the amount of uncovered head should be minimal.

With the above description it is evident that whilst anteversion would be important with the rotation of the limb, the neck shaft angle is important when the limb is abducted or adducted. With over three hundred degrees of movement possible in the average

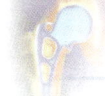
hip in all directions it is not difficult to envisage why minimal changes in either of the two would alter biomechanics and stability in one extreme or other of movement.

RELATION OF THE FEMORAL MEDULLA TO THE TROCHANTER AND THE FEMUR

The femoral medulla is an extended hourglass with a short upper bowl and a long lower bowl. The medullary cavity starts at the level of the lesser trochanter and flows down to the level of the condyles.

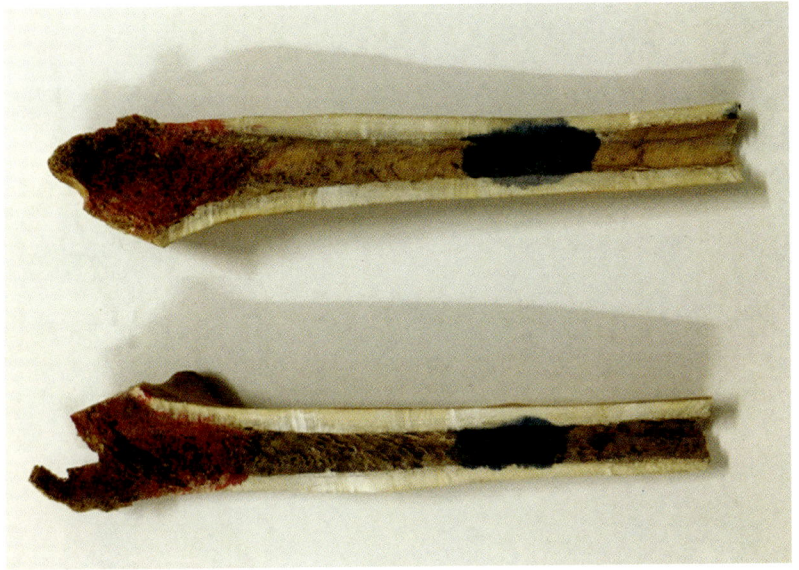

Both above and below it blends with the cancellous bone which is abundant both in the trochanteric area and the condylar area of the femur. The narrowest part of the medullary canal is the isthmus.

The medullary canal is present slightly medially nearer to the lesser trochanter that to the greater trochanter and whilst one reams the femur from upwards, the direction should be straight going deep into the back of the flare of the greater trochanter to identify the trochanter and to avoid making a false passage and perforating the cortex.

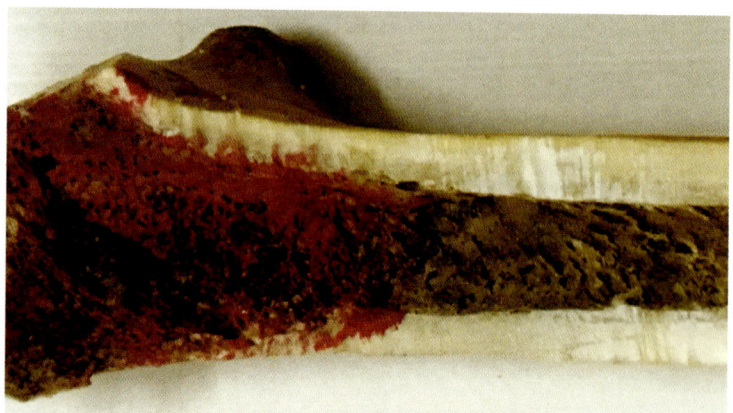

THE PELVIS

Again there are three aspects which are important. The orientation of the acetabulum with relation to the coronal plane or version, the orientation in relation to the sagittal plane referring to the shallowness or depth of the cavity and the various amounts of bone thickness all around the acetabulum.

ACETABULAR VERSION

The normal acetabulum is retroverted by about 12 to 15 degrees. Retroversion means that as the patient is lying supine; the

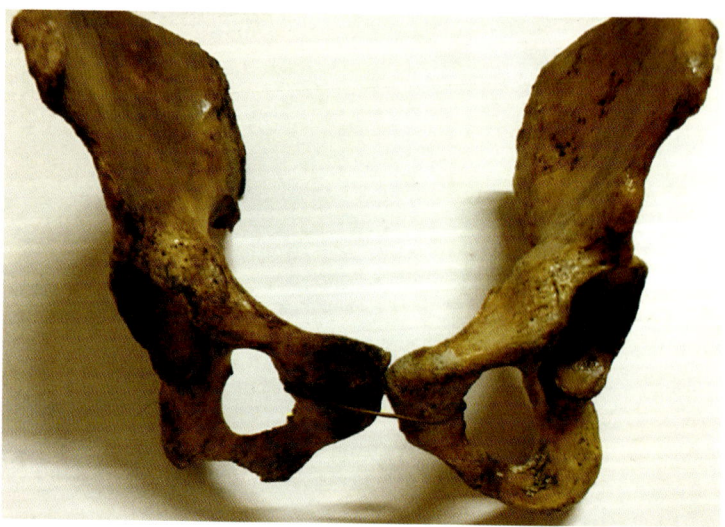

acetabulum does not fully and directly face the wall on the side. It is tilted 15 degrees backwards towards the floor. This is compensated by the normal anteversion of the femur, which is responsible for a full anatomical covering of the femoral head in an average individual; with the limb in neutral to slight external rotation.

If the acetabulum were to face more forwards it would go from neutral to anteversion. Likewise if it were to point more posteriorly retroversion would increase.

In a normal individual it does not matter if physiologically the acetabulum is a bit more neutral or retroverted than normal, but with an artificial hip, with a much smaller ball for the head, even small changes or malpositioning will lead to a marked uncovering of the head and consequently be a detriment to the stability of the head.

ACETABULAR DEPTH

The depth is the distance from the flare of the outer acetabular margin to the innermost portion of the acetabulum. Normal acetabuli are spheroidal with a considerable depth, but in patients with old CDH, or septic dislocations of childhood, the normal femoral pressures are absent during the period of growth and remodeling; and consequently the acetabular roof slopes out laterally; leaving a shallow acetabulum.

In most cases if there is a persistent dislocation of the head, it would migrate upwards and its constant pressure on the ileum would form a false acetabulum, just above the superior lip of the acetabulum.

In certain old untreated CDH patients; this false acetabulum may be really well formed and deep as compared to a pretty shallow or even nonexistent normal cavity.

It is important to note that as the ileum is traced upwards, there is a lateral flare of the bone.

Consequently, with a false acetabulum; not only is this lying superiorly, it also lies laterally causing the femur to adduct. Thus a shortening in such a hip is more marked than it actually is, because the true shortening caused by the acetabulum being higher up is accentuated by the apparent shortening due to the position of the hip.

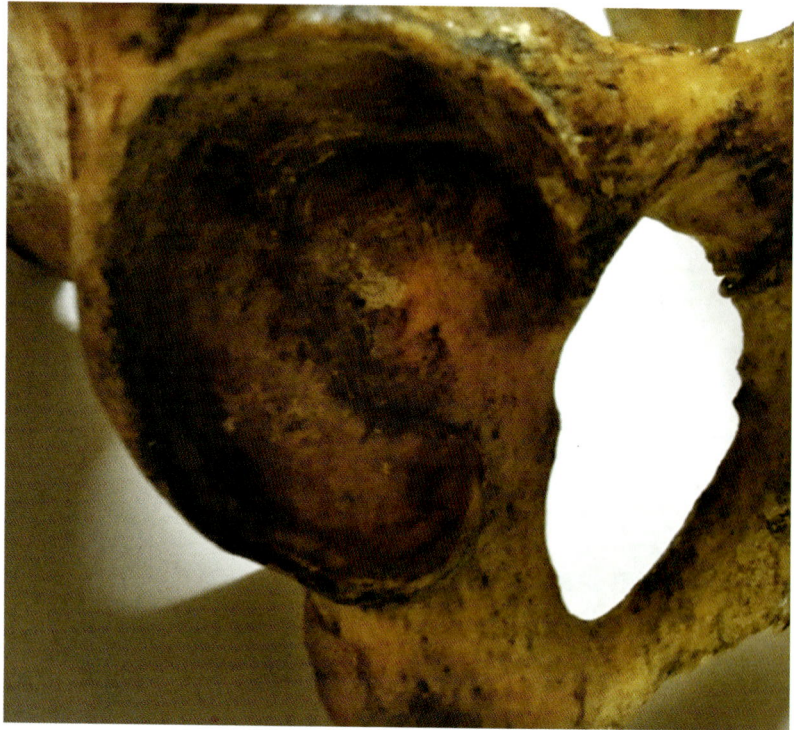

When one attempts to replace such hips, one must resist the temptation of placing the cup high up anywhere near the false acetabulum. All attempts must be made to locate the true acetabulum, and deepen it sufficiently to reach the true anatomic and mechanical axis.

Conversely there may be many pathological conditions with an acetabulum is too deep. This is called a *protrusio* and is most common in rheumatoid hips. The fulcrum of the hip gets reduced and so do the movements, and after a certain stage there are practically no movements in the joint.

Protrusion can also be a consequence of the relentless wear in a Hemi Arthroplasty, or in osteomalacia where the acetabular floor is weak. Anatomically when one is replacing the hip, it is imperative that the new socket is placed sufficiently superficially to get the correct lever arm length to avoid unequal force distribution and reduction in the range of movement. How is this achieved? Either by reinforcement implants, bone cement

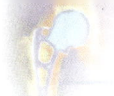
or bone grafts, techniques of which are described in detail in the subsequent chapters of this book.

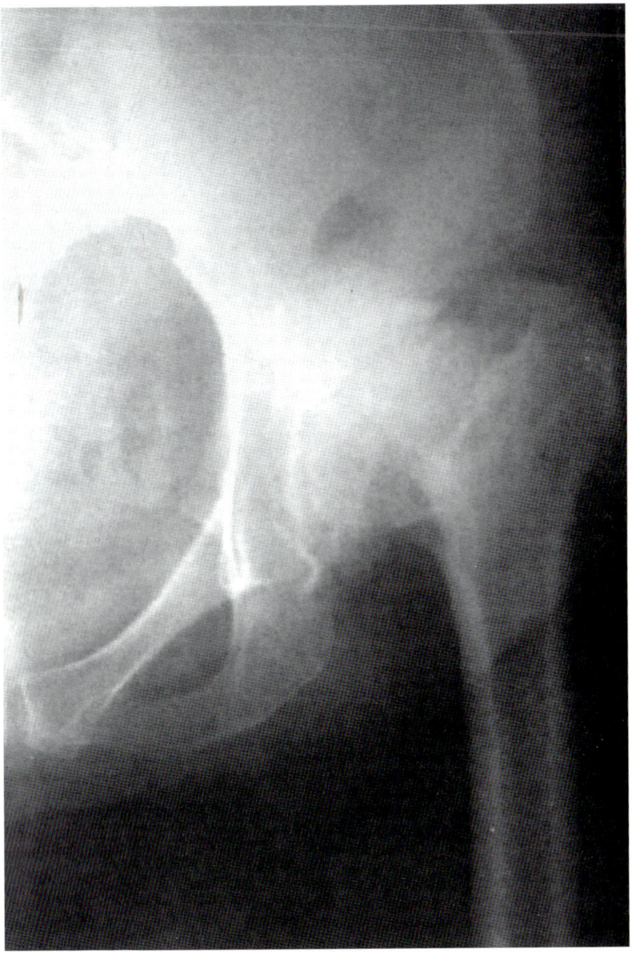

ACETABULAR WALL THICKNESS

When one imagines the acetabulum as a cup one has to know that this cup does not have uniformly thick walls all around. The wall thickness varies depending on the load and the pressures transmitted through it.

By cross sectioning the pelvis at various levels, by drilling multiple holes in the acetabulum and measuring them by a depth gauge it can be found that the acetabulum is quite weak

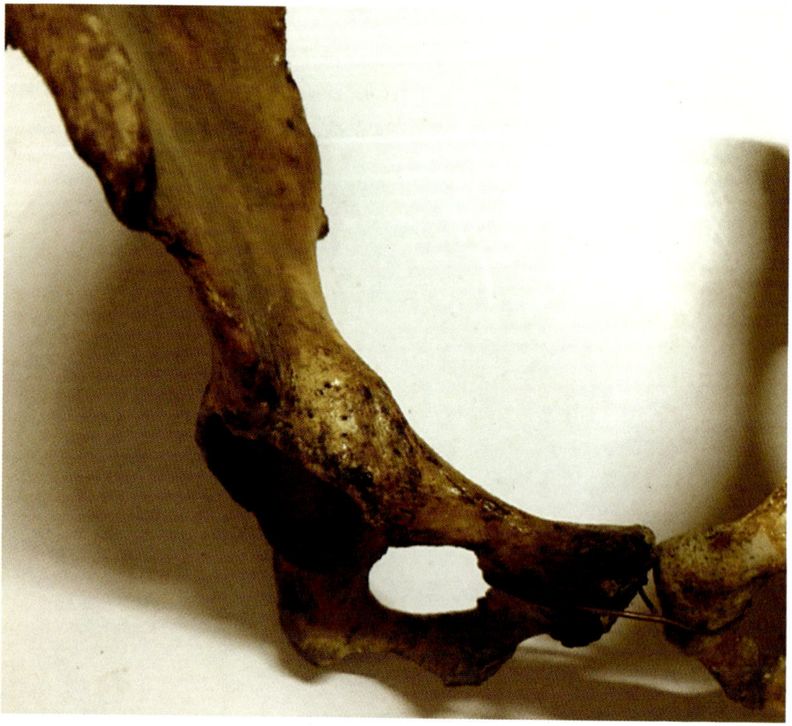

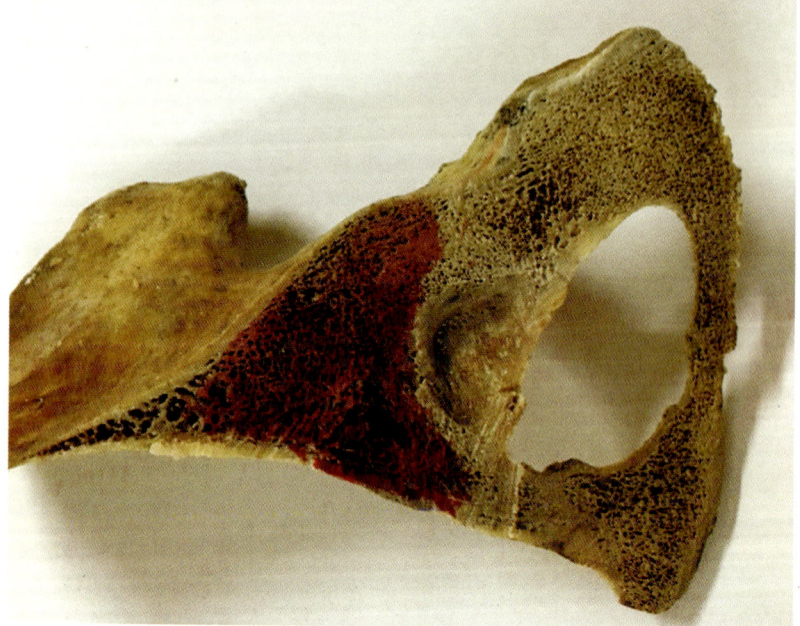

inferiomedially especially around the foveolar area and in some cases may be egg shell like.

Conversely the roof area which bears the brunt of weight transmission when a person walks; is correspondingly thicker. The thickest portion is the pelvic flare wherein the ileum ischium and the Pubis blend.

Charnley used this fact by making the largest pilot hole here and Ring used this part to affix his acetabular components with a screw or peg type cup.

In cases of protrusio and acetabular wall deficiencies, it is this part that has to be reinforced to allow a normal transmission of forces across the joint.

2

Surgical Approaches to the Hip

CLASSIFICATION OF APPROACHES

Anterior

Smith-Peterson
Short anterior bikini
Ilioinguinal

Extensive (anterior lateral and posterior)

Extended Smith-Peterson
Judet and Letournel
Ruedi Trans trochanteric.

Lateral

Modified Watson Jones
Hardinge
Trans Trochanteric Charnley
Lateral transgluteal

Posterior

Posterolateral
Southern

Medial

Ludloff

SMITH-PETERSON'S APPROACH TO THE HIP

History

Marius Nygaard Smith-Petersen (1886–1953), a pioneer hip surgeon described this approach in 1917. He began his orthopaedic career under E.G. Brackett, prior to which he has worked in physiology and neurosurgery. Dr. Smith-Petersen started private practice in Boston, Massachusetts in 1923. He served as Assistant Instructor in Orthopaedic Surgery at Harvard Medical School from 1920–1930, as Instructor in Orthopaedic Surgery at Harvard Medical School from 1930–1946, as Clinical Professor of Orthopaedic Surgery at Harvard Medical School from 1935–1946 and as Chief of Orthopaedic Service at Massachusetts General Hospital from 1929–1946 and as consultant to The Surgeon General from 1942–1945. He was internationally known for the development of the Smith-Petersen nail and hip nailing techniques and for hip-mold arthoplasty. He was awarded the Grand Cross of the Order of St. Olav by the King of Norway. He was a brilliant surgeon and a gifted professor.

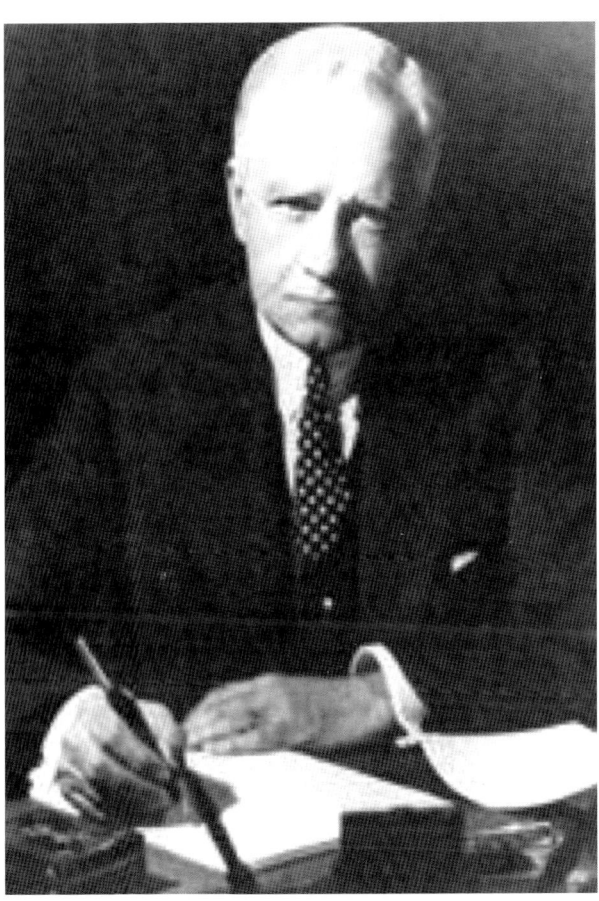

Plane

Between Tensor Fascia Lata and Gluteus Medius posteriorly;
And Sartorius and Rectus Femoris anteriorly.

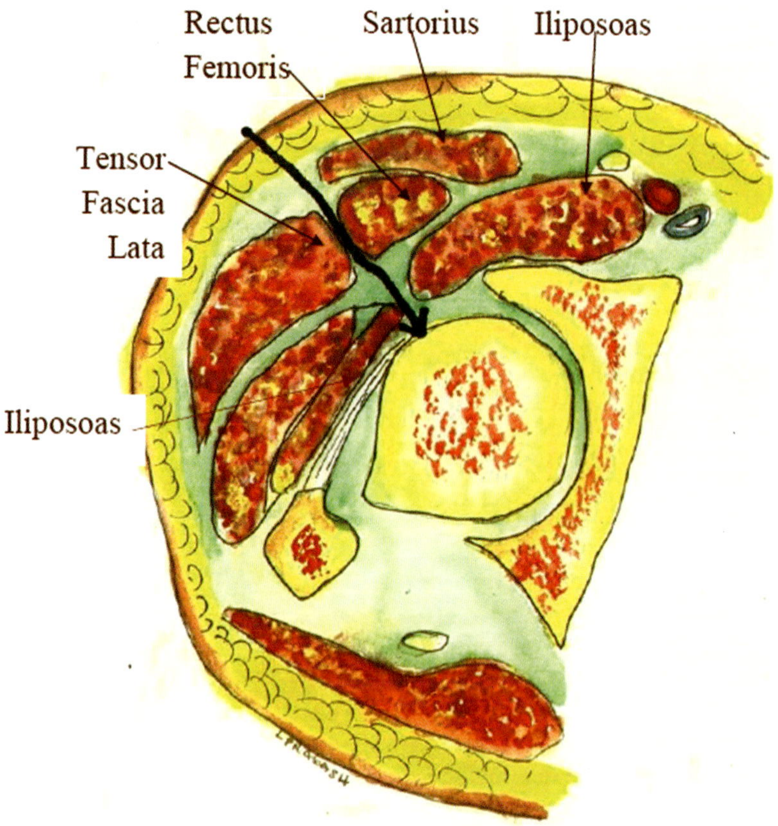

SMITH-PETERSON'S APPROACH

Access Provided

Inner and outer table of ileum
Anterior and superior acetabulum
Femoral head and neck
Proximal femoral shaft.

Dislocation

The hip joint is dislocated anteriorly.

Position and Draping

Supine with sandbag under the hip
Leg is draped free

Drape passes around upper thigh to expose anterio superior iliac spine to gluteal tubercle.

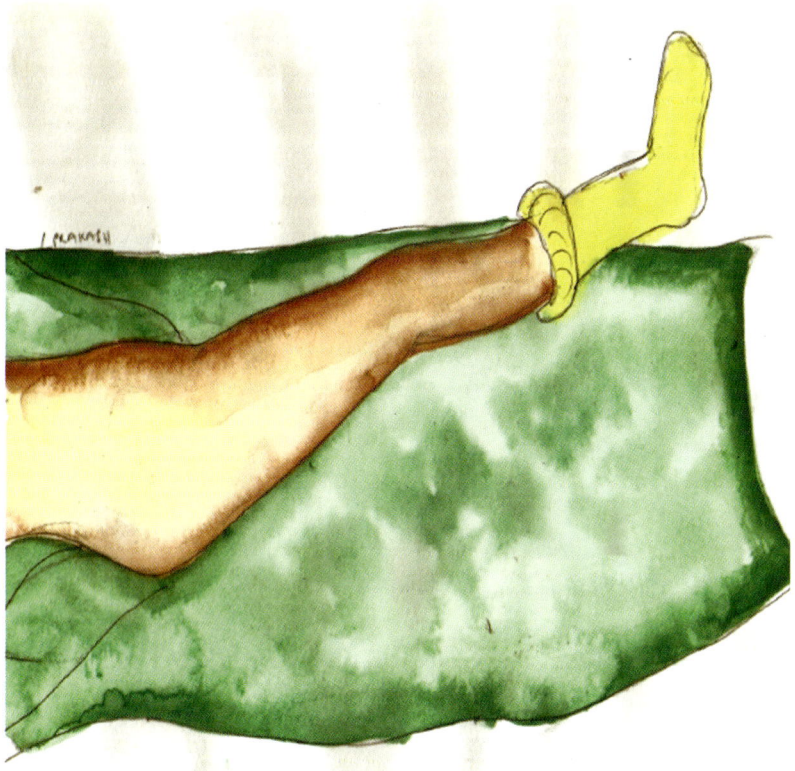

Incision

Midpoint of the incision is anterio superior iliac spine.

This is extended superiorly along the iliac crest and inferiorly as a straight line leading towards lateral patellar border.

Depending on the exposure needs, the skin incision can be extended upwards or downwards.

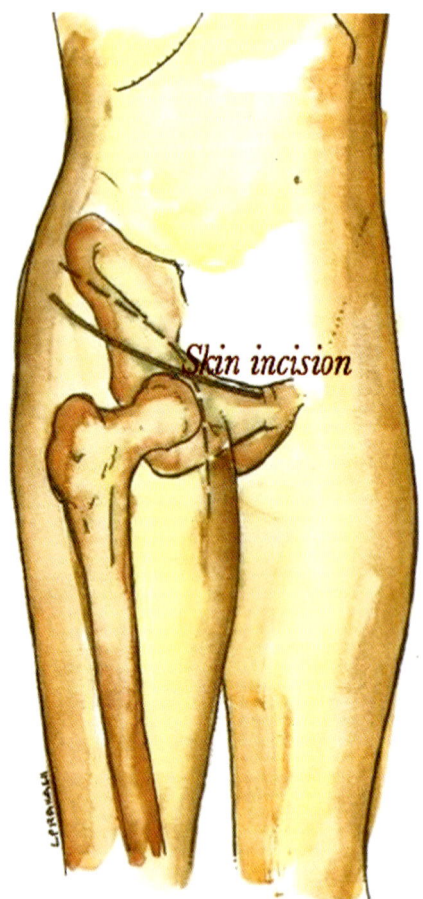

Smith petersons approach

Dissections

After skin and subcutaneous fat are cut, deep Fascia over anterosuperior iliac spine and over anterior thigh is incised.

A longitudinal incision is made over Tensor Fascia Lata and the cleavage between it and Sartorius is developed.

This is deepened, Rectus Femoris is identified and the plane between Gluteus Medius and Rectus Femoris is opened up.

The ascending branch of lateral circumflex vessels is now located and ligated, to allow dissection to be carried above to ASIS.

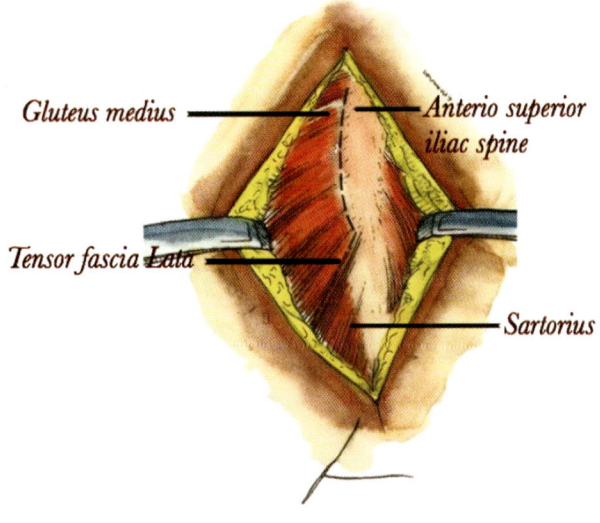

Anterior iliofemoral approach

Deep to the lateral edge of Rectus Femoris, the hip capsule is visualized. Detaching the reflected head of Rectus Femoris, increases the degree of exposure of superior acetabulum.

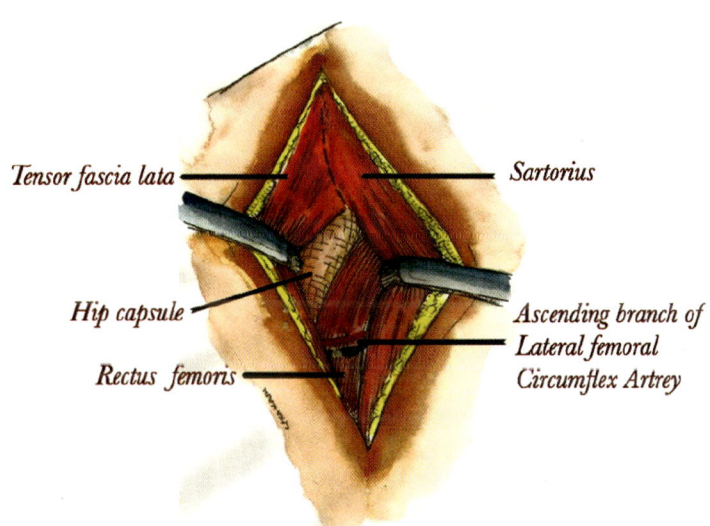

Anterior iliofemoral approach

Muscles over lateral pelvic wall are subperiosteally stripped as far posteriorly as required, and one can go right up to the sciatic notch.

Increased exposure can be obtained by detaching the attachment of Rectus Femoris from the anteroinferior iliac spine.

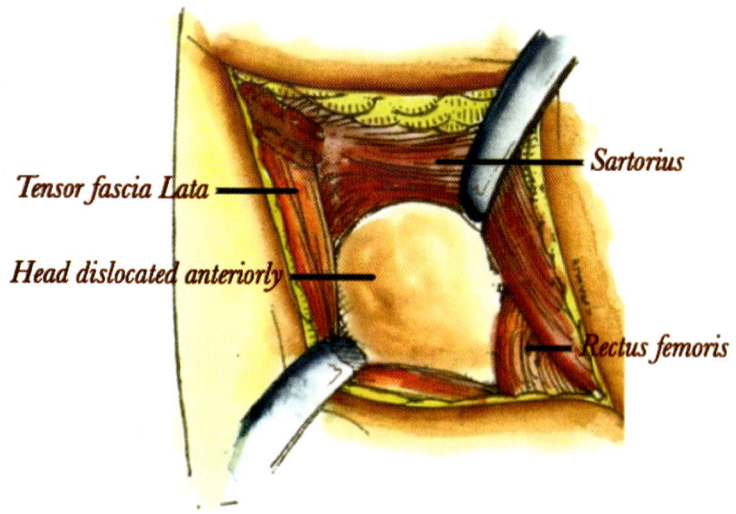

Tensor fascia Lata

Head dislocated anteriorly

Sartorius

Rectus femoris

Femoral head is dislocated by internally rotating the limb

Adduction and external rotation of the hip stretches the hip capsule which is cut with a 'T' shaped incision.

Gluteus Medius can be stripped off the lateral pelvic wall for additional exposure.

External rotation and adduction will dislocate the hip after capsular incision.

Indications

Pediatric Hip Exposures

Congenital dislocation of the hip where both femoral and acetabular surgeries can be combined.

Pelvic Osteotomies

Traumatic anterior dislocation, and acetabular injuries involving anterior column of pelvis.

Arthrodesis or Total Hip Replacement in selected cases.

Tumours of the anterior hip.

Advantages

Excellent proximal femoral and anterior acetabular exposure.

Gluteal release in high riding hips especially CDH.

Posterior blood supply to head of femur is preserved.

Bone grafts can be simultaneously and easily removed.

Disadvantages

Restricted femoral medullary exposure.

Detachment of glutei and TFL, necessitates prolonged protection.

Lateral femoral cutaneous nerve injury is common.

THE SHORT ANTERIOR BIKINI APPROACH

History

Edgar Somerville described this approach in 1953. He was an outstanding figure of the generation that developed paediatric orthopaedic surgery in the UK in the postwar years. Somerville first made his name as co-author with Girdlestone of the second edition of the book "Tuberculosis of Bones and Joints' (1952).

The children whom he treated were examined personally once a year in Oxford at clinics which soon became study sessions on skeletal development.

Miniaturized radiographs, meticulously mounted on a large cardboard sheet, told the story of each child's hip. Like frames from a slow-motion cinematograph, the yearly films were used to teach the importance of the fourth dimension in paediatric surgery.

Plane

Between Tensor Fascia Lata and Gluteus Medius medially; and Sartorius and Rectus Femoris laterally.

Access Provided

Limited direct access to the hip joint alone.

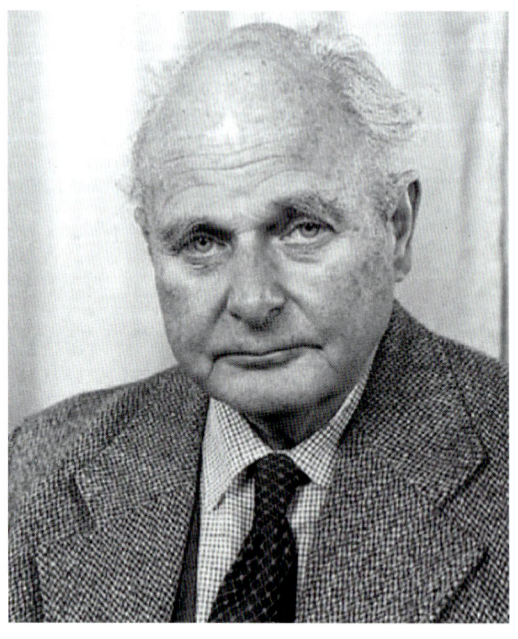

Dislocation

The hip joint can be technically dislocated anteriorly, but a complete dislocation to the extent of viewing of the acetabulum is difficult with this approach.

Position and draping

Supine with sandbag under the hip
Leg is draped free

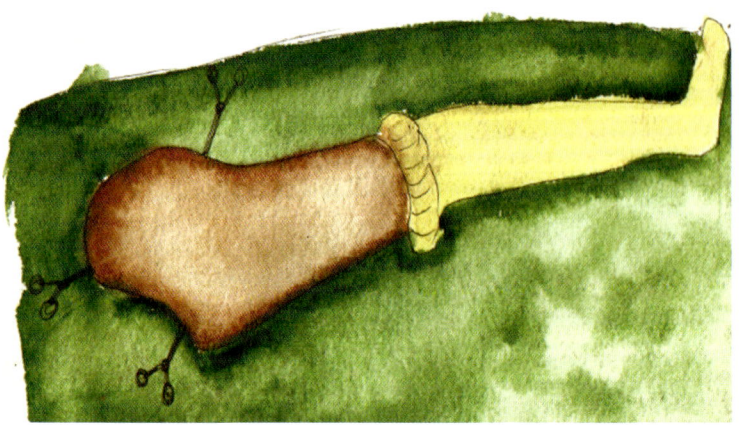

Drape passes around upper thigh to expose anterio superior iliac spine to gluteal tubercle.

Incision

Short oblique incision 4 cm below ASIS.

Dissections

After skin and subcutaneous fat are cut, deep Fascia over anterosuperior iliac spine and that over anterior thigh is incised.

The incision between TFL and Sartorius is developed. Branches of lateral circumflex vessels are ligated. Rectus Femoris is elevated to expose the anterior capsule.

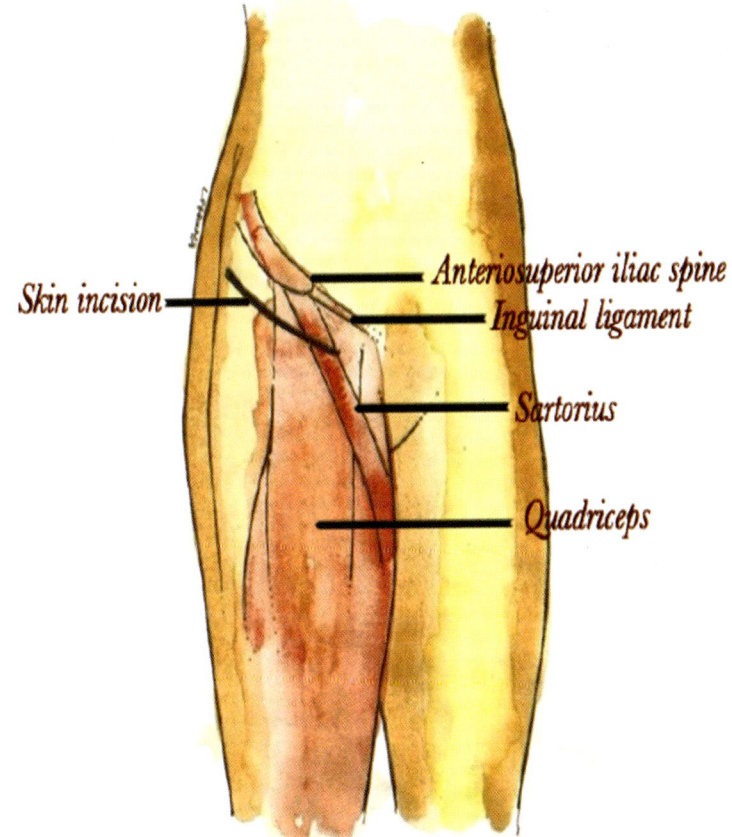

Skin incision

Anteriosuperior iliac spine

Inguinal ligament

Sartorius

Quadriceps

Short anterior approach to the hip

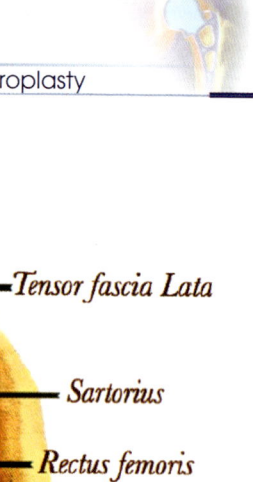

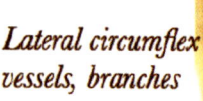

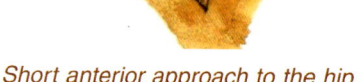

Hip capsule — Sartorius

Lateral circumflex — Rectus femoris
vessels, branches

Tensor fascia Lata

Short anterior approach to the hip

Inferior blunt dissection allows access to Iliopsoas tendon and lesser trochanter.

Indications

Access to anterior hip capsule, without detachment of hip abductors.

Psoas tenotomy and anterior capsular releases.

Biopsy and septic arthritis.

Advantages

Small scar, cosmetic incision.

Reduced morbidity due to preservation of gluteal origin.

Disadvantages

Limited exposure.

Difficult to dislocate hip.

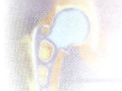

ILIOINGUINAL APPROACH

History

Judet described this approach in 1964.

Henri Judet was one of the first to practice orthopedics exclusively in France. His reputation was authoritative at the time. He devoted considerable time on research and developed numerous surgical techniques for congenital hip dislocation, clubfeet, and other birth defects. His sons John and Robert started their clinic, The clinic *"Jouvenet"* which became a Mecca of orthopaedic surgery. It was located at 6 square Jouvenet in Paris' 16th arrondissement.

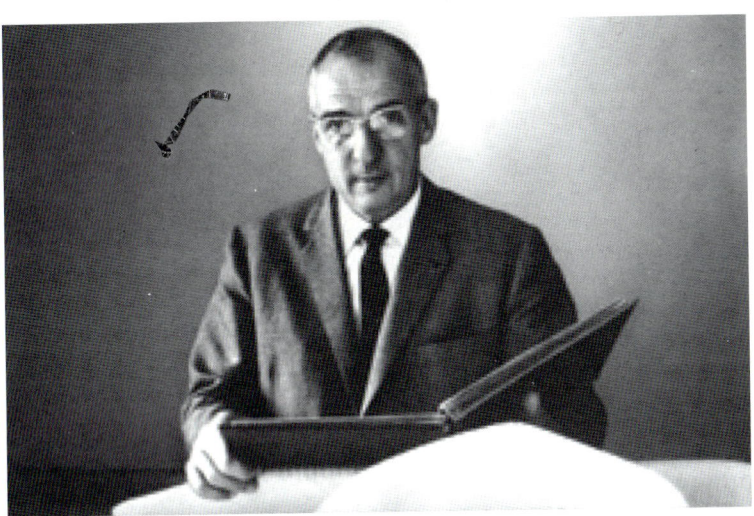

Robert Judet

Plane

Between Iliopsoas and the pelvic wall

Access provided

A decent and extensive acetabular exposure giving access to
Interior of hemi pelvis
Iliac crest
Exterior of pelvic crest
Sciatic notch inferio-medially
Symphysis pubis anteriorly
Ala of sacrum posteriorly.

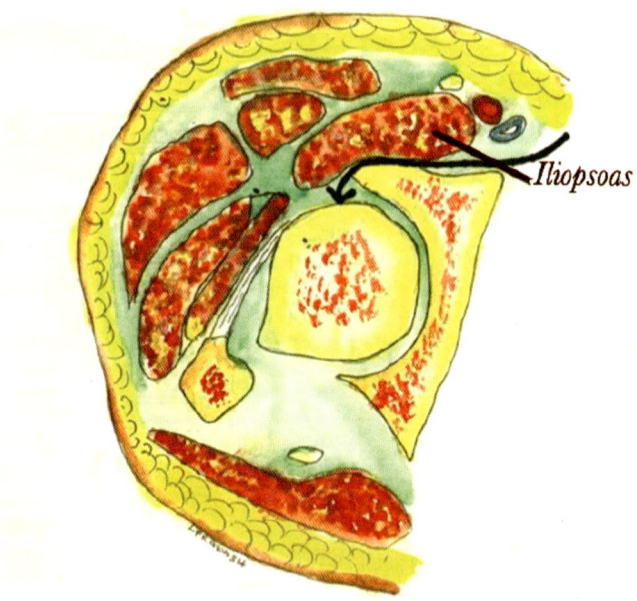

Anterior ilioinguinal approach

Dislocation

Hip can be dislocated superiorly, anteriorly or posteriorly depending on the requirements of the area of acetabulum to be exposed.

Position and draping

Supine with sand bag under buttock.

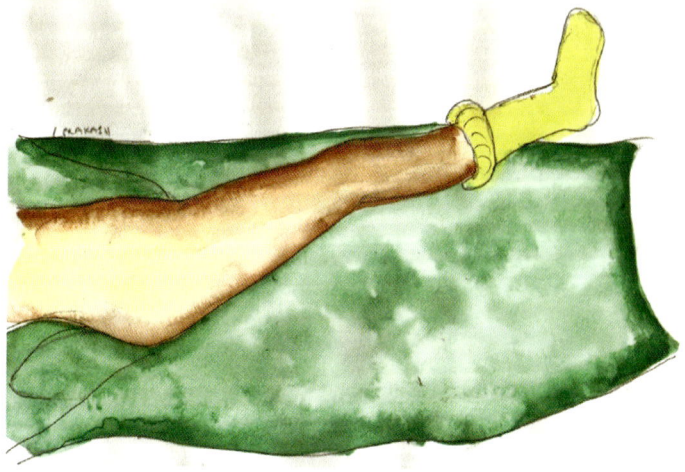

Incision

Long incision from posterior iliac crest to Symphysis Pubis, which is curved distally.

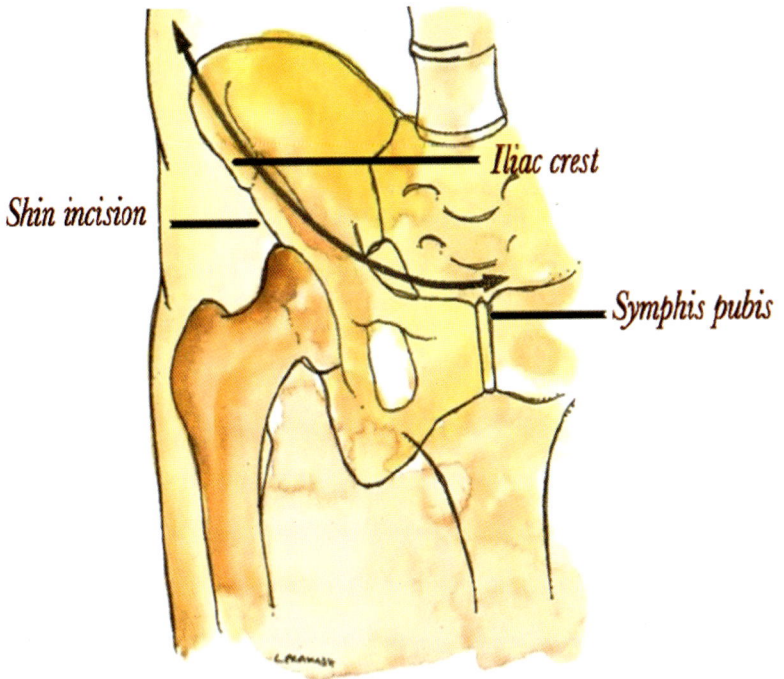

Ilioinguinal approach

Iliac crest is exposed and structures can be stripped off the pelvis both from outer and inner tables.

Dissections

On the inner side, either abdominal muscles are gently erased off the iliac crest or the anterior third of the iliac crest is osteotomized and then snapped inwards, breaking the inner table and allowing a sub periosteal dissection of the Iliacus muscle.

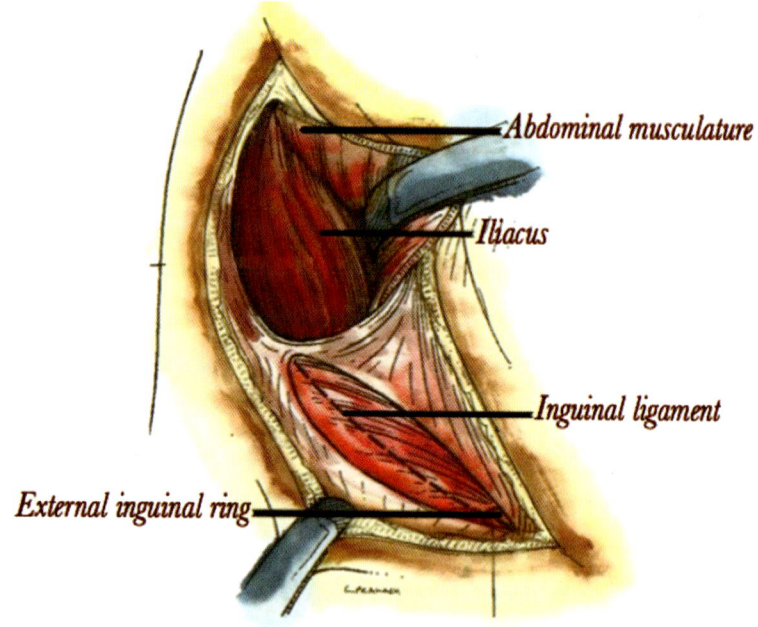

Ilioinguinal approach to the hip

This stripping can be carried as far back as the sacroiliac joint if required.

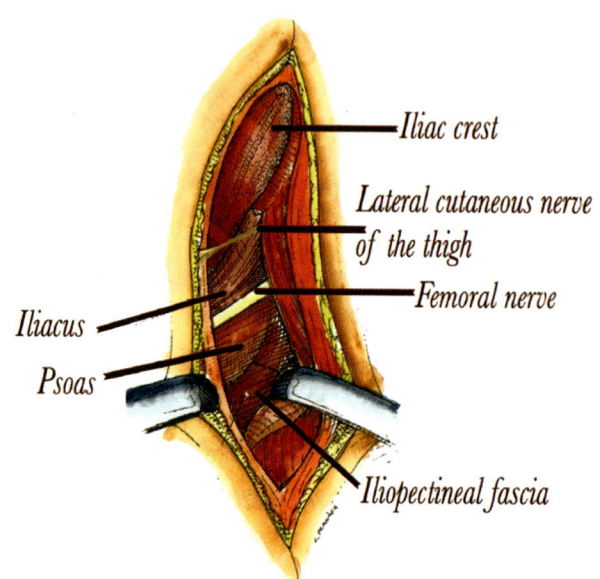

The aponeurosis of external oblique is divided from ASIS along the iliac crest. The lateral cutaneous nerve of the thigh is now identified and protected.

At this stage, starting from the conjoint tendon, the inguinal ligament is detached from its origins, leaving a dense fibrous strip for reattachment.

The Iliopsoas muscle mass and femoral nerve come into view. The Iliopectineal head is identified and detached from pelvis, allowing mobilization of Iliopsoas muscle mass along with the femoral nerve.

By passing a loupe of soft tape or rubber catheter, these can be retracted in either direction.

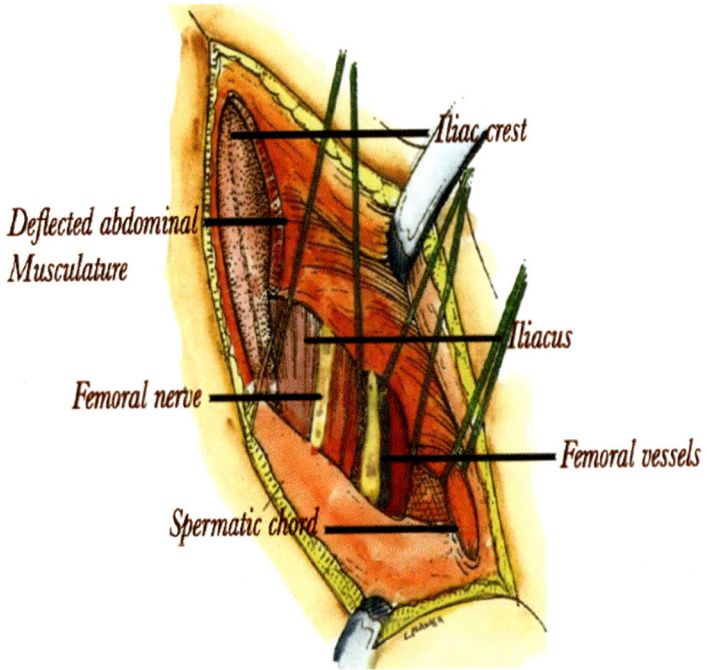

This now exposes three bundles of structures. Laterally is the Iliopsoas, and medially is the spermatic chord (in the male). Between them lies the femoral neurovascular bundle. These three can be retracted carefully in either direction to expose the whole of pubic ramus.

Should there be a need to expose the contra lateral Pubis the incision can be carried across the midline, and the whole anterior brim of the pelvis can be exposed by this approach.

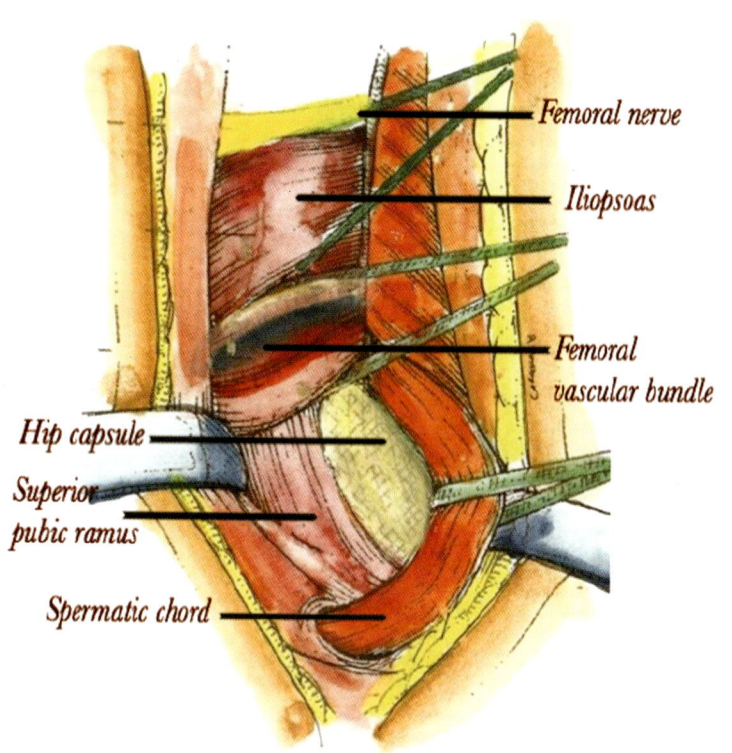

Indications

Pelvic fractures, except those involving sacrum.

Fractures of the anterior column.

Superior pubic ramus fractures.

Floating Symphysis Pubis or disruption of Symphysis Pubis.

Advantages

Good field of exposure from one side to the other especially in anterior column fractures.

Good clean cosmetic scar.

Disadvantages

Difficult and technically demanding operation

Lateral cutaneous nerve is in danger and irritating complications occur if it is cut.

External iliac and femoral vessels have to be carefully protected.

RUEDI APPROACH

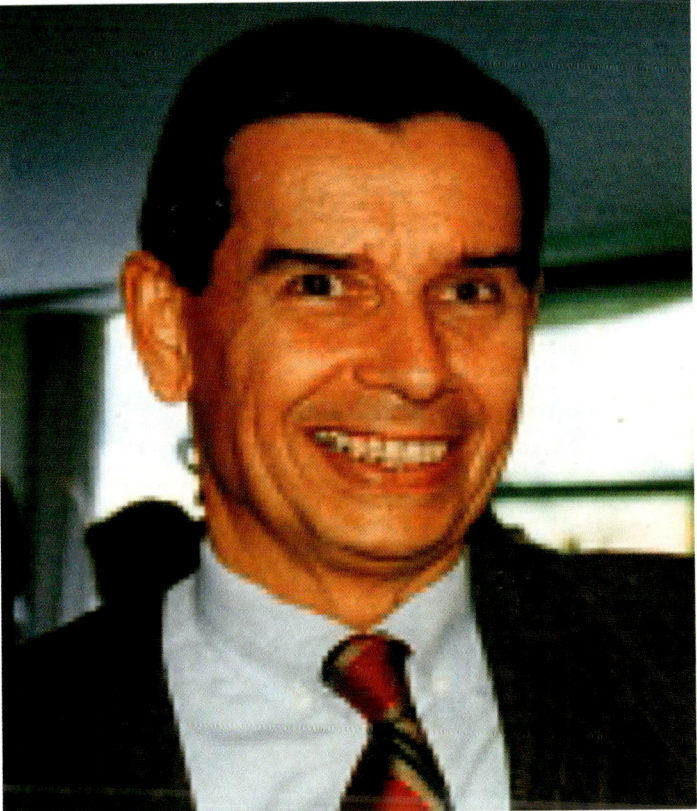

Surgeons confronted with acute trauma are frequently under great pressure to act quickly. Only a few have an infallible three-dimensional memory as regards the different approaches necessary for treating fractures by internal fixation. Thus there is a real need for a reference book on the approaches to the extremities. This is true both for the emergency situation and for the "evening before" preoperative planning.

THOMAS RUEDI, was one of the early AO teachers, founder members and a gifted trauma surgeon. He is also a wonderful artist and an unusual illustrator. This modification of Judet's approach was described by Ruedi in 1968. He has authored numerous AO books and manuals, many of them illustrated by himself and these books form essential reading for all trauma surgeons across the world.

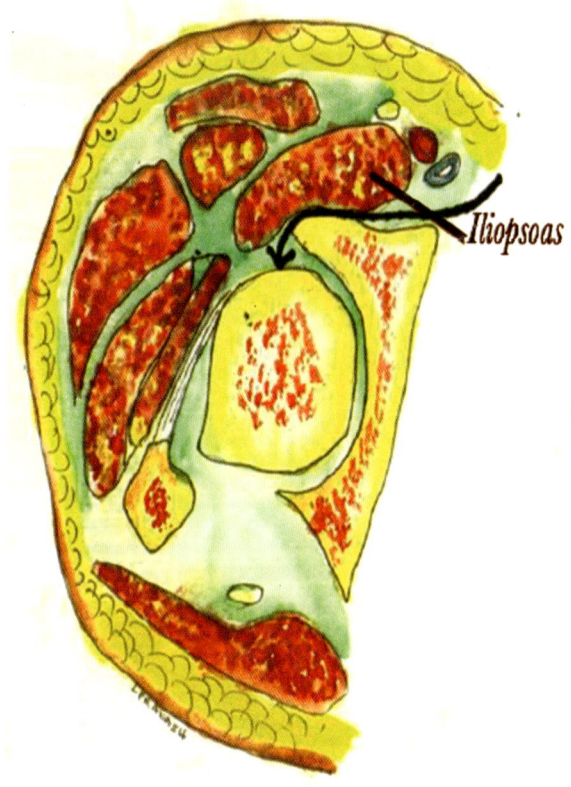

Iliopsoas

Plane

Between Iliopsoas and the pelvic wall, after osteotomy of Anterio Superior Iliac spine.

Access provided

One of the most extensive acetabular exposures giving access to Interior of hemi pelvis.

Iliac crest

Exterior of pelvic crest

Sciatic notch inferio-medially

Symphysis Pubis anteriorly

Ala of sacrum posteriorly.

Dislocation

Hip can be dislocated superiorly, anteriorly or posteriorly depending on the requirements of the area of acetabulum to be exposed.

Position and Draping

Supine with sand bag under buttock.

Incision

Long incision from posterior iliac crest to Symphysis Pubis, which is curved distally.

Osteotomy of ASIS along with anterior half of iliac crest.

Fascia along the inferior border of inguinal ligament is incised.

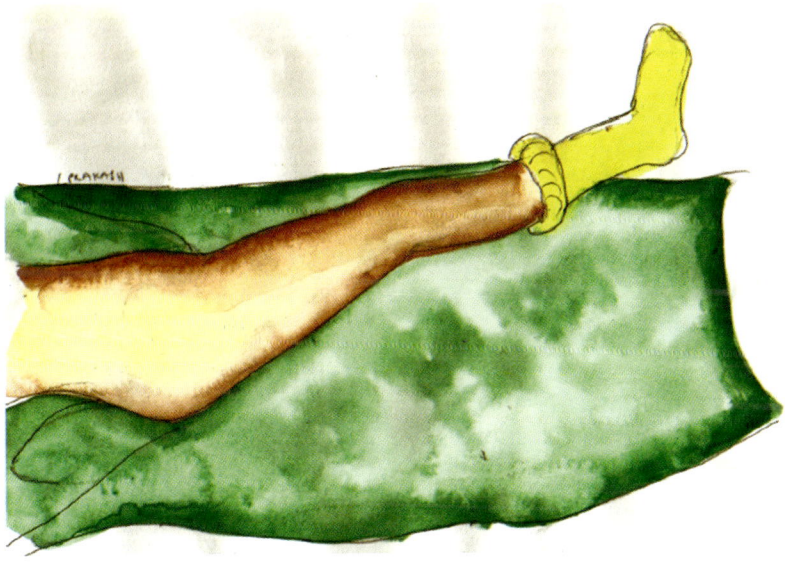

The iliac sliver, ASIS, inguinal ligament, and external abdominal musculature are retracted superiorly and medially.

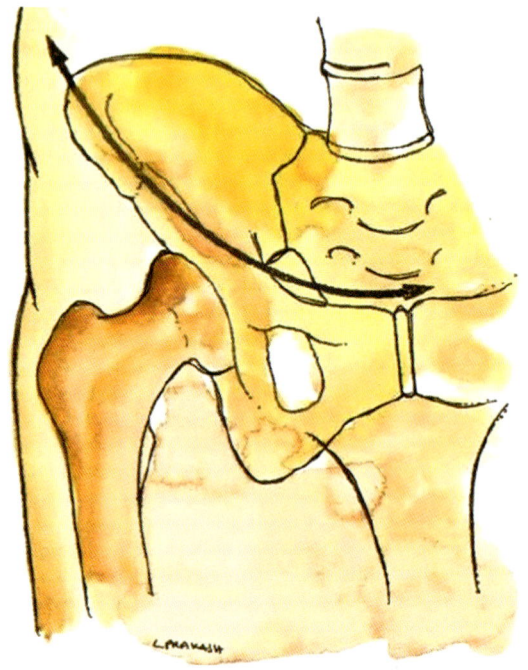

Ruedi approach is a little inferior

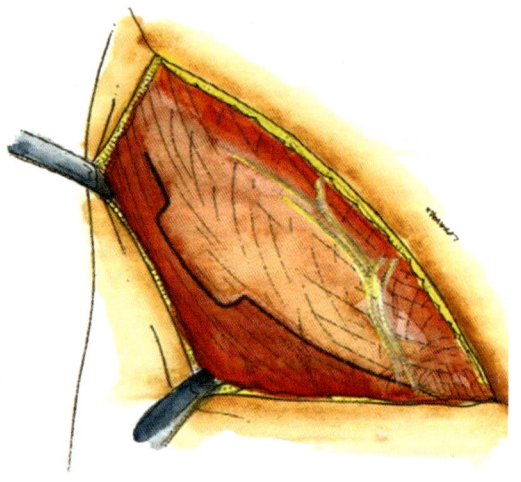

Deep incision before ASIS osteotomy

The lateral cutaneous nerve of the thigh is identified and protected. Iliopsoas muscle mass and the femoral neurovascular bundles are identified and separated as with Judet approach.

In males, the spermatic chord is protected, and the superiomedial aspect of pubic ramus is stripped leaving a decent strip for reattachment.

In complex pelvis injuries the approach can be extended to the other side of midline, to expose the whole anterior brim of pelvis.

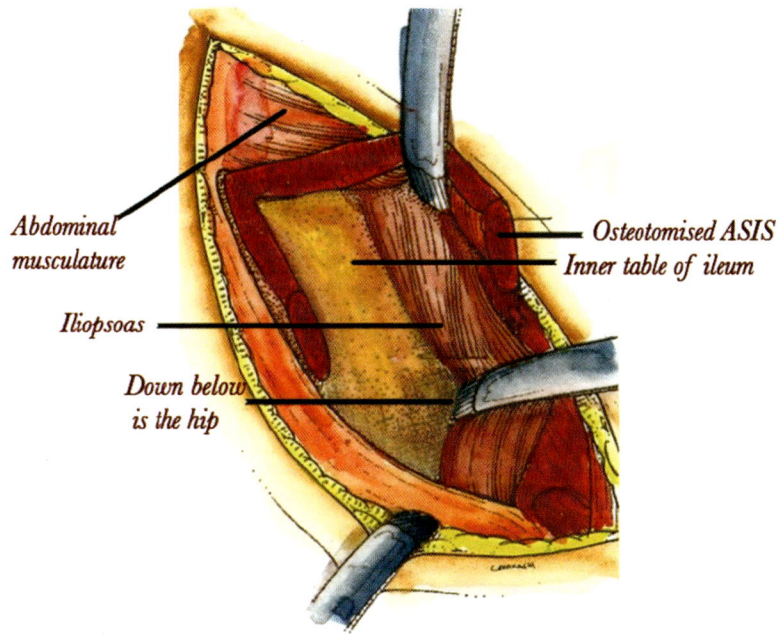

Abdominal musculature

Osteotomised ASIS

Inner table of ileum

Iliopsoas

Down below is the hip

Indications

Pelvic fractures, except those involving sacrum.

Fractures of the anterior column.

Superior pubic ramus fractures.

Floating Symphysis Pubis or disruption of Symphysis Pubis.

Advantages

Excellent field of exposure from one side to the other especially in anterior column fractures.

Good clean cosmetic scar.

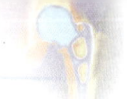

Disadvantages

Difficult and technically demanding operation

Lateral cutaneous nerve is in danger and irritating complications occur if it is cut.

External iliac and femoral vessels have to be carefully protected.

EXTENDED ILIOFEMORAL APPROACH BY JUDET AND LETOURNEL

History

Émile Letournel, born in 1927 was an outstanding French surgeon of his times. He joined Judet in 1954, and was a pioneer in the study of acetabular fractures.

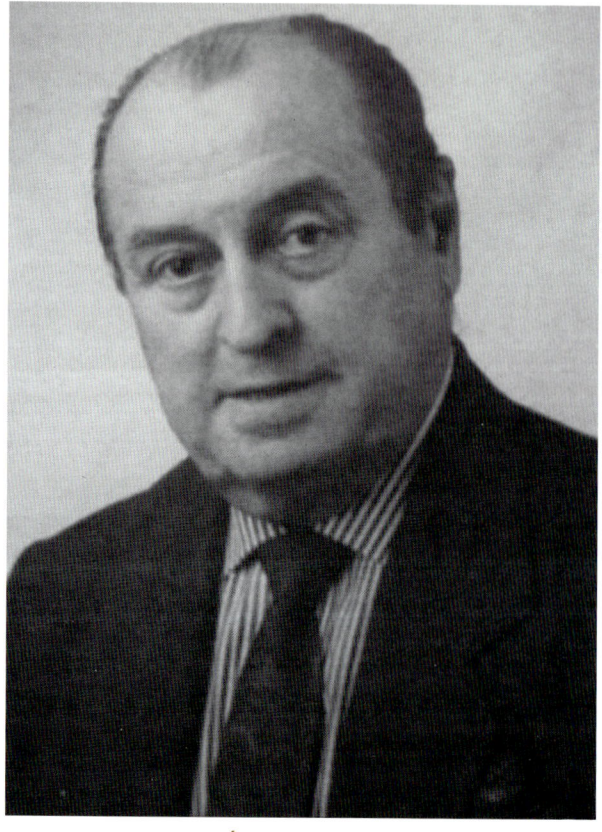

Émile Letournel

Professor Letournel was recognized as the conclusive source of extensive experience and innovative techniques in the management of severe pelvic and acetabular trauma. His lifelong contributions to the understanding of complex acetabular fractures and the techniques required to treat these difficult injuries have defined the fundamental principles of these injury patterns. He described this approach in 1964.

Plane

Between Sartorius and Tensor Fascial Lata inferiorly

Subperiosteal elevation of Gluteus Medius and Minimus muscles.

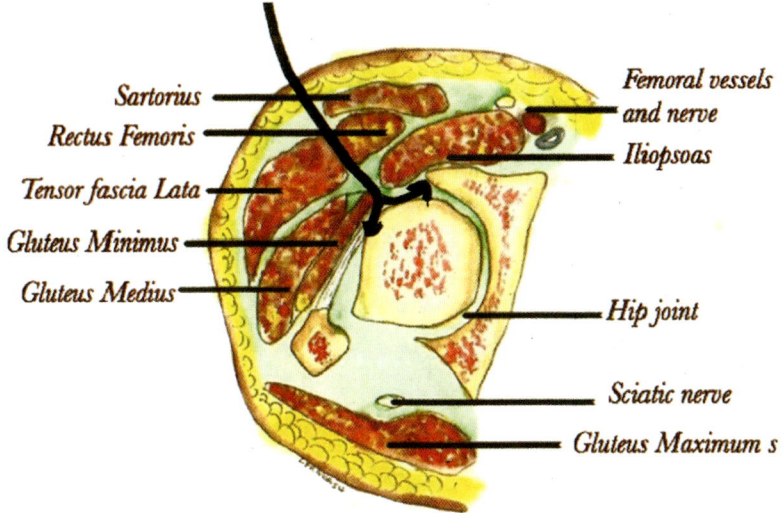

Access

Posterior acetabular column
Superior dome of acetabulam
Anterior column as far back as iliopubic eminence

Dislocation

In any direction needed except inferior

Position and Draping

Lateral position

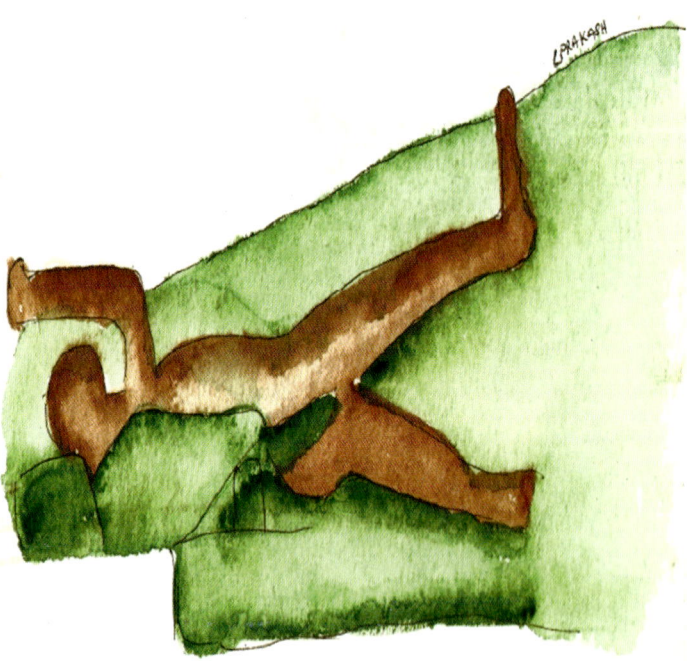

Appropriate attachments on the operating table ensure a fixed lateral position.

K wire with tensioned Ilizarov Half Ring in the distal transcondylar area to give good traction. (The original Letournel method advocates a stienman pin and stirrups.)

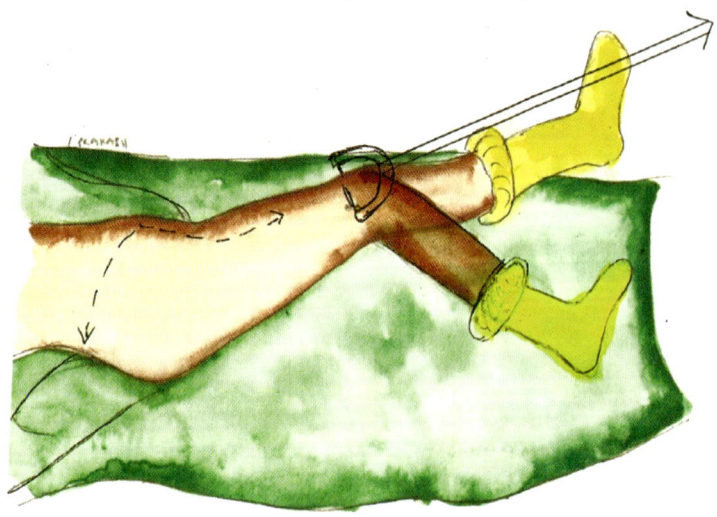

The knee should be draped free and kept flexed to avoid stretching of the sciatic nerve.

Incision

Along the anterior 80% of the iliac crest up to the ASIS

Curves to 90 degrees at ASIS to go towards patella

Exposure up to a little below mid thigh allows relaxation of structures and a better acetabular exposure.

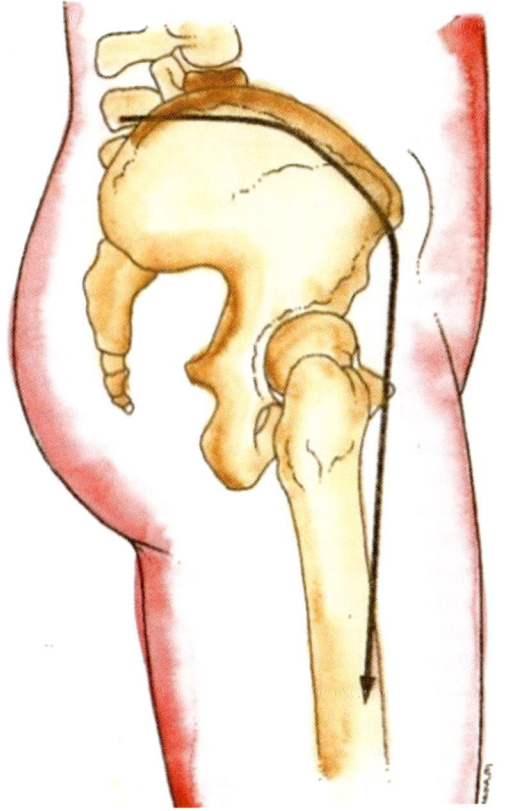

Skin incision for extended iliofemoral approach of Judet and letournel

Dissections

Sub periosteal detachment of the Gluteus Medius and Minimus from the outer wing of the ileum, right up to the sciatic notch, allowing them to be retracted posteriorly.

The superior gluteal neurovascular bundle is identified and protected.

The short lateral rotators are now detached with sufficient flaps for reattachment.

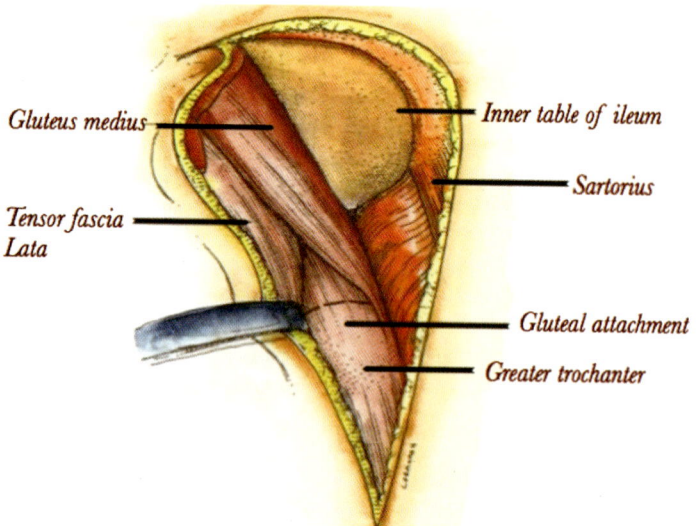

Order of detachment of rotators is Piriformis, superior gamellous, obturator internus, inferior gamellus and the quadrates Femoris.

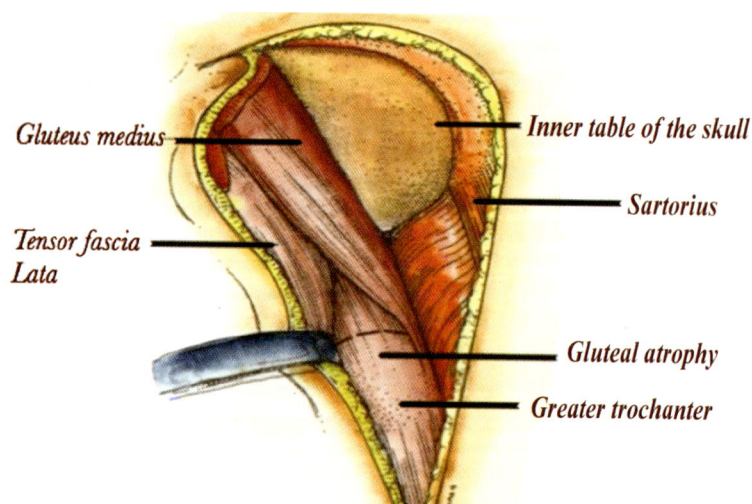

Division and medial retraction of both heads of Rectus Femoris

Abdominal muscles are either detached from iliac crest of the crest is osteotomised to deflect the bone with muscles.

Flexion of the hip at this stage relaxes all the muscles and an extensive approach is achieved.

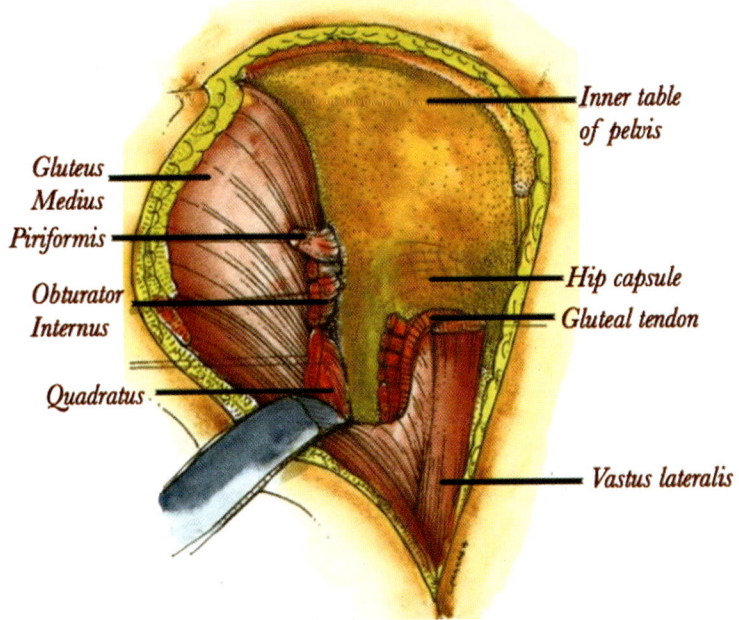

Gluteus Medius

Piriformis

Obturator Internus

Quadratus

Inner table of pelvis

Hip capsule

Gluteal tendon

Vastus lateralis

Extended iliofemoral approach

Indications

Pelvic fractures, involving both columns.

Fractures of the anterior column, superior dome

Advantages

An extensive large exposure that can be extended in either direction.

Disadvantages

Anterior column exposure is limited to its superior parts.

Detachment of glutei needs proper reattachment and post operative protection.

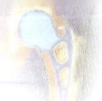

ANTERIOR APPROACHES

History

Watson-Jones in 1936 described an easy anterior approach with a more acceptable scar than the original Ollier's approach on which it was based.

Louis Xavier Édouard Léopold Ollier was born in Vans, Ardèche, France, where both his father and grandfather had been doctors. He initially studied natural science at Montpellier; in 1849 he was assistant in Botany in the faculty of Medicine. He then became an intern of Lyon Hospital in 1851, graduated in medicine with distinction in 1856, and in 1857 obtained his doctorate at Paris based on histological studies of 400 malignant tumours.

In 1860, aged only 30, Ollier became the Chief surgeon at the Hôtel-Dieu in Lyon, one of the oldest hospitals in Europe. When France was invaded by the Germans in 1870 he became head of the Lyons Ambulance. A meticulous and thorough surgeon, he soon attracted patients from all over the world.

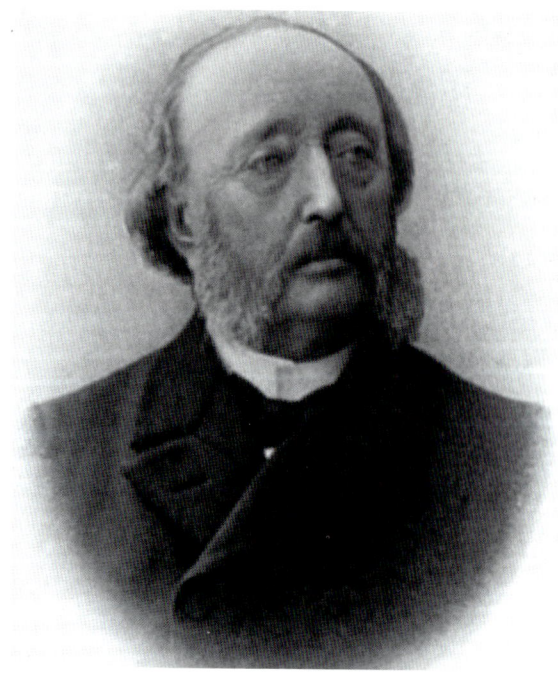

In 1877 Ollier was appointed professor of clinical surgery and in 1894, Ollier was made commander of the Légion d'Honneur. Ollier died in Lyons in 1900 at the age of 70.

Ollier was revered for his role in the development of orthopaedic surgery in France, A monument was erected in his memory in the square outside his home and in and the Museum of pathological anatomy at the University of Lyon, which now bears his name.

Ollier was one of the first surgeons to employ an audit on his operative procedures, stating "It is in the certification and criticism of old results that is to be found the true consecration of operative methods which are intended to be used for purposes of conservative surgery".

The U shaped incision for anterolateral hip approach was described by him in 1881.

Ollier's original approach involved osteotomy of the greater trochanter after the U shaped incision. This approach has been abandoned for the more cosmetic linear skin incisions and easier transtrochanteric approaches. Here a few drawings show the approach, but the current anteriolateral Watson Jones approach is described more fully subsequently.

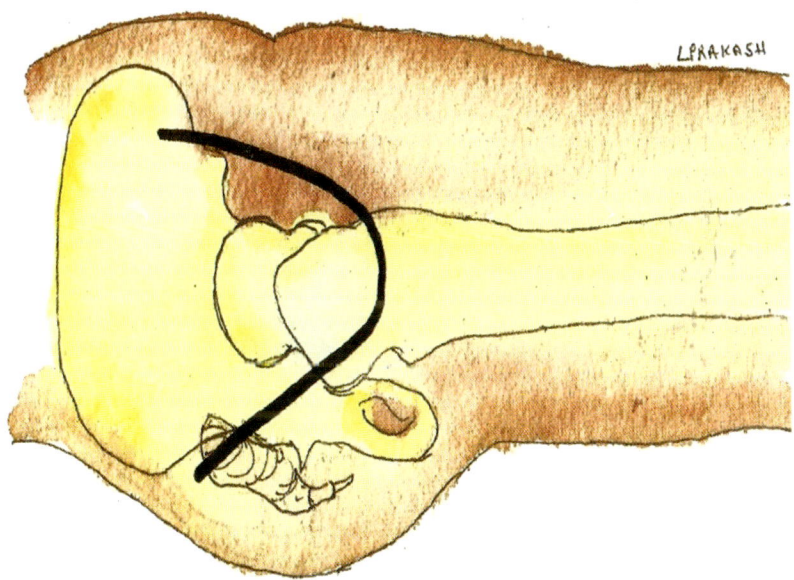

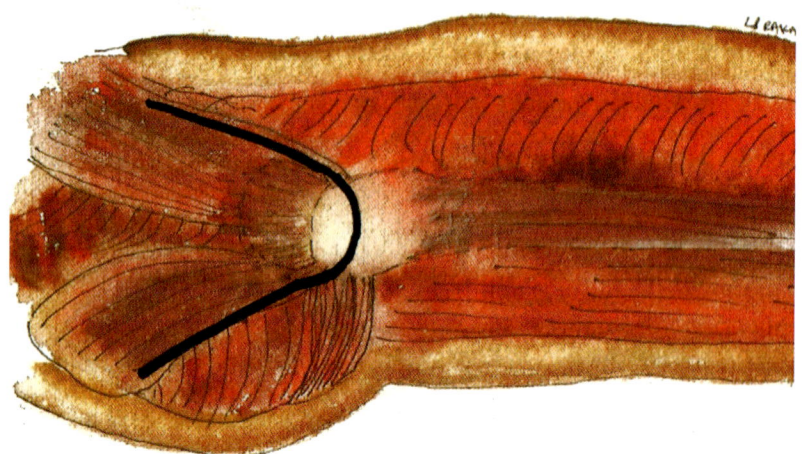

After trochanteric osteotomy, it is deflected superiorly along with the abductors to expose the superior capsule.

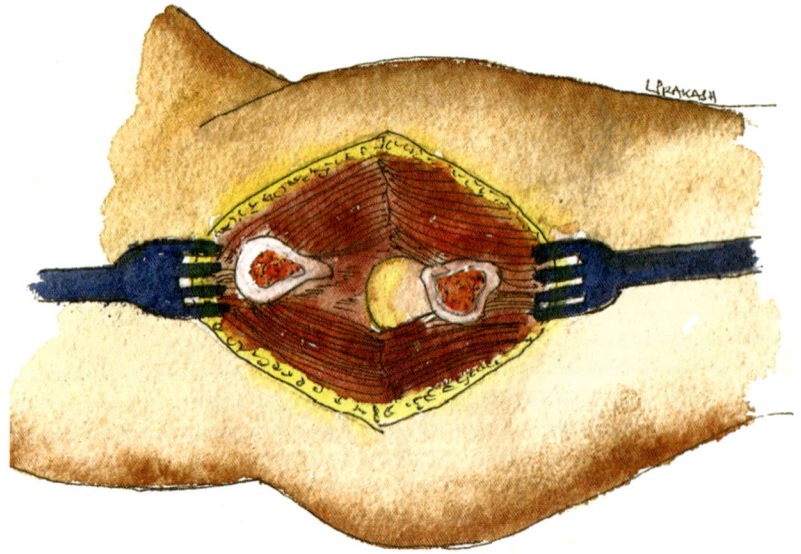

Sir Reginald Watson-Jones has often been described as the pioneer scientist of the new era of orthopaedics in Britain.

Watson-Jones was born on March 4, 1902, to a schoolteacher and his wife. He graduated from the University of Liverpool in

1922 with a Bachelor's degree in Science and went on to receive his medical education at the university's Medical School. In 1926 he became one of the first surgeons to receive the MCh Orth degree.

Following his education in Liverpool, he continued his training in London, where he met and impressed Sir Robert Jones, eventually becoming his protégé.

Shortly after the start of his orthopaedic career, Reginald Jones adopted his mother's maiden name and became Reginald Watson-Jones to distinguish himself from the many other Joneses practicing medicine in England at that time, including his mentor. Also, that period saw the beginning of a seemingly inexhaustible writing talent when The Journal of Bone and Joint Surgery, accepted his first paper for publication in 1930. He would eventually publish two to three papers every year in numerous journals for decades.

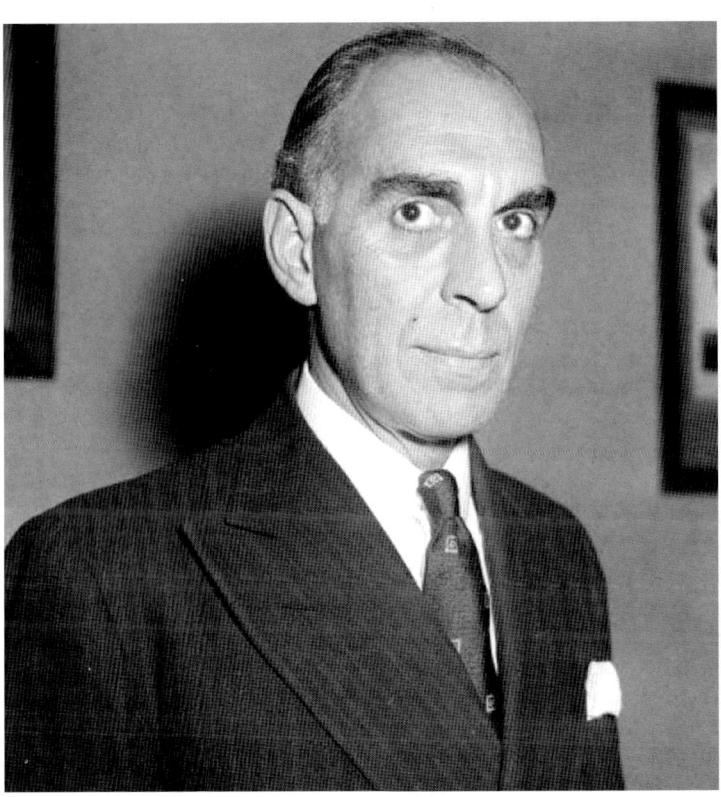

Watson-Jones' excellent surgical abilities, combined with the exposure he received from his hospital appointments, allowed his practice to thrive. He eventually had a Packard limousine with chauffeur, a butler, a personal secretary and an office staff of five, according to his J.B.J.S. obituary.

Plane

Between Tensor Fascia Lata and Gluteus Medius and Minimus.

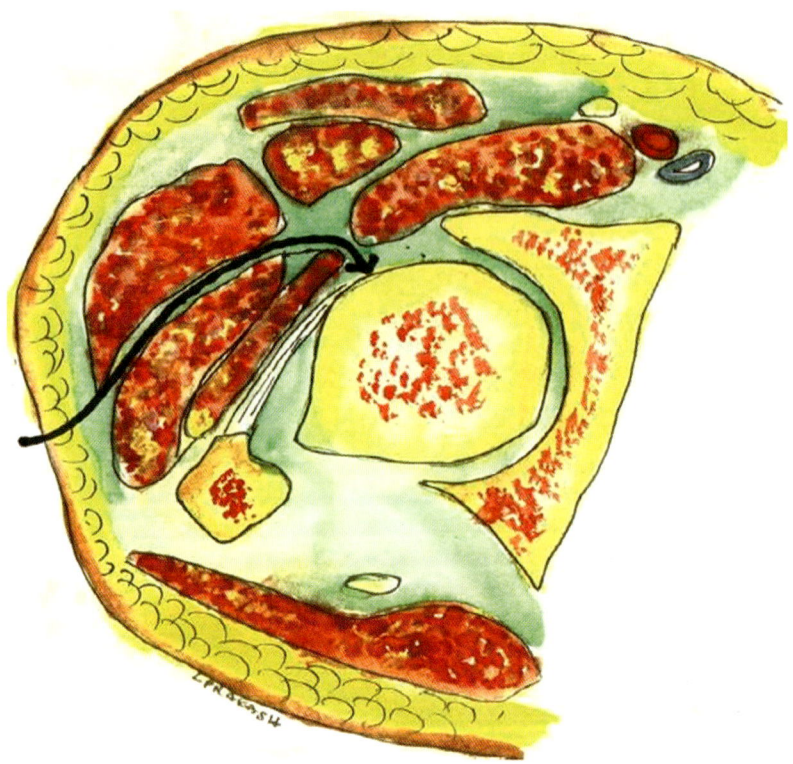

Access Provided

Lateral pelvic wall

Anterior capsule of hip joint

Acetabulum

Proximal femur

Dislocation

Anterior

Position and Draping

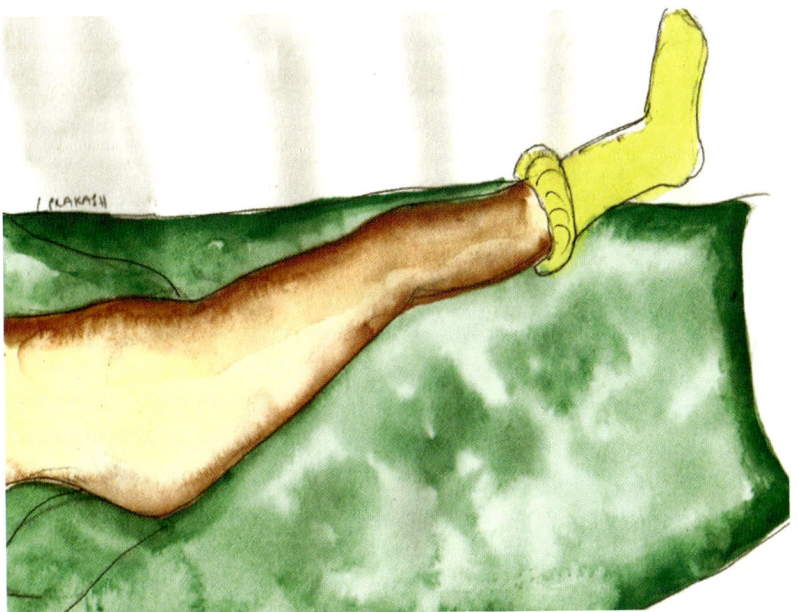

Supine with two small sand bags or rolled towels under both the buttocks. The leg below the knee is draped free as the flexed knee acts as the fulcrum for dislocating and reducing the hip joint.

Incision

From a little above ASIS curving over trochanteric flare, descending straight down to thigh.

Dissections

Fascia Lata is cut along the posterior border of trochanteric flare. This is split longitudenaly parallel to the femur downwards and in the direction of ASIS upwards.

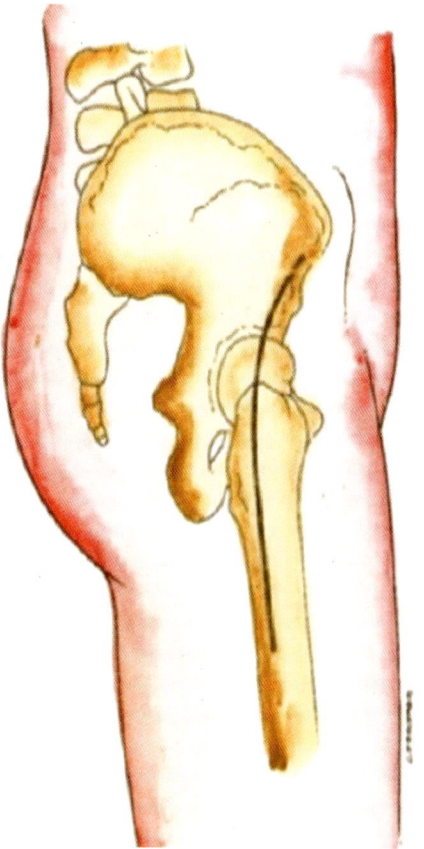

Modified watson jones approach

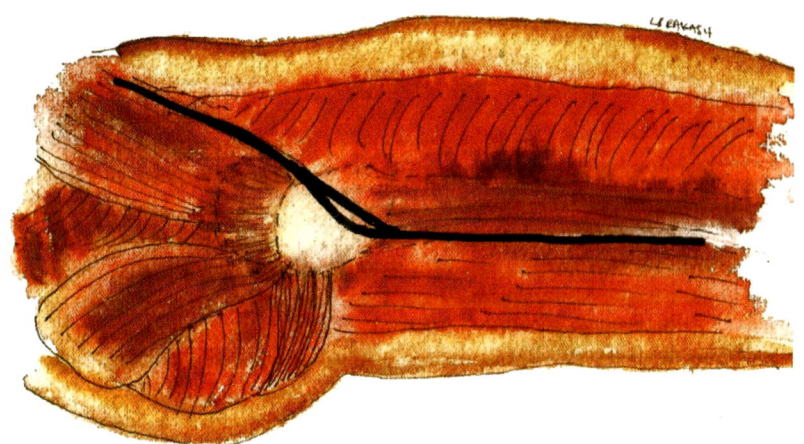

After clearing off the adipose tissue from Vastus Lateralis, the gap between Gluteus Medius and Tensor Fascia Lata is identified.

Bleeders are cautrized on the way and Gluteus Medius and Minimus attachmnts from greater trochanter are cut, leaving decent stubs for reattachment.

The Rectus Femoris is now elevated to visualize the anterior capsule of the hip. By externally rotating the hip, the capsule is stretched for incision to expose the hip joint.

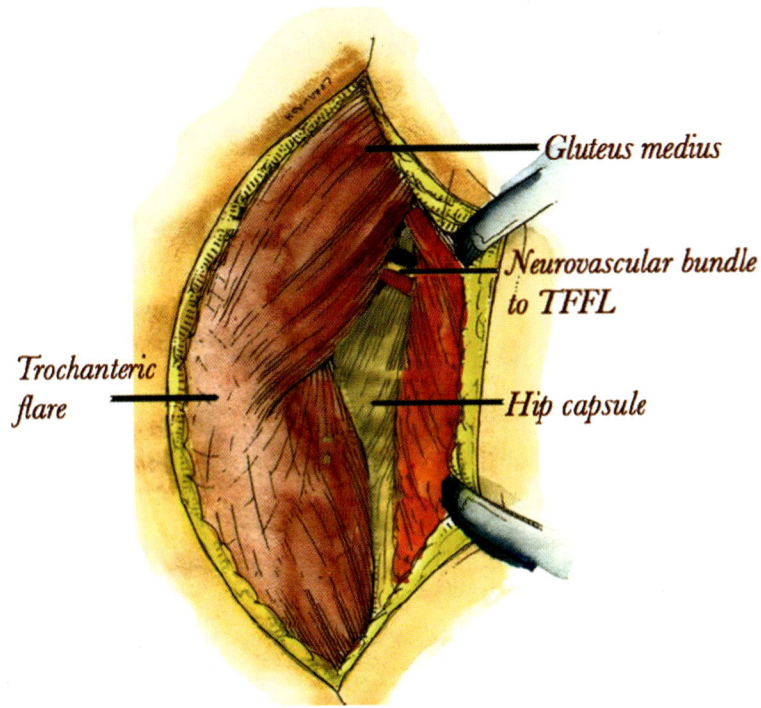

Gluteus medius

Neurovascular bundle to TFFL

Trochanteric flare

Hip capsule

The vessels and nerve to Tensor Fascia Lata are preserved to the maximum extent.

A 'T' shaped incision in the capsule exposes the hip joint. By using the flexed knee and leg as the long arm of the lever, abduction and external rotation of the flexed knee dislocated the hip.

In osteoarthritic hips or deeply seated heads, it may not be possible to dislocate the hip easily. One must desist from forcible attempts to dislocate the head at this stage, because it may lead to a spiral fracture of femur.

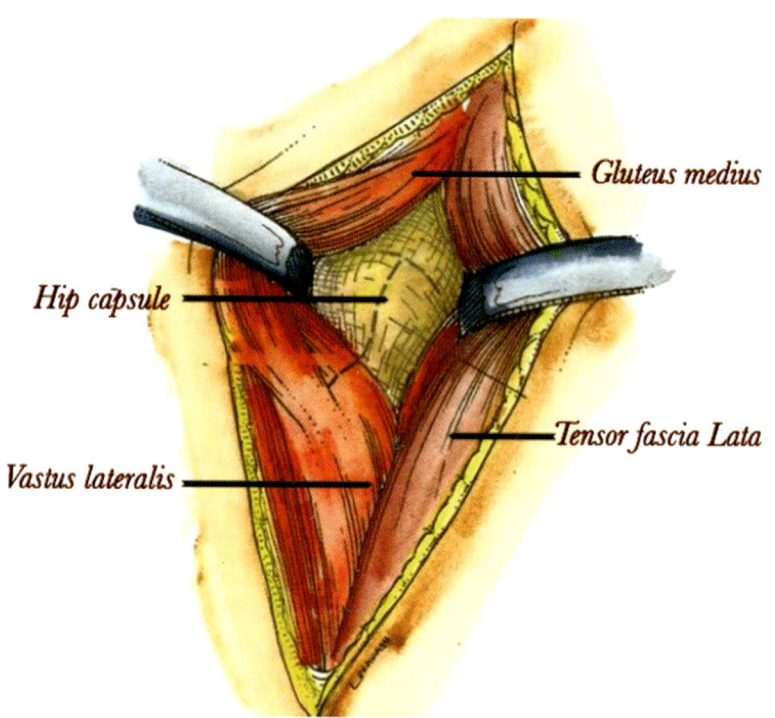

If the exposure is made for total hip replacement, it may be a good idea to cut the neck, and remove the head, after retracting the trochanter.

Indications

Open reduction and internal fixation of fractures of neck of femur.

Hemiarthroplasty and bipolar.

Total hip replacement.

For capsular release with psoas tenotomy.

The approach is not recommended for Revision Arthroplasties.

Advantages

Preservation of abductor mechanism allows rapid rehabilitation and weight bearing.

Orientation of femoral stem is easier as the anterior border of lesser trochanter can be used to decide the version of the stem.

No vital structures in the way, except way superiorly.

Disadvantages

Damage to neurovascular bundle to Tensor Fascia Lata.

Rather limited exposure to acetabulum for reaming and screw placement in cementless hips.

Poor exposure of femoral neck.

This approach was popularized by Maurice Müller for his total hip replacement procedure.

Maurice Müller, a pioneering hip surgeon, was named surgeon of the century by SICOT in 2002.

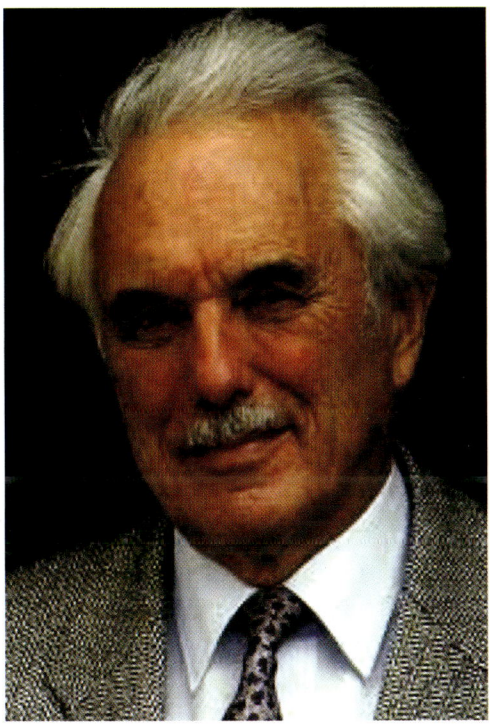

Maurice Edmond Müller

Born on 28 March 1918, Müller was a surgeon, inventor, scientist, designer, biomechanical engineer, and a very skilled magician. I have had the pleasure of watching him do startling magic tricks.

He was born and had his early schooling in Biel Switzerland. He had his medical studies in various Swiss universities, and finally received his M.D. from University of Zurich in 1946.

After spending his initial years serving the poor in Ethopia, he returned to Switzerland to work in its various hospitals. He was professor at University of Berne, and chief orthopaedic surgeon at Inselspital in Berne.

His interest in internal fixation of fractures stemmed from observing the results of Gerhad Kuntchner and Robert Danis, the pioneers of intramedullary and plate fixation. After developing his own instrumentation and implant designs, he founded the AO foundation with three other Swiss colleagues in 1958.

In the early sixties he developed a strong interest in hip replacements and visited Sir John Charnley in Wrightington, UK. After spending some time there, he returned with a set of instruments and began performing hip replacements in Berne. Though extremely pleased by the results of hip replacements per se, he was a tad dissatisfied with a high post-operative dislocation rate, which he attributed to a small head size used in Charnley hips and the lateral trans trochanteric approach, which in his opinion considerably weakened the abductor mechanism.

In 1963, he modified the Charnley system to produce hips with 28mm head diameter and began using them by the anteriolateral Watson Jones approach. This was named the Charnley–Müller hip. By 1964, when Charnley expressed dissatisfaction with the use of his name for a design and approach which were not essentially his, Müller modified the hip further, straightening the stem, and using a head diameter of 32 mm.

In 1967, he founded another company Protek AG to market his Müller hips. He was a rich man by his retirement and became a great patron of arts, donating close to eighty million Swiss

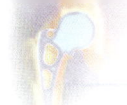

franks for the cause of building an art museum dedicated to a Swiss painter.

One of the lesser known facts about Müller is that apart from his medical writings, he has also published a few articles in magic magazines, explaining certain card trick secrets that he had conceived.

TRANS GLUTEAL LATERAL APPROACH

History

First described in 1954 by Osborene and McFarland, the cleavage was through the Gluteus Medius proximally and vastus lateralis distally. This was later modified by Hardinge for total hip replacement.

BRYAN LESLIE MCFARLAND 1900–1963

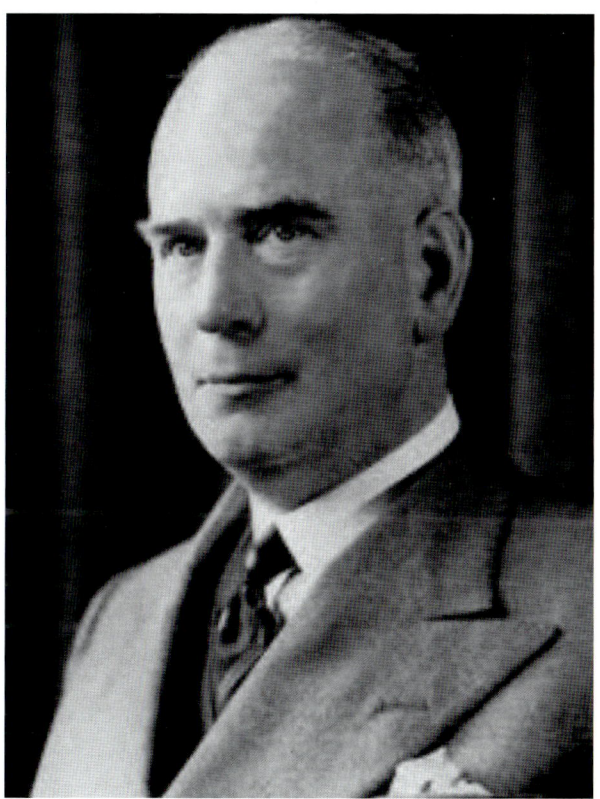

Professor Bryan McFarland was Director of orthopaedic studies and professor of orthopaedic surgery in the University of Liverpool, past president of the British Orthopaedic Association, vice-president of the Royal College of Surgeons of Edinburgh, and president of the International Orthopaedic Society.

Born and brough up in Liverpool, Bryan's life was spent on Merseyside, first at the Wallasey Grammar School and then the medical school of the University of Liverpool. He was one of the first candidates to become master of orthopaedic surgery in 1926; gained the fellowship of the Royal College of Surgeons of Edinburgh in 1928; and 20 years later was elected Fellow of the Royal College of Surgeons of England in recognition of clinical and academic achievement. The determination to serve crippled children was evident during his house surgeon's appointment at the Leasowe Children's Hospital. At the age of 25, he became assistant consultant to the Royal Liverpool Children's Hospital, and later to the Alder Hey Children's Hospital. He was assistant orthopaedic consultant to the David Lewis Northern Hospital from 1928 to 1933 when he became full consultant orthopaedic surgeon to Robert Jones's own hospital, the Royal Southern.

In earlier years, Bryan's teaching of undergraduate and postgraduate students was overshadowed by the powerful personality of the late Professor McMurray, whom Bryan served loyally and faithfully as clinical lecturer; but on elevation in 1948 as director of orthopaedic studies, and later in the professorial chair of the University, his magnitude of vision blossomed and his great qualities of surgical, achademic and scientific brilliance emerged.

The distinction he added to this historic school of orthopaedics will be treasured with pride and affection by M.Ch. (Orth.) graduates not only in Great Britain but in other countries throughout the world.

An excellent marksman, he was passionate about wild fowl hunts He would leave home at three A.M. to arrive in Anglesey before dawn for wild fowl shooting. It was not until after the age of 40 that he became an enthusiastic fisherman, but so thorough was his preparation and practice that he could equal the skill of any professional angler.

Mr. Kevin Hardinge is a practicing consultant orthopaedic surgeon in Manchester. He has worked in Wrightingtom with Sir John Charnley and in Exeter with Mr. Robin Ling. He is still active in orthopaedics in Manchester. An M.Ch. Orth. from Liverpool, he described his classical transgluteal approach based on Osborne and MacFarland's incision in 1982

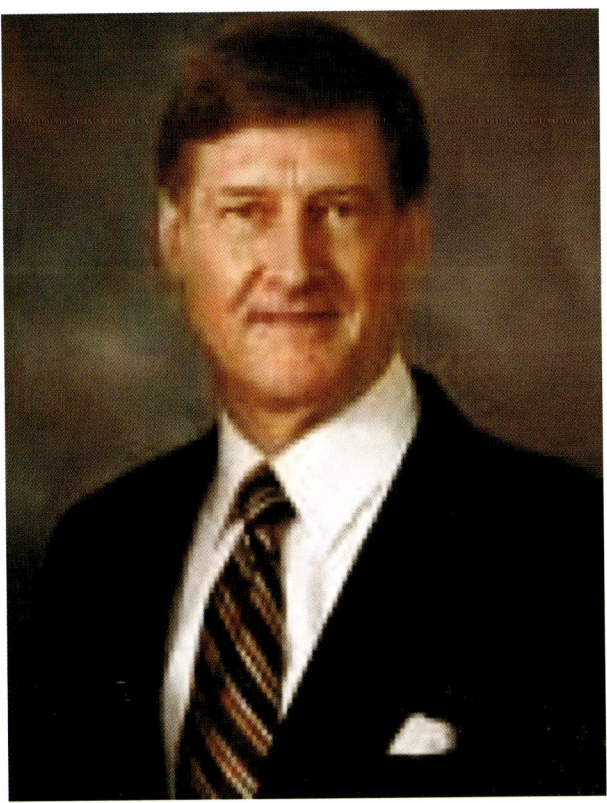

Mr. Kevin Hardinge

Plane

Single flap of Gluteus Medius, its periosteal attachment and vastus lateralis are lifted as a single layer from the anterior part of the trochanter.

Access provided

Excellent 360 degree approach to the acetabulum.
Decent approach to proximal femur.

Dislocation

The hip is dislocated anteriorly by externally rotating the limb using the flexed knee as a fulcrum.

Position and draping

The positioning depends on the surgeon's familiarity and comforts, and the patient can be in either supine or lateral position. If supine, the operative hip is raised with a small pillow. In lateral position, the patient is strapped to back rests and sand bags, to keep the pelvis steady during the entire surgery.

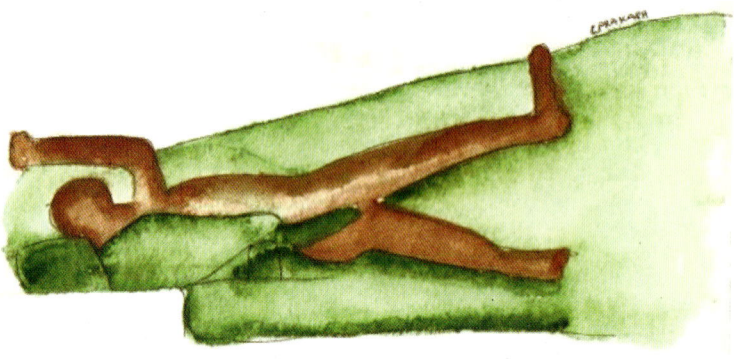

The limb is draped free and the knee should flex comfortably to provide a good lever arm for generous internal and external rotations of the hip joint during the surgery.

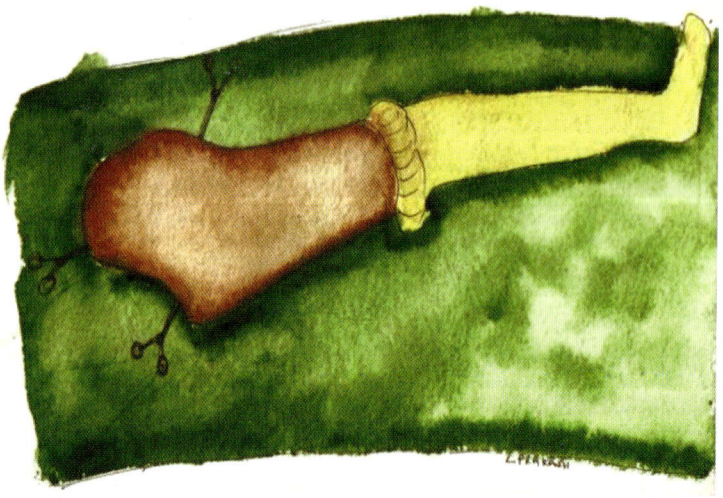

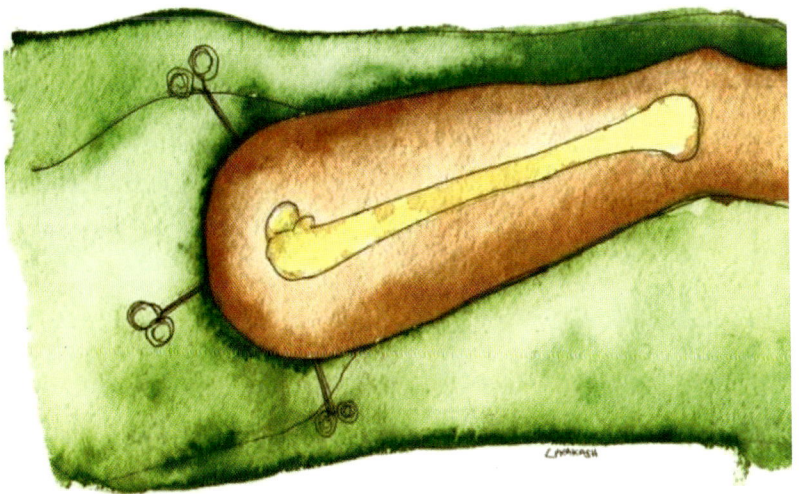

Incision

Straight mid lateral incision, extending 5cm up and down from the mid point of the greater trochanter.

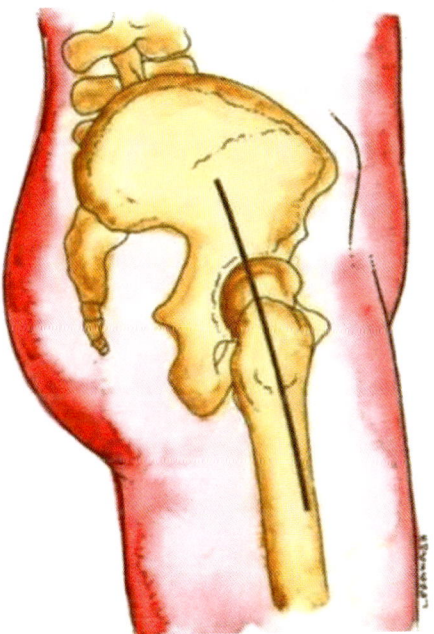

Straight incision for a Hardinge approach

Dissections

Subcutaneous tissue is incised in the same line as skin.

Glistening white Tensor Fascia Lata is identified over greater trochanter, and using a cutting diathermy a bone deep incision is made on the posterior margin of greater trochanter.

The attachment of Gluteus Medius to the greater trochanter is visualized by full internal rotation of the hip.

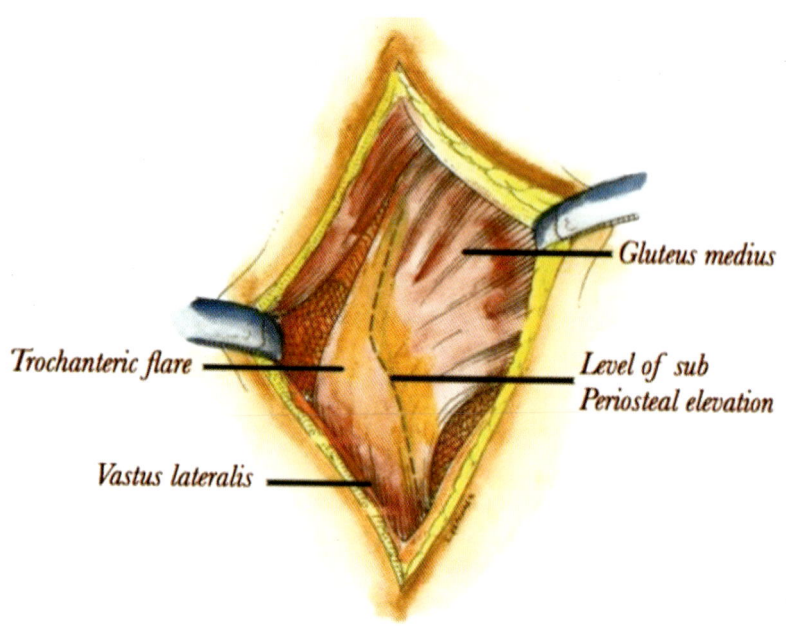

The whole width of Gluteus Medius is identified, and the muscle is split in line of its fibres at the junction of its anterior and middle thirds.

Now using a very sharp chisel, the entire subperiosteal flap on the anterior aspect of the trochanter, starting with Gluteus Medius proximally, and the Fascia of the vastus lateralis distally is lifted as a single flap and deflected anteriorly.

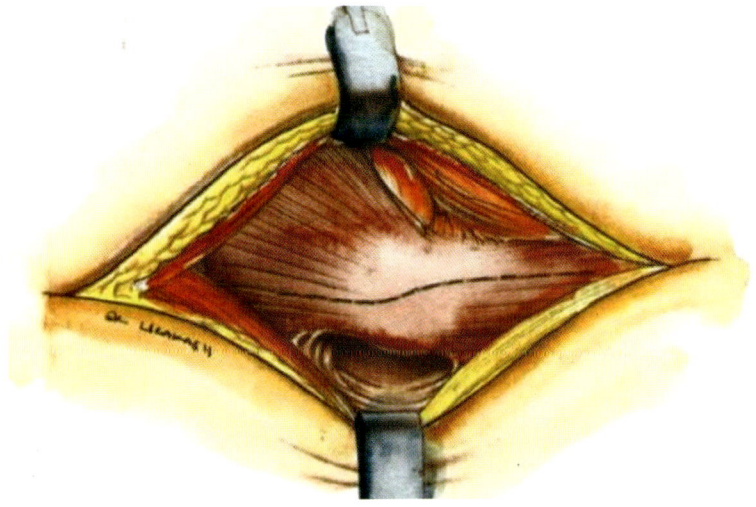

The entire gluteal structures are lifted as one flap

The tendon of Gluteus Medius is now detached, and the hip capsule below is cut with a 'T' shaped incision.

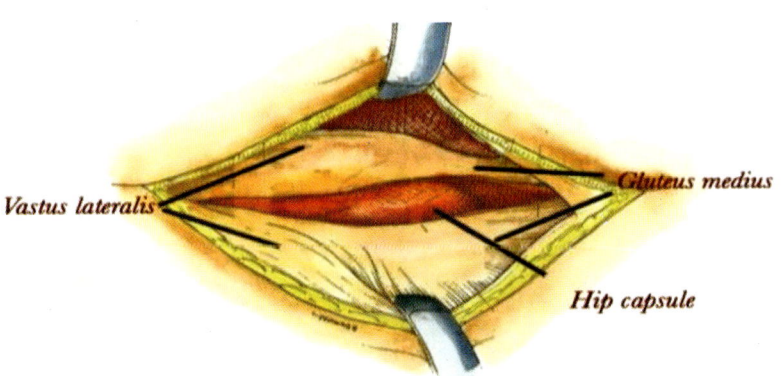

Level of cleavage in Harding

The transverse branch lateral circumflex femoral artery has to be located deep within the vastus lateralis and cauterized, to avoid persistent bleeding.

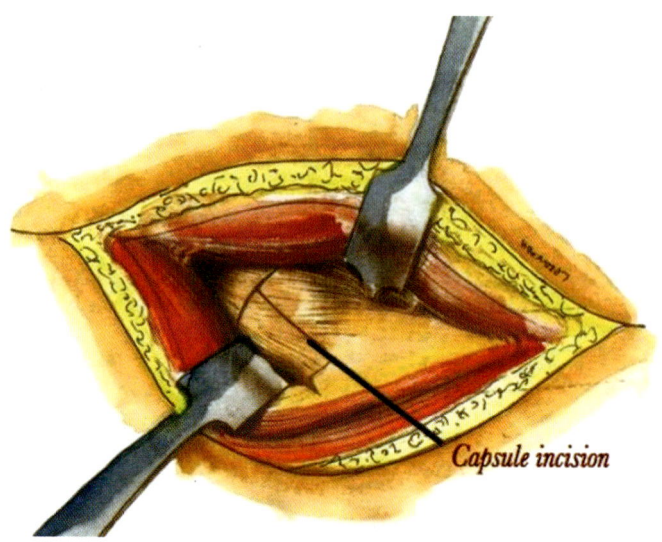

Capsule incision

Judicious placement of Homman Retractors allows a full vision of the capsule, and a fairly extensive capsular dissection can be done.

Note that the hip can be dislocated by internal rotation. An easy method is to keep the flexed knee on the opposite thigh. If the head does not come out, additional capsular releases may be performed.

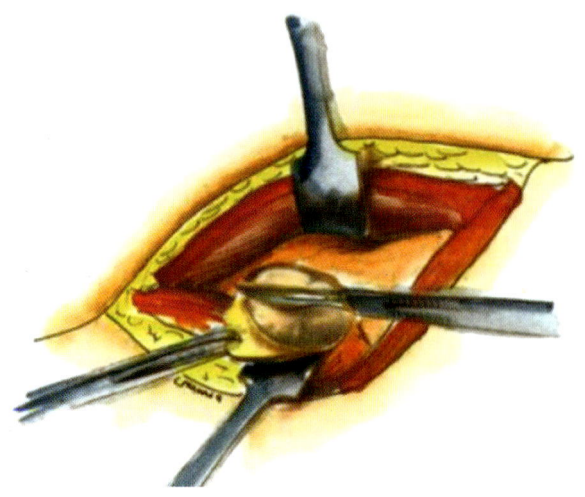

Capsular excision to expose head

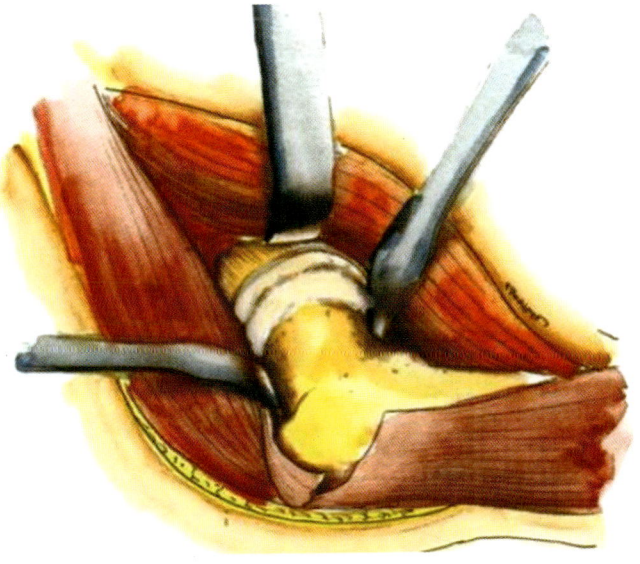

External rotation to dislocate the head

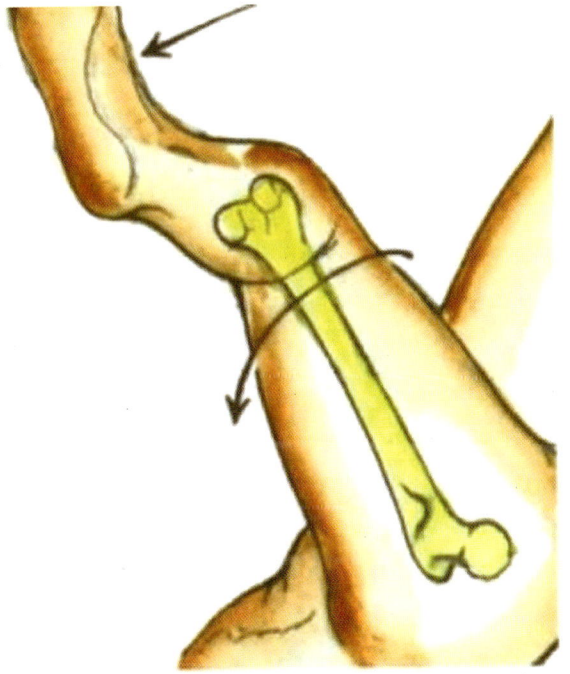

External rotation will dislocate the head

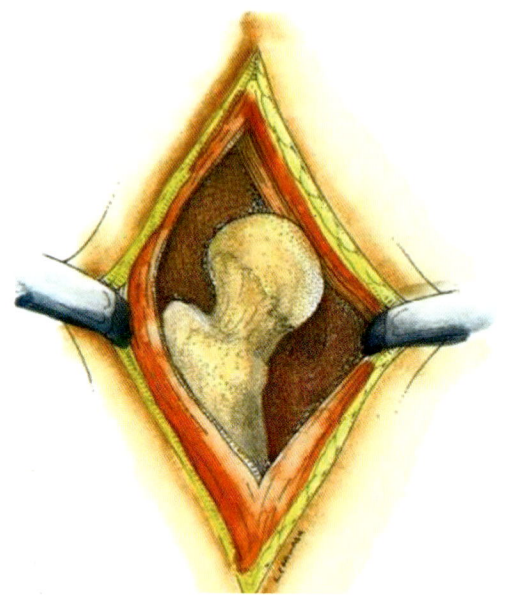

Head dislocated in the Hardinge approach

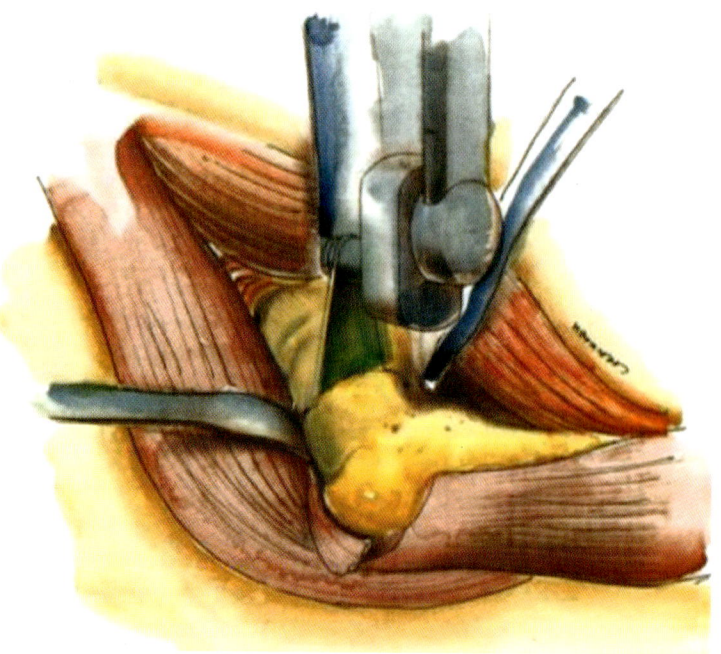

In case the hip and is fused, neck is osteotomized first

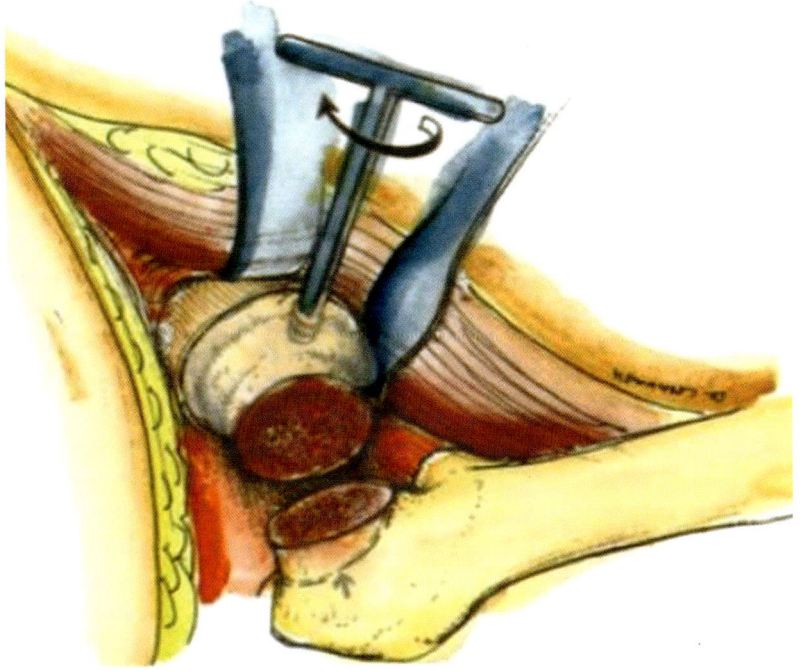

The cut head is removed with a cork screw

Indications

Hemi arthroplasty

Total Hip replacement

Revision hip replacement.

Advantages

Excellent exposure.

Supine position allows perfect cup placement.

Preservation of greater trochanter allows rapid return to work.

Disadvantages

Slightly increased blood loss.

Gluteal weakness post operatively.

CHARNLEY'S TRANS TROCHANTERIC APPROACH

History

Sir John Charnley (1911–1982)

He is probably the greatest hip surgeon of all times and it was his ceaseless toil that produced the Total Hip Replacement. I quote from Mr. Wroblowsli's article about him.

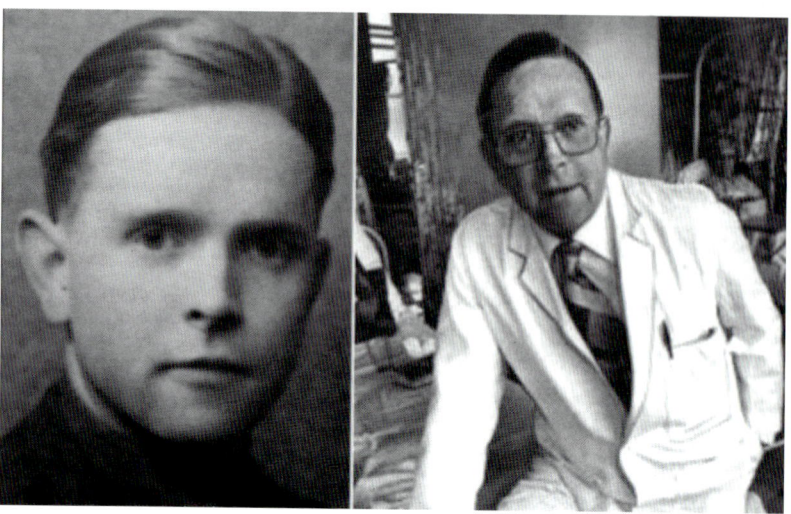

Charnley's contributions to orthopaedic sciences and surgery are so vast that it would be difficult to do justice when attempting to present more than a mere outline. Three aspects form a main theme: trauma, fusion of joints by compression methods, and total hip arthroplasty.

The Closed Treatment of Common Fractures, first published in 1950, went to three editions and three reprints, the third one 40 years after the volume was first published! Justice will not be done by attempting even to summarize the volume, which has become, as intended by Charnley, the vade mecum of a practising trauma surgeon. Charnley's objective is clearly stated in the preface to the first edition: ...*An attempt is here made to re-emphasize the non-operative method, and to show that far from being a crude and uncertain art, the manipulative treatment of fractures can be resolved into something of a science.*

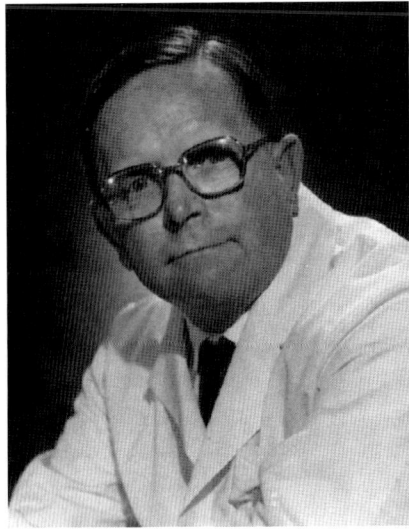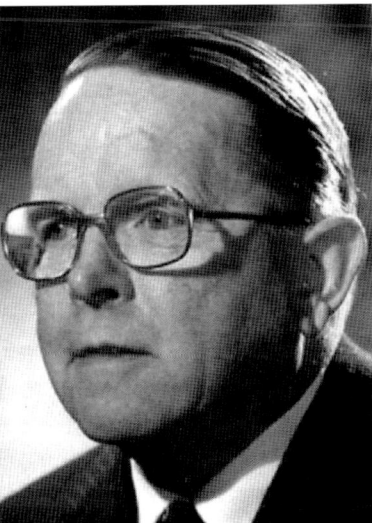

Yet Charnley was not slow to admit that certain fractures, as of the tibia, proved difficult and had to be treated by internal fixation.

In 1961 Charnley wrote: *There is a tendency to imagine that serious research nowadays can only come out of a laboratory, and the contributions from the pure act of thinking on clinical facts ended with the great clinicians of the past. In the training of young surgeons... the attempt to foster the habit of making clinical observations and questioning accepted beliefs ought to start from the earliest moment.*

Published in 1953, Compression Arthrodesis is a monumental work on the physiology, principles and practice of cancellous bone union under compression. *'A few observations on the human body are often of more value than a large series of experiments on animals. It has rightly been said that every surgical operation is a biological experiment.'*

Although not as popular a method of treatment as it used to be before the advent of total joint arthroplasty, the principles remain valid and are almost certainly the basis of formation of the Association for the Study of Osteosynthesis, the *Arbeitsgemeinschaft fur osteosynthesefragen Group with their very detailed description of operative treatment and compression fixation of fractures.*

Few individuals are capable of changing their practice by advocating diametrically opposite views and remain successful.

Charnley did just that—from arthrodesis to arthroplasty—from abolition of all movement to restoring all of it.

From 1962 onwards, Charnley committed his energies to hip replacement surgery with a full-time practice at Wrightington Hospital. And here began his breathtaking and monumental work in arthroplasty.

Charnley himself did suffer trials and tribulations when developing his hip replacement methods, but he never gave up. Finally, in November 1962, the Charnley hip replacement became practical reality and has become the gold standard for this form of treatment. Clinical and radiographic success of this procedure is now approaching 50 years of follow-up.

Total dedication to all aspects demanded by this type of surgery consumed Charnley's time. Development of the clean air enclosure, total body exhaust suits and the instrument tray system are the essential aspects to reduce deep infection in this type of surgery.

Prospective documentation, the establishment of a Centre for Hip Surgery and the collection of numerous post-mortem specimens bequeathed by his patients in order to study the histology of the bone–cement interface, show clearly how far seeing Charnley's ideas were.

Charnley's contribution to orthopaedic surgery was recognized both nationally and internationally with numerous awards, including a knighthood in 1977.

Plane

Trans trochanteric

Access Provided

A very wide access for both acetabulum and upper femur in all directions.

Dislocation

Anterior or posterior depending on the surgeon's choice.

Position and Draping

Once again, depending on the surgeon's choice, the patient can be placed supine or in lateral position. A slightly increased hip maneuverability in lateral position makes it the position of choice in revision arthroplasty.

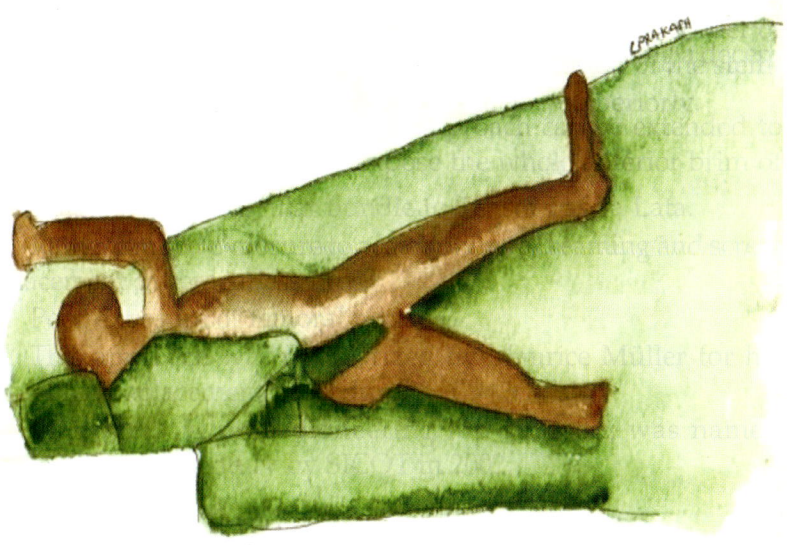

The leg is draped free for easy hip maneuverability.

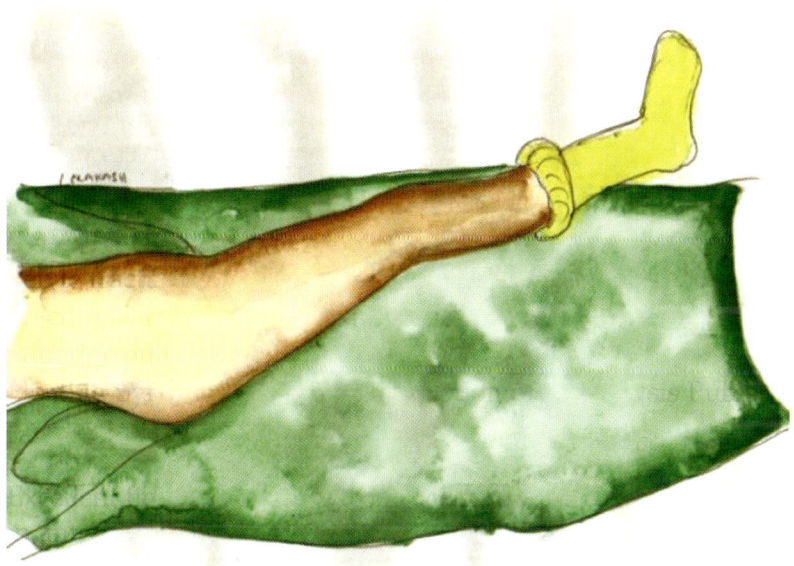

Incision

Straight incision centred over trochanter extending 5 cm proximally and distally.

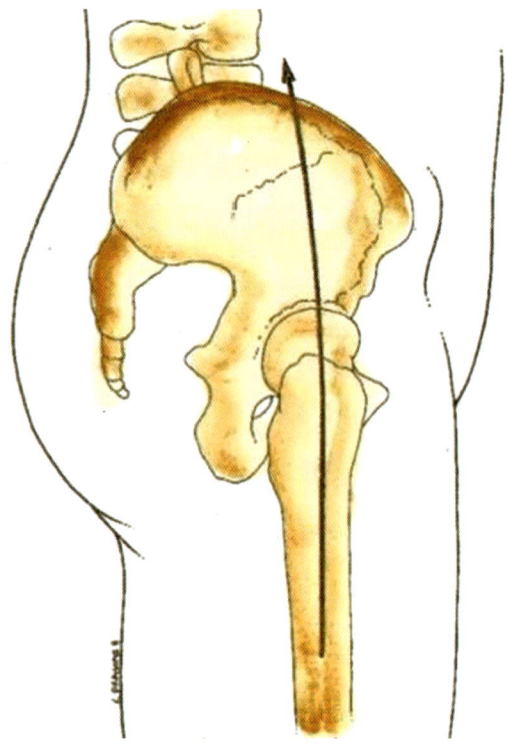

Charnley's Trans Trochanteric approach

Dissections

The Fascia Lata is divided in skin line. The gap between Tensor Fascia Lata and Gluteus Medius is explored till the hip capsule.

The posterior margin of the Gluteus Medius is now identified and a curved forceps is introduced directly over the capsule coming from the anterior to posterior fibres of Gluteus Medius.

The limb is internally rotated and abducted to guide the tip of the curved forceps to emerge correctly.

The anterior half of the origin of the vastus lateralis is now erased with a cutting diathermy, going bone deep and a part of vastus lateralis is now deflected out.

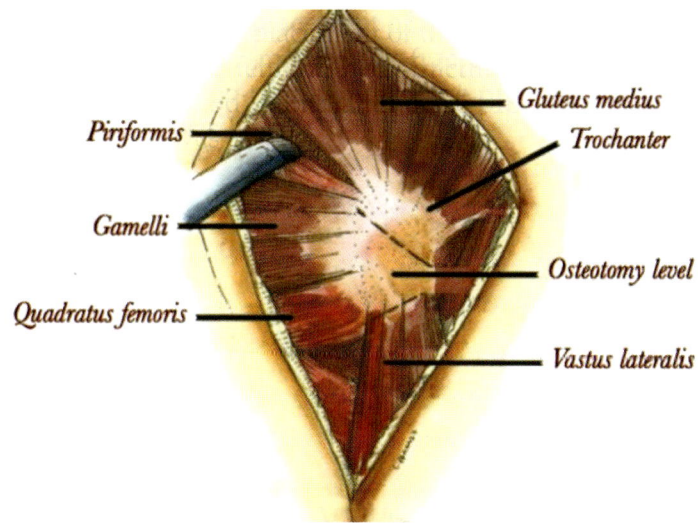

Osteotomy level in Charnley approach

The trochanteric osteotomy is now performed. The curved artery forceps may be used to pull out a Gigli saw which can then be see sawed. Else a Stienman pin pushed into the trochanter, gives a wedge-shaped Chevron osteotomy for better reattachment.

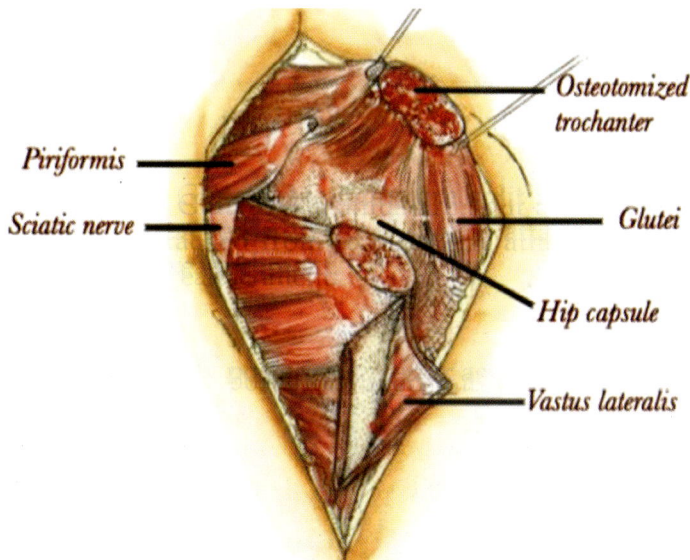

Trochanteric osteotomy gives a really wide exposure

Some surgeons use small sharp chisels, while others use power saws. The important point to remember is to include the posterior aspect of the greater trochanter as well. The piece should not be too small to make reattachment difficult.

Deflection of the osteotomized trochanter exposes piriformis which is divided to reach the hip capsule.

The capsule is cut or excised to expose the hip. Dislocation is easy by external rotation and abduction.

The trochanter is reattached either by tension band wires or by a couple of lag screws.

The following drawings redrawn from Charnley's book describe the master's steps. No text is needed to explain them, as a picture is well worth a thousand words.

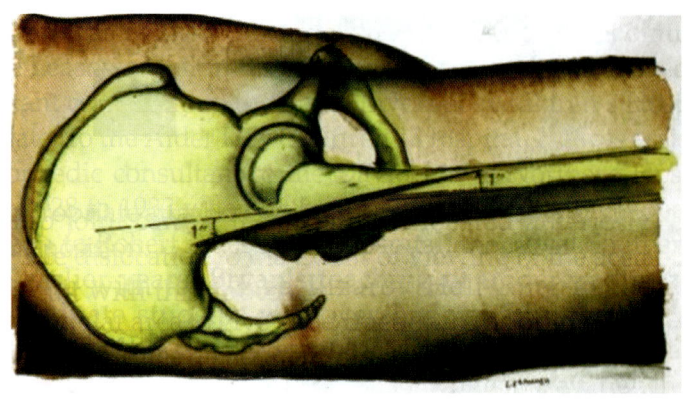

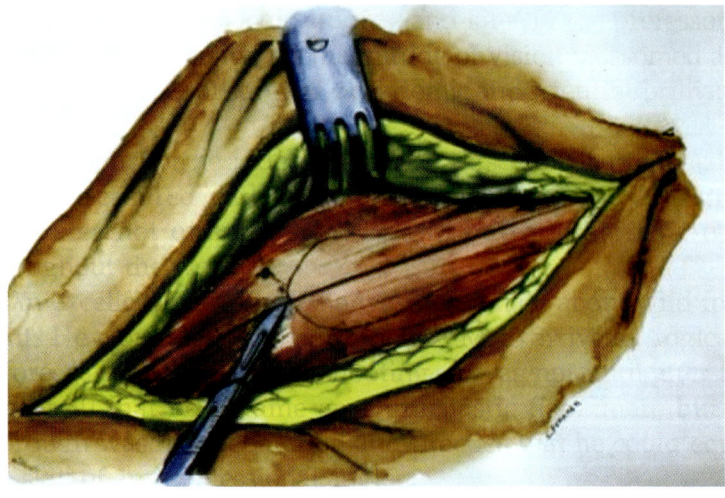

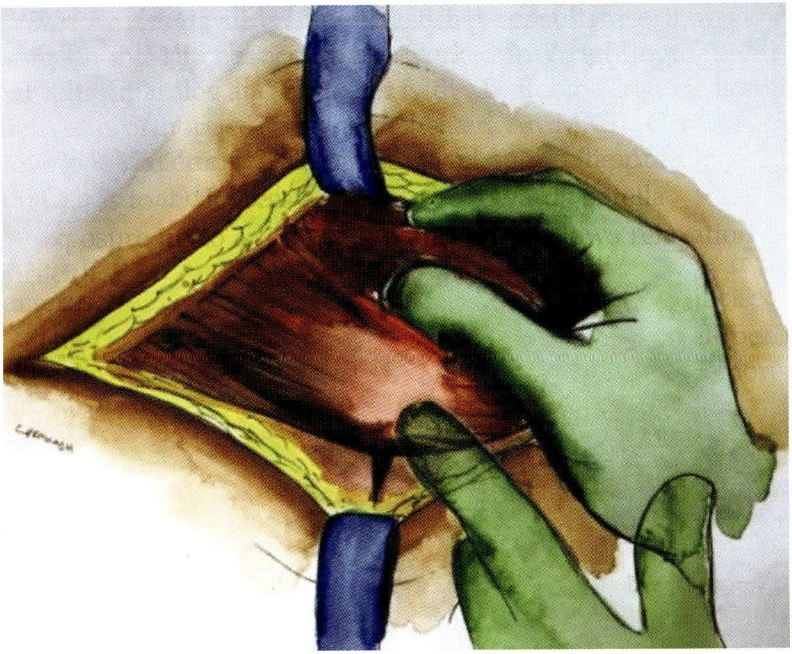

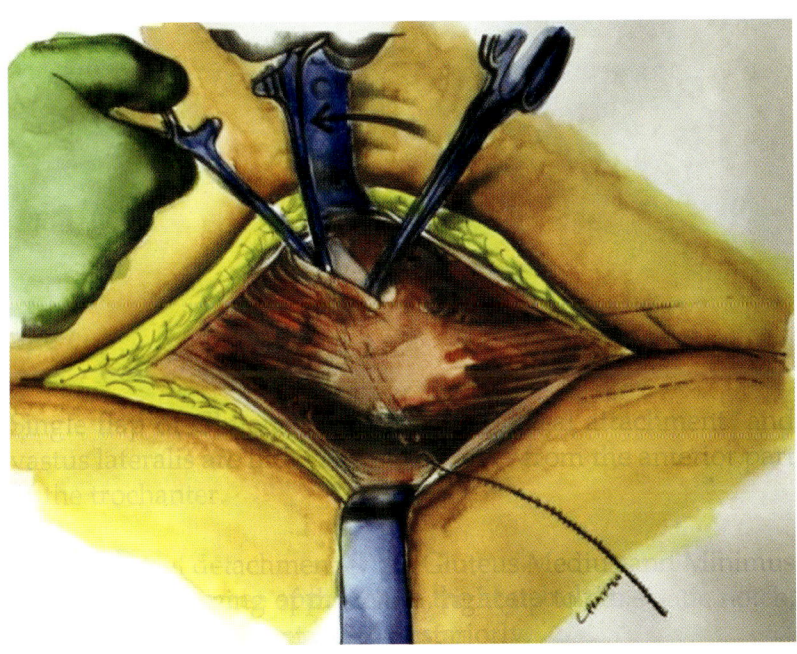

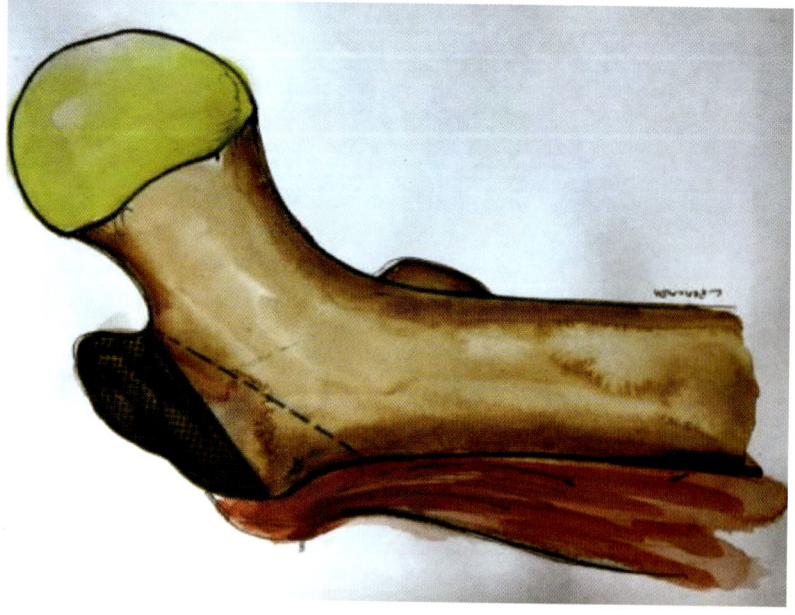

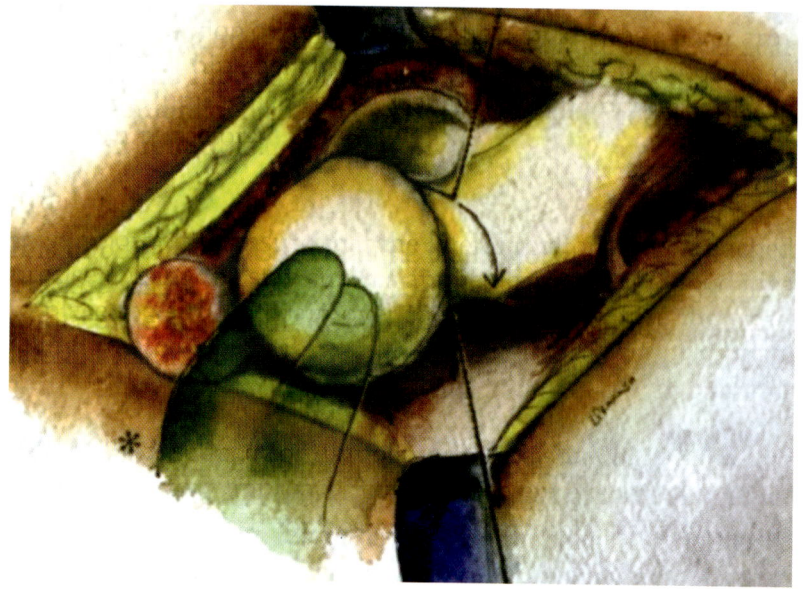

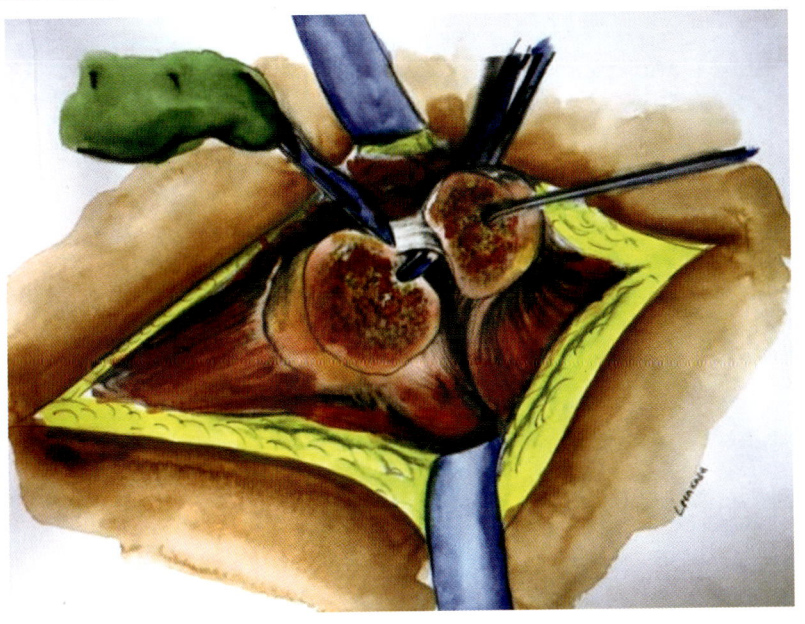

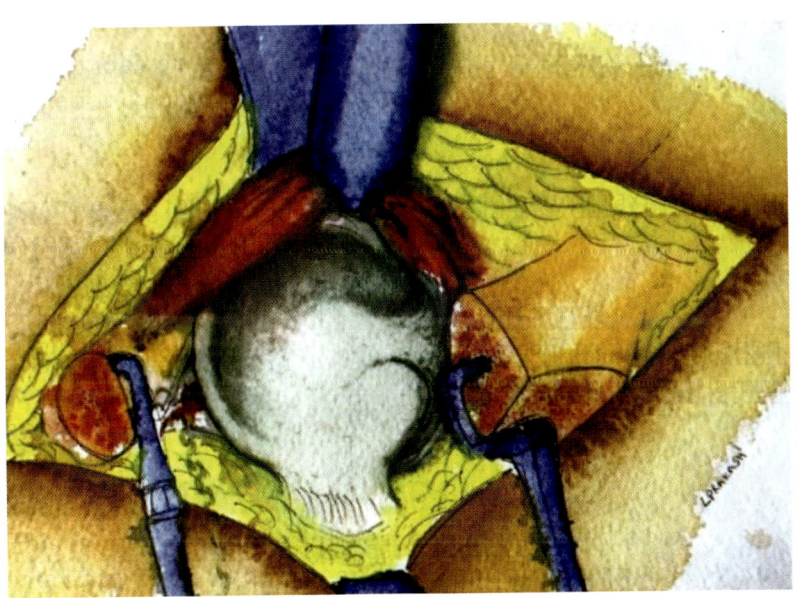

Indications

Primary and revision hip replacements, especially difficult and complex hips.

Advantages

Widest exposure of hip.
Gluteus Medius and Minimus remain undamaged.
Distalization of the trochanter can tighten the abductor lever arm and improve post-operative function.

Disadvantages

Increased blood loss
Slower recovery
Trochanteric problems, non unions and bursitis.

EXTENDED TRANS TROCHANTERIC APPROACH

History

This approach was described by Rüedi in 1984 along with his AO colleagues, and was principally meant for complex pelvi acetabular injuries.

Plane

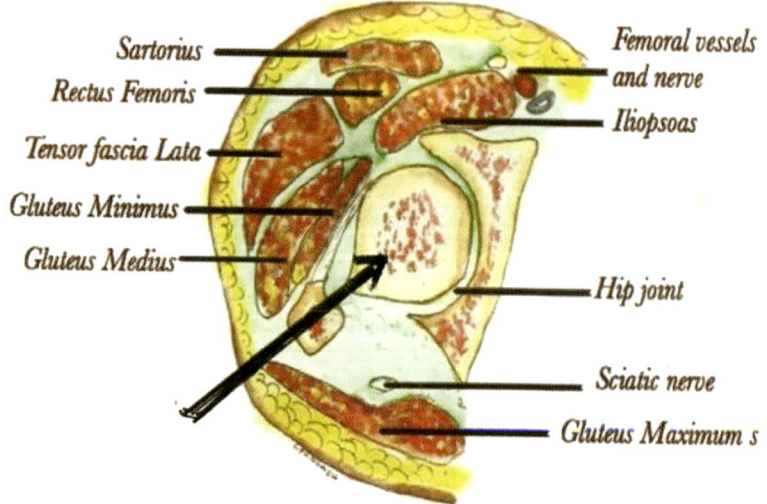

Sartorius

Rectus Femoris

Tensor fascia Lata

Gluteus Minimus

Gluteus Medius

Femoral vessels and nerve

Iliopsoas

Hip joint

Sciatic nerve

Gluteus Maximum s

Anatomical planes for hip approach

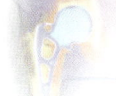
Trans trochanteric approach, where stripping muscles from pelvis exposes the pelvis from anterior column right up to iliopubic eminence.

Access provided

Posterior column
Superior acetabular dome
Anterior column
Iliopubic area

Dislocation

Anterior, posterior, or inferior, depending on the fracture type and fixation needs.

Position and draping

In lateral position, the patient is strapped to back rests and sand bags to keep the pelvis steady during the entire surgery. The limb is draped free and the knee should flex comfortably to provide a good lever arm for generous internal and external rotations of the hip joint during surgery.

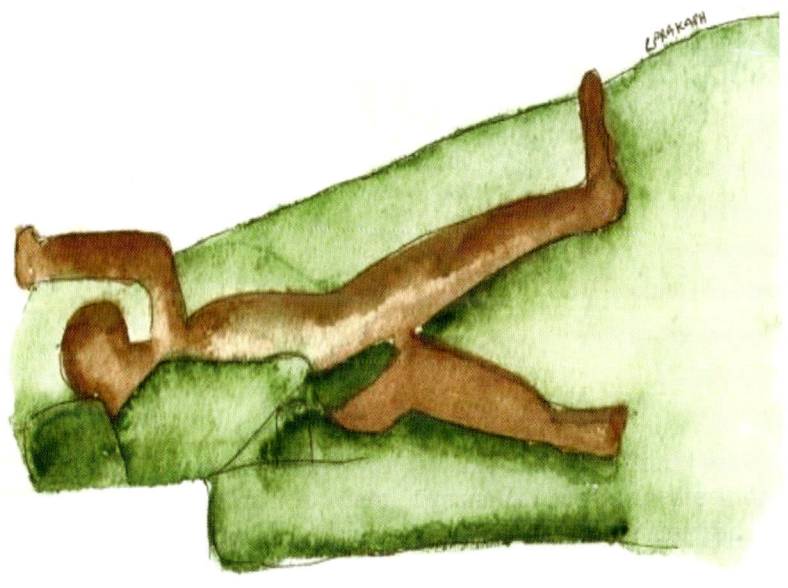

A distal femoral pin traction on an Ilizarov half ring or a Bohler's stirrup will allow traction to be applied when needed.

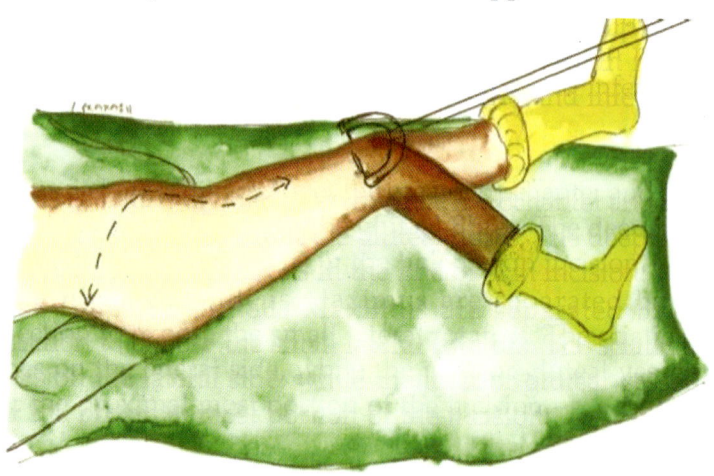

Incision

The three landmarks to be kept in mind are Iliac crest, posterior border of trochanteric flare, and lateral border of patella.

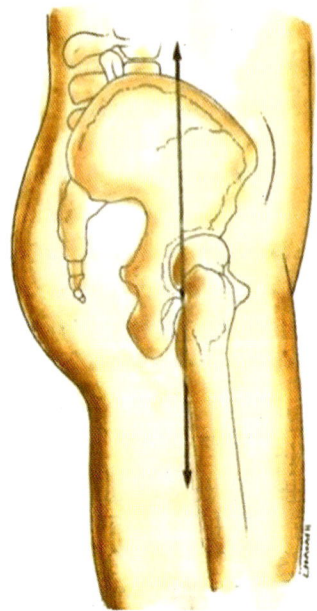

Extensive trans trochanteric approach

The skin incision is a straight line centred over Greater trochanter extending almost equally upwards and downwards.

Dissections

Subcutaneous fat and Fascia are dissected a little more extensively in the proximal part of the incision than the distal part. The Gluteus Medius is exposed as far as iliac crest.

A high skein incision allows it to be retracted in a thick flap to allow a 'T' incision in the Gluteus Medius dividing the iliotibial tract towards front and back a little below the iliac crest.

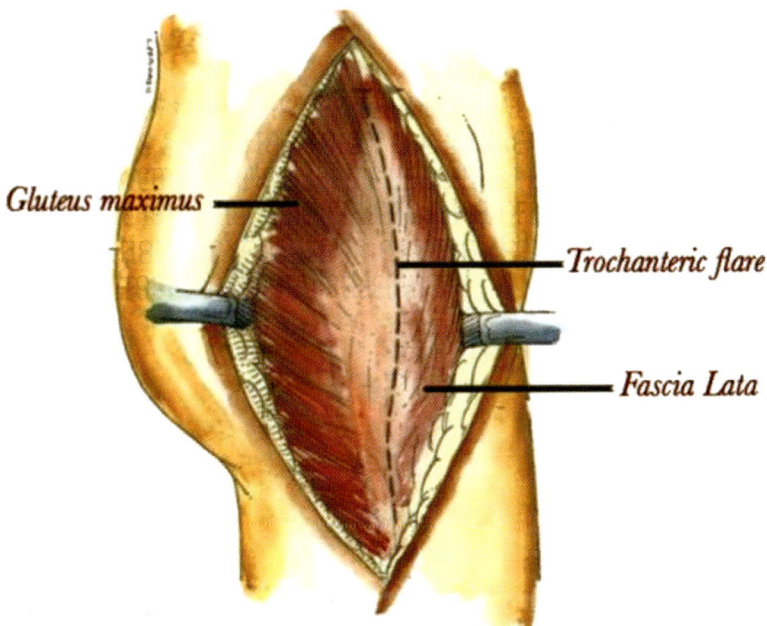

Deep Fascia is raised as flaps from the underlying muscles. The posterior flap contains the Gluteus Maximus. Iliotibial tract is detached from upper Gluteus Medius.

Gluteus Medius, short lateral rotators and vastuis lateralis are identified.

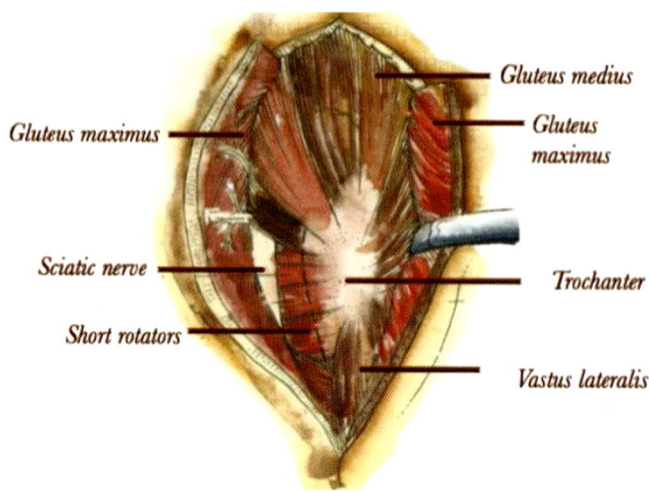

Gluteus maximus is split

Greater trochanter is now osteotomized, to allow Gluteus Medius and Minimus to be sub periosteally elevated from ASIS to sciatic notch.

The superior neuro vascular bundle is identified and protected. This is the only remaining supply for the remaining muscle belly and the muscle mass has to be frequently replaced back till it perfuses red again.

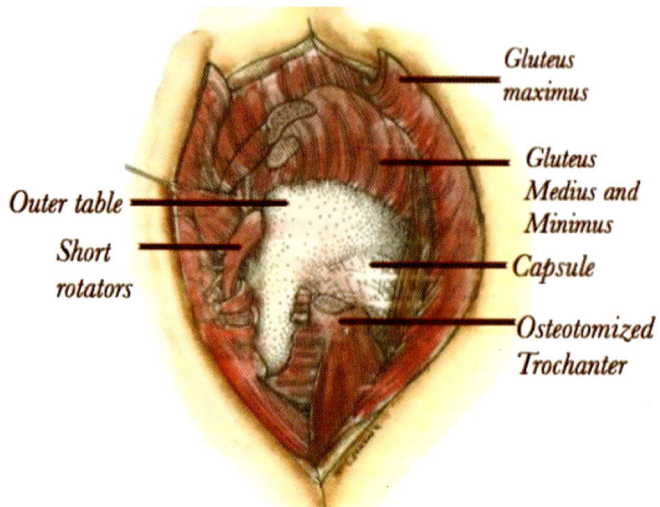

Reudi's approach

Small lateral rotators are now detached from posterior border of greater trochanter leaving sufficient mass for reattachment. Their posterior retraction protects sciatic nerve.

Anterior column is accessed by dividing the straight and reflected head of Rectus Femoris.

Osteotomy of iliac crest will give additional access if needed.

Flexion of the hip and sub periosteal erasure of iliacus muscle from inner table allows palpation of inner surface of acetabulum to check reduction.

The iliac crest is reattached with lag screws, and trochanter with screws, clamps or wires. The lateral rotators are reattached before closure.

Indications

Pelvic fractures, including those involving sacrum.
Fractures of the anterior column.
Superior pubic ramus fractures.
Floating Symphysis Pubis or disruption of Symphysis Pubis.

Advantages

Excellent field of exposure from one side to the other, especially in anterior column fractures.

Good clean cosmetic scar.

Disadvantages

Difficult and technically demanding operation
Superior gluteal vessels have to be carefully protected, and the muscle mass repeatedly perfused intraoperatively.

Increased blood loss.

Osteotomies have to be fixed back.

POSTERIOR APPROACHES

History

Von Langenbeck in 1874, and Kocher in 1887 described posterior approaches with minor differences. Frequency of foot drop and sciatic injuries made these approaches unpopular until 1950, when Gibson described his variation. In 1957, Moore described his modification for insertion of his prosthesis. From the 1960s, the direct posterolateral approach has become the most popular approach for most hemi arthroplasties and total replacements of hip.

Bernhard Rudolf Konrad von Langenbeck, nephew of the anatomist and surgeon Konrad Johann Martin Langenbeck, studied in Göttingen, where he received his doctorate in 1835. He began his career as a lecturer in Physiology and Pathological Anatomy in Göttingen in 1838.

Langenbeck became an extraordinary professor in Göttingen, and in 1842 was called to the chair of surgery in Kiel, where he was also director of the Friedrich Hospital.

Later he became the physician to the general staff – General-Stabsarzt – and then Physician General (Generalarzt) and consulting surgeon, and that same year, he was raised to the nobility.

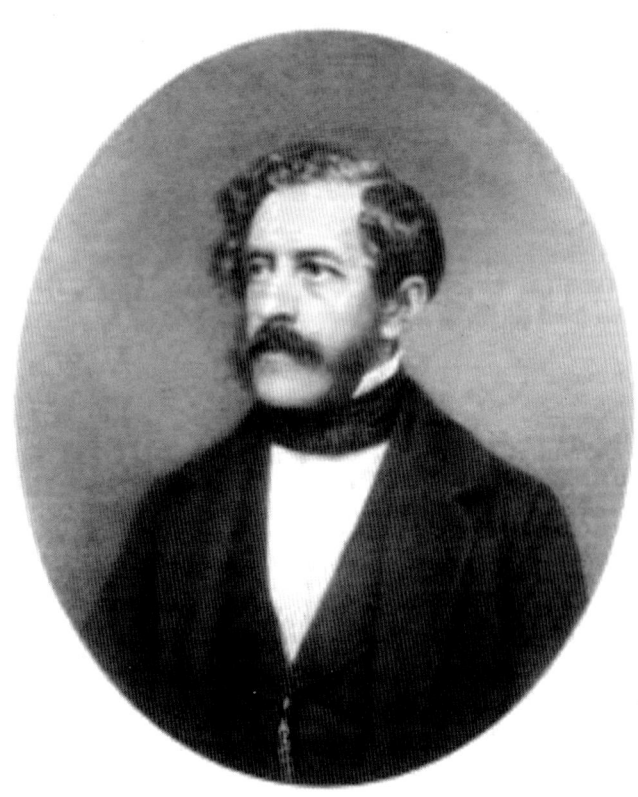

Bernhard Rudolf Konrad von Langenbeck His experiences from the field hospitals were laid down in numerous papers. His fields of interest were resection of joints as well as gunshot wounds and their treatment.

He was a great innovator and developed several surgical instruments. In surgery, apart from his hip approach, he made important contributions in the development of plastic surgery, and manipulations of the contracted knee joint in contractures with percutaneous tenotomies. He is also remembered for his operation of cleft palate published in 1861.

For years, Langenbeck was the undisputed leader of German surgery and is best known today as the "father of the surgical residency". He developed a system by which new medical graduates would live at the hospital as they gradually assumed a greater role in the day-to-day care and supervision of surgical patients. Among his most well-known "house staff" were such illustrious surgeons as Christian Albert Theodor Billroth and Emil Theodor Kocher.

The brilliance of his house-staff model was acknowledged by Sir William Osler and William Stewart Halsted, who quickly co-opted this concept into the teaching system of the Departments of Medicine and Surgery respectively at the Johns Hopkins University Hospital in the late 19th century. From orthopaedics to ENT, from maxilofacial to arthrolysis, from medical training to apprenticeship, from design to instruments making, his contributions to the field of medicine were phenomenal. In 1864 he was knighted for his services during the Danish war. He was a highly recognized and very popular teacher, drawing large flocks of students to the University of Berlin during his tenure.

Emil Theodor Kocher (1841–1917, Bern) was the Swiss surgeon who won the 1909 Nobel prize for Physiology or Medicine for his work on the thyroid gland.

After qualifying in medicine at the University of Bern in 1865, Kocher studied in Berlin, London, Paris, and Vienna, where he was a pupil of Theodor Billroth. In 1872 he became professor of clinical surgery at Bern, remaining as the head of the surgical clinic for 45 years.

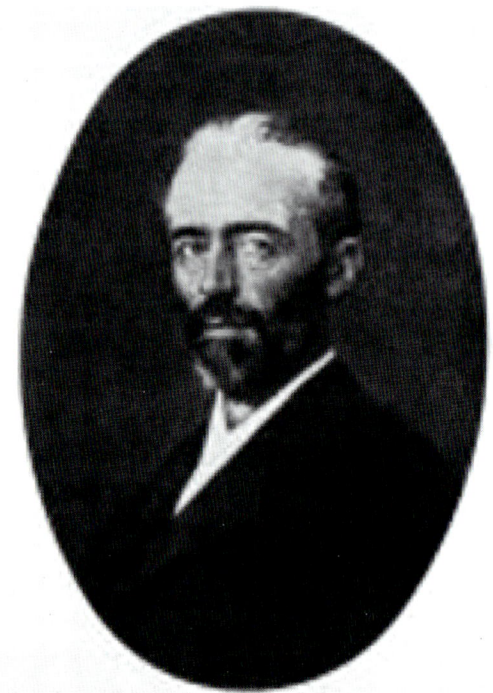

Emil Theodor Kocher

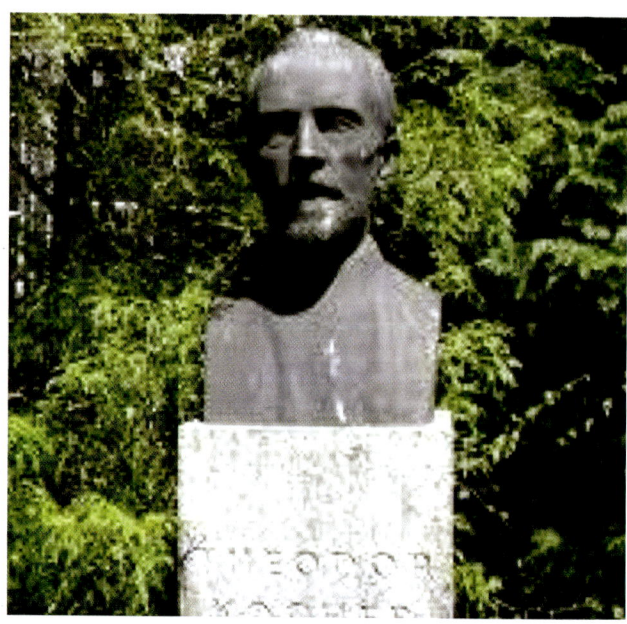

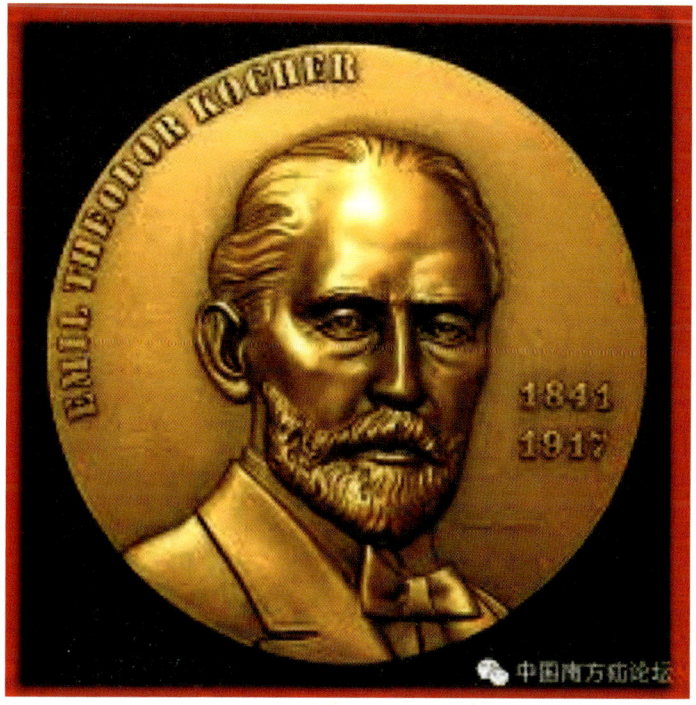

There, Kocher became the first surgeon to excise the thyroid gland in the treatment of goitre (1876). In 1883, he announced his discovery of a characteristic cretinoid pattern in patients after total excision of the thyroid gland; when a portion of the gland was left intact, however, there were only transitory signs of the pathological pattern.

His other surgical contributions include a method for reducing dislocations of the shoulder and techniques for surgery on hip, stomach, lungs, tongue, cranial nerves and for hernia. In surgical practice, he adopted the principles of complete asepsis introduced by Joseph Lister. He also devised many new surgical techniques, instruments, and appliances. The forceps and incision (in gallbladder surgery) that bear his name remain in general use.

Austin Tally Moore (1899–1963) was an orthopaedic surgeon in South Carolina. He performed one of the first total hip replacements in 1940, but it was the hemiarthroplasty which he first performed in 1942 to which he lent his name.

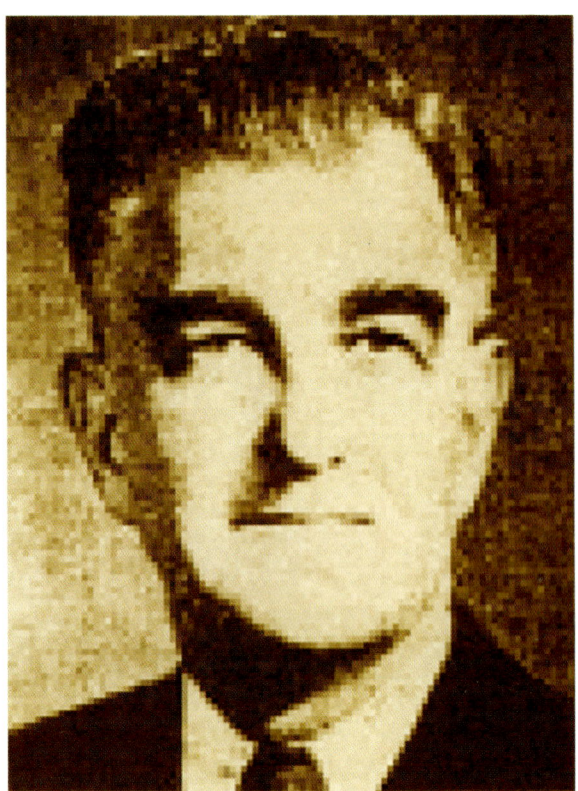

Dr. Austin T. Moore

After completing his medical school in 1924 from South Carolina, he worked in various hospitals till 1939, when he founded Moore Clinic in Columbia. He was also was the surgeon of the psychiatric hospital in the city of Columbia, which had 7,000 beds. Fractures of the neck of the femur are frequent among older patients who are often in bad general state.

Moore devised a revolutionary process of fixing the femoral head in such fractures, whereby the metal head would be carried by a stem driven into the medullary canal of the femur. In 1952, he designed an improvement that featured a fenestrated stem to allow bone ingrowth. Both designs were produced in collaboration with *Howmedica Inc.* (at the time, *Austenal Laboratories*, now merged with *Stryker® Corporation*).

These were the first hip arthroplasty products that were widely distributed. They eventually became legendary and are still widely used for replacement of the femoral head and neck, especially following femoral neck fractures in the elderly. He described his method of implanting the prosthesis in J.B.J.S. in 1957 (the year I was born).

MOORE'S SOUTHERN APPROACH

Plane

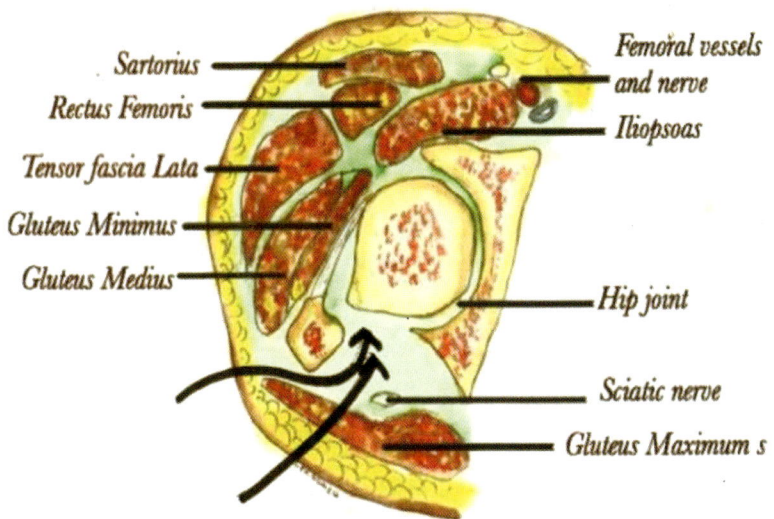

The fibres of Gluteus Maximus are split and small lateral rotators are detached from trochanteric attachment leaving enough bits for reattachment.

Access provided

Hip joint, especially posterior superior aspect.
The sciatic nerve.
Neck of femur.
Lesser Trochanter.

Dislocation

Posterior.

Position and Draping

The original Moore's position was semi prone with sand bags under the affected ASIS. Later modifications placed the patient in the lateral position, stabilized in place by supports, clamps and sand bags.

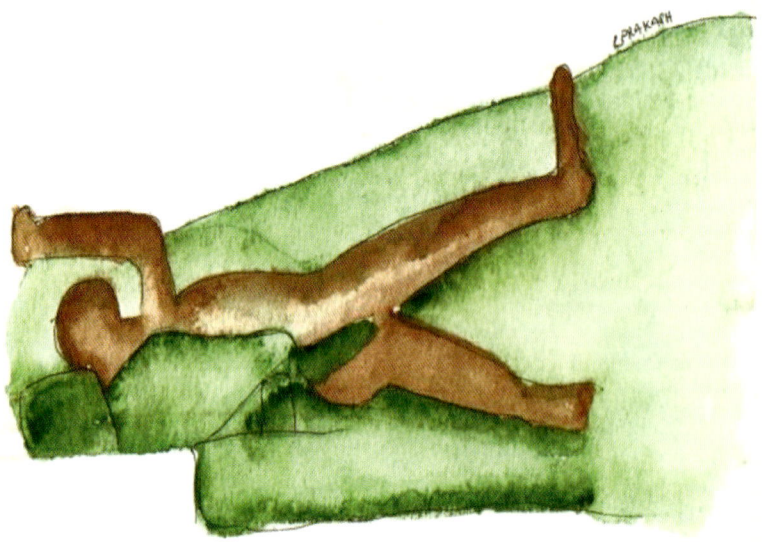

Incision

Begins three inches below the posterosuperior iliac spine, extends to trochanterioc flare and then curves along the lateral border of thigh.

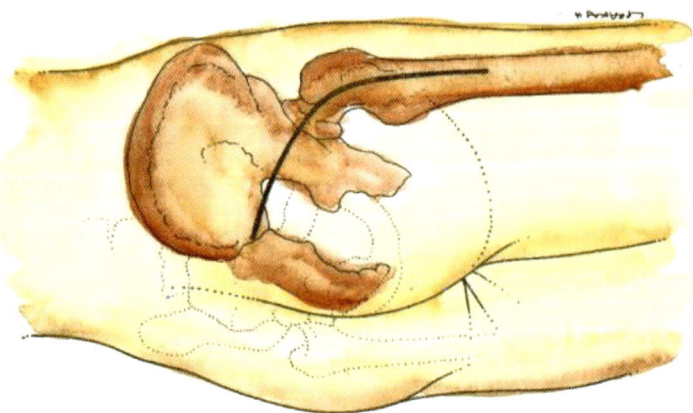

Dissections

The Fascia Lata is divided over the greater trochanter and carried in both directions in the line of skin incision.

The fibres of gluteus maximus are separated by blunt dissection to expose the small lateral rotators. The sciatic nerve comes on the lateral side, while the inferior gluteal vessels are near the proximal most portion of the incision.

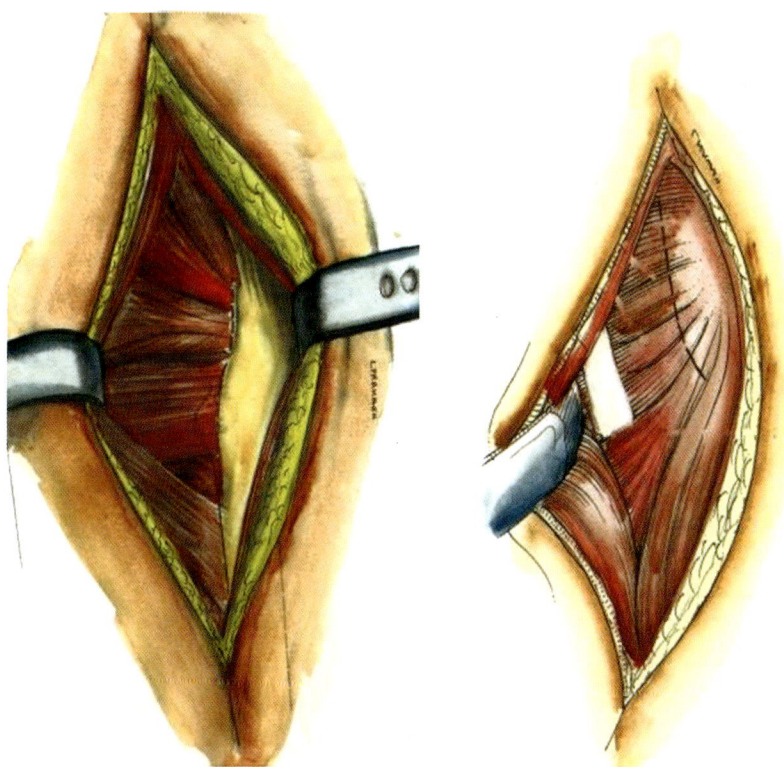

The small lateral rotators are now divided close to their insertion into the trochanter, leaving enough attachments for repair.

This exposes the hip joint capsule, which can be incised in a 'T' fashion. The femoral head and neck will be visible at this stage.

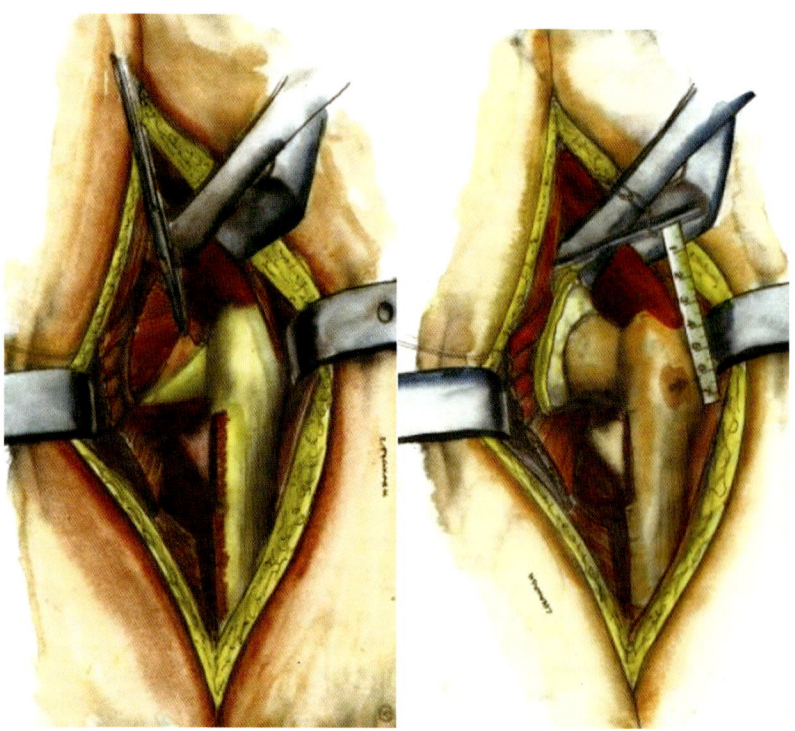

Internal rotation of the leg, using the bent knee as a lever arm, dislocates the hip easily and provides a complete exposure of the acetabulum, which can be visualized using properly placed Homman retractors.

Closure

It is important to ensure that the lateral rotators are reattached precisely using the stay sutures applied earlier. It is a good idea to place the suction drain over the joint, then suture the small lateral rotators above it.

Indications

Originally described for unipolar arthroplasty, this remains the most satisfactory approach for that problem even today.

It can also be used for posterior column pelvis and posterior acetabular fractures.

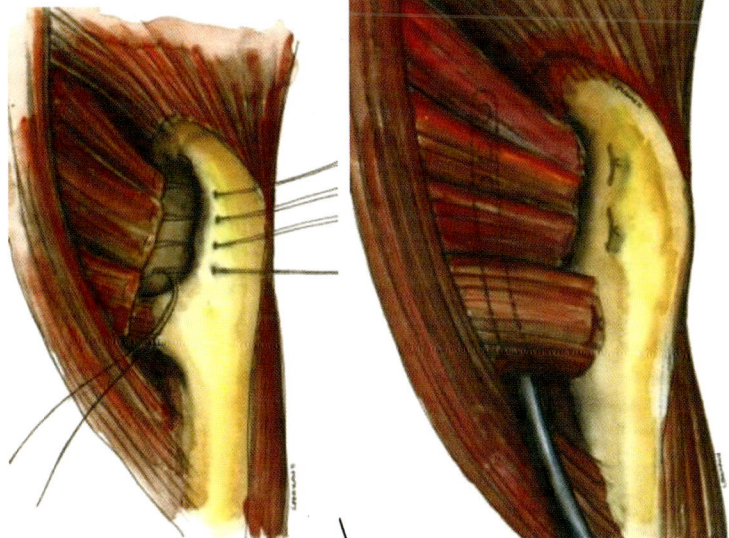

Advantages

Easy and quick exposure through almost bloodless fields and planes.

Easy dislocation of the hip.

This is probably the best approach for unipolar and bipolar hips.

Provides an excellent access to the posterior lip and the posterior column of the acetabulum.

Disadvantages

Sciatic nerve injury and foot drop due to neuropraxia in case of excessive lateral exposure.

Injury to inferior gluteal vessels.

Dependant incision with associated problems.

Slightly higher risk of post-operative infection and dislocation.

Acetabular exposure is a little less adequate that lateral approaches.

THE STANDARD LATERAL APPROACH

This is the preferred and most commonly used approach for total hip replacements, and is a modification of Moore's approach with a slightly more lateral straight incision. This has the advantage of making the approach less dependent and avoids post-operative oedema. It provides the same excellent approach as the Classic Moore's Southern approach, but at the same time has a lesser rate of post-operative complications.

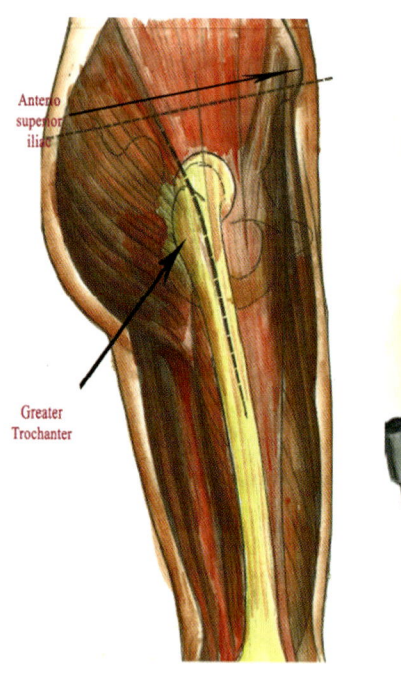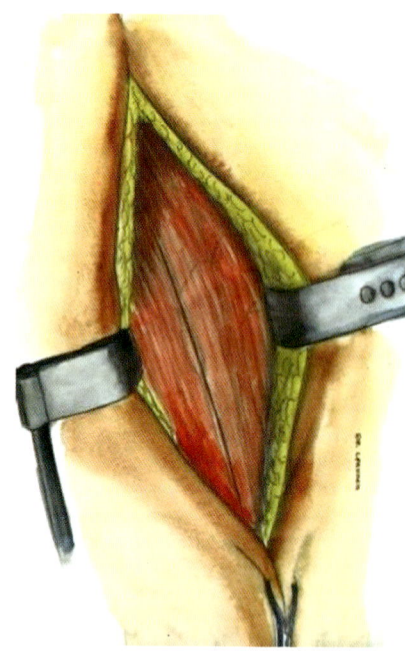

Plane

The fibres of Gluteus Maximus are split and small lateral rotators are detached from trochanteric attachment leaving enough bits for reattachment.

Access Provided

Hip joint, especially posterior aspect.
Neck of femur
Lesser Trochanter.
Acetabulum

Dislocation

Posterior.

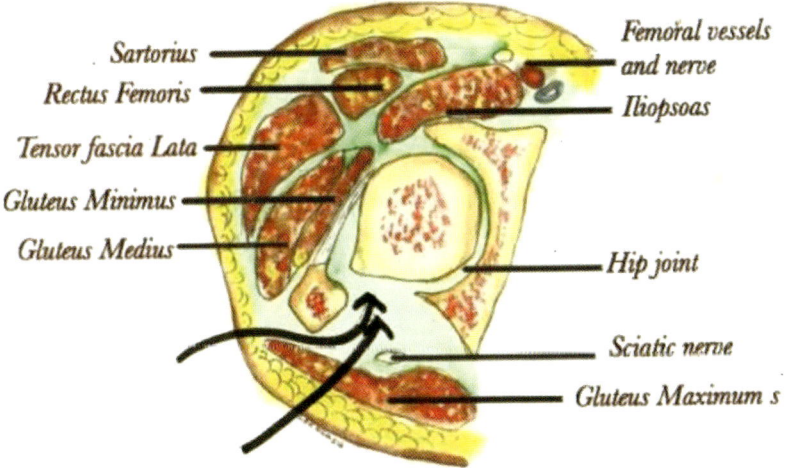

Sartorius

Rectus Femoris

Tensor fascia Lata

Gluteus Minimus

Gluteus Medius

Femoral vessels and nerve

Iliopsoas

Hip joint

Sciatic nerve

Gluteus Maximum s

Position and Draping

A lateral position with sand bags and table attachments to keep the patient stable. The leg is draped free for manipulations and dislocations.

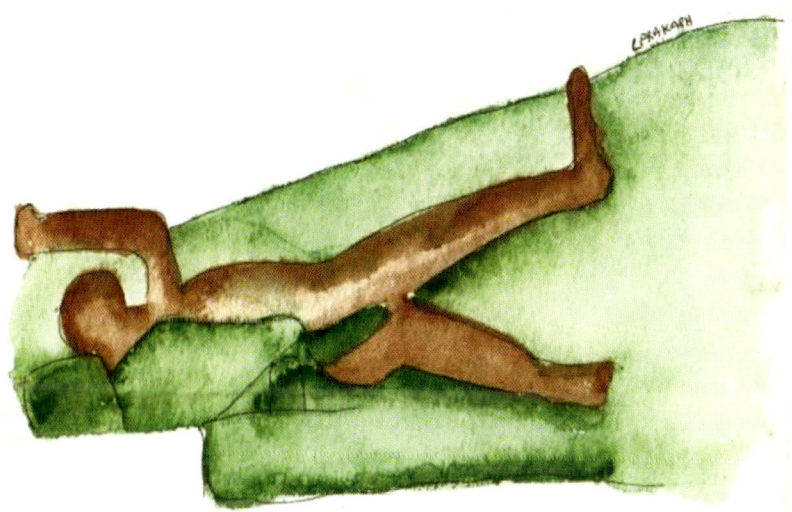

The knee is flexed and kept flexed throughout the procedure to ensure that sciatic nerve is kept relaxed during the entire period.

Incision

Straight midlateral or slightly posterolateral incision centred on posterior aspect of greater tyrochanter extending superiorly to iliac crest about 7.5 cm below trochanteric flare. In revisions, the incision can be extended both superiorly and inferiorly.

Dissections

The Fascia Lata is divided over the greater trochanter and a finger inserted to separate it from the gluteal fibres. The deep incision is carried in both directions in the line of skin incision.

The fibres of Gluteus Maximus are separated by blunt dissection to expose the small lateral rotators. The sciatic nerve comes on the lateral side, while the inferior gluteal vessels are near the proximal most portion of the incision.

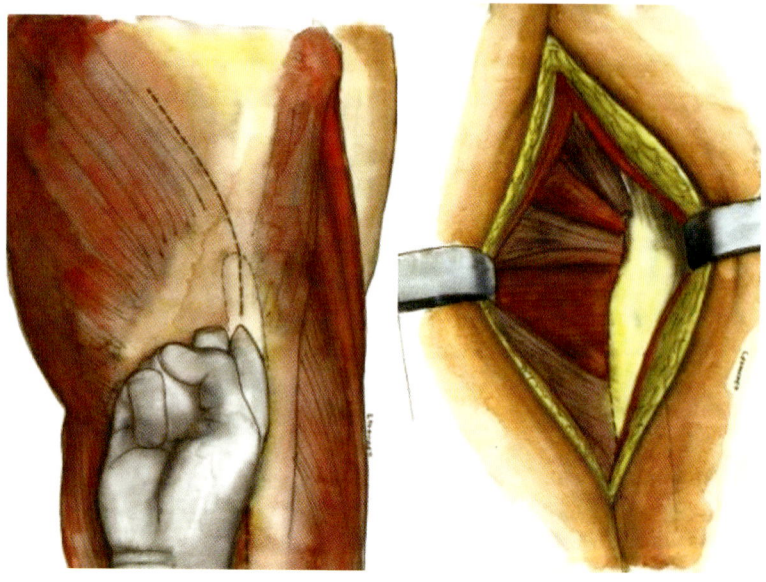

Sciatic nerve may not always be visualized, but its position should be always kept in mind. The fatty areolar tissue over the small lateral rotators is cleared by pushing it with a pad.

The hip is now internally rotated and this stretches the attachment of the lateral rotators and these can be now detached, leaving adequate bits for reattachment. Stay sutures in the lateral rotators allow the whole belly to be retracted

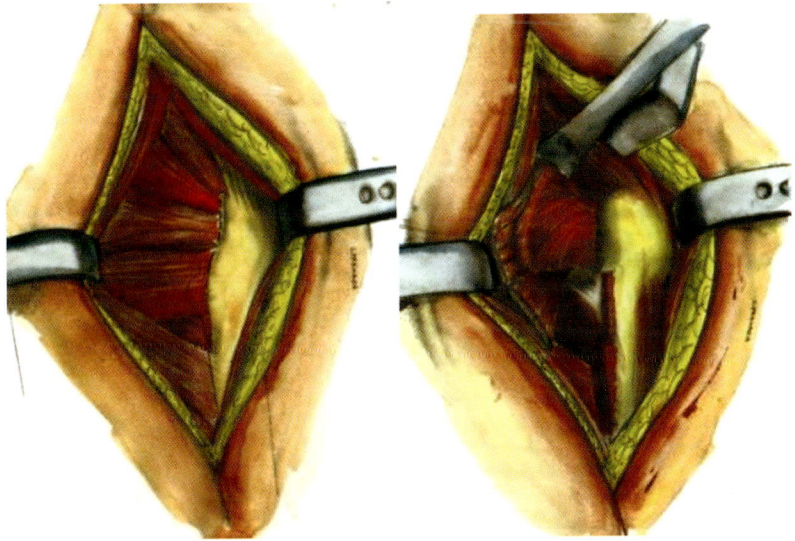

This unit of small lateral rotators retracted posteriorly acts as a soft tissue sleeve to protect the sciatic nerve. The medial circumflex femoral artery (at the uppermost part of the exposure) needs to be identified and either ligated or coagulated.

If additional exposure is desired, Gluteus Maximus is detached from its femoral attachment.

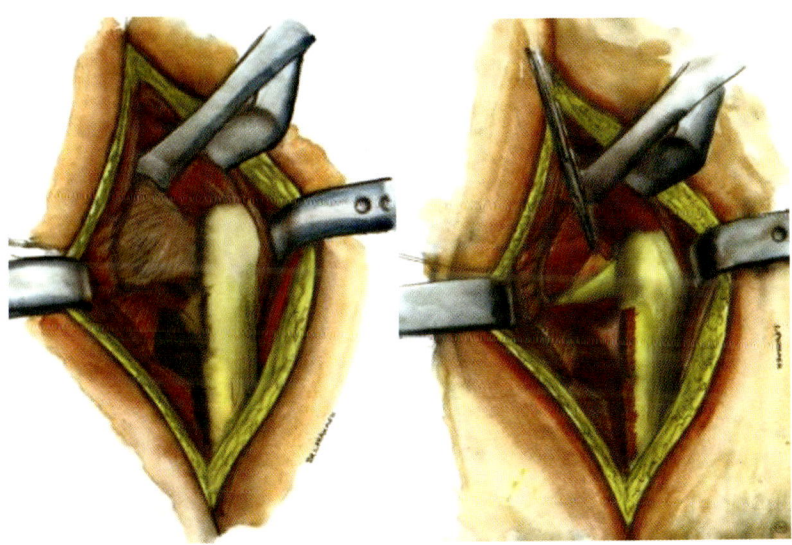

At this stage the capsule is incised along the femoral neck and the hip is exposed.

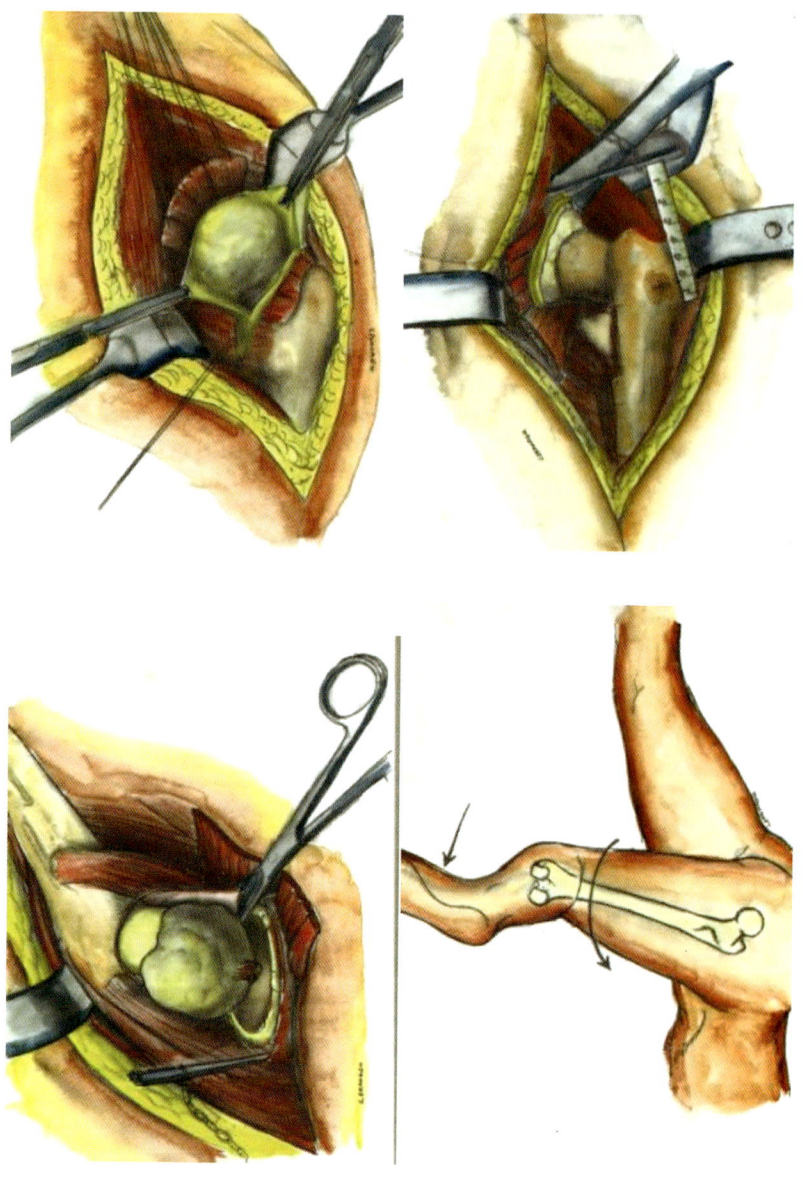

The hip is dislocated by flexion adduction and internal rotation of the hip.

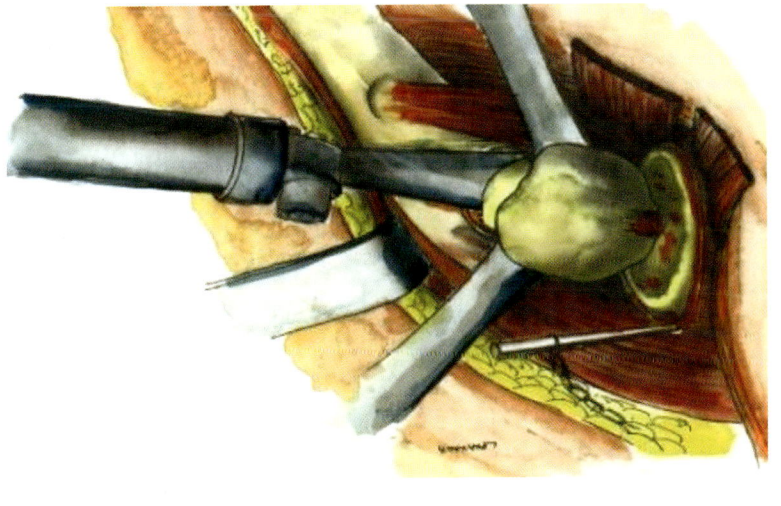

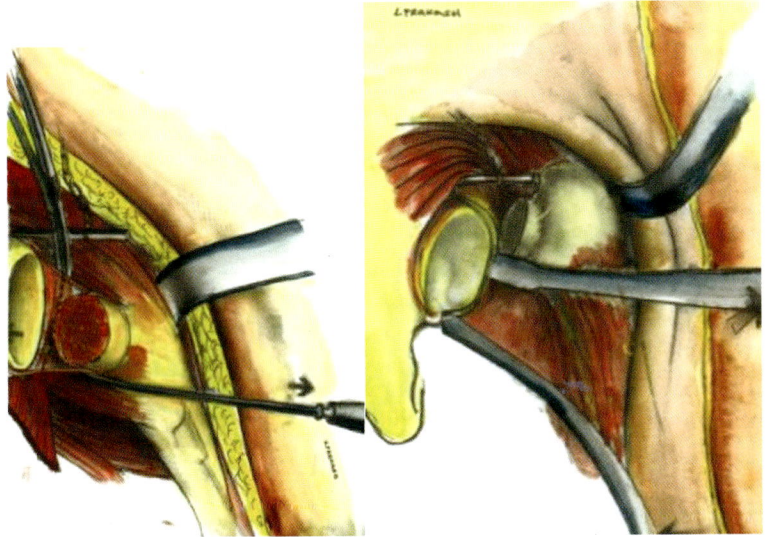

Appropriate and judicious placement of Homman retractors will expose the whole of acetabulum.

Indications

Monopolar, bipolar, and total hip replacements
Revision hip replacements.

Fracture with posterior dislocation of the hip, especially with trans acetabular posterior column fractures.

Exploration of sciatic nerve.

Drainage of septic arthritis of the hip joint.

Advantages

Easy quick approach through relatively bloodless fields and planes.

Easy dislocation of hip, with extreme maneuverability.

Decent exposure for acetabular reaming.

Disadvantages

Increased risk of dislocation and infection.

Positionally dependant area subject to tissue oedema and associated complications.

MEDIAL LUDLOFF APPROACH

History

Karl Ludloff (1864–1945) studied in Jena, Würzburg, Munich, and Strassburg. He received his doctorate in Jena in 1894 and

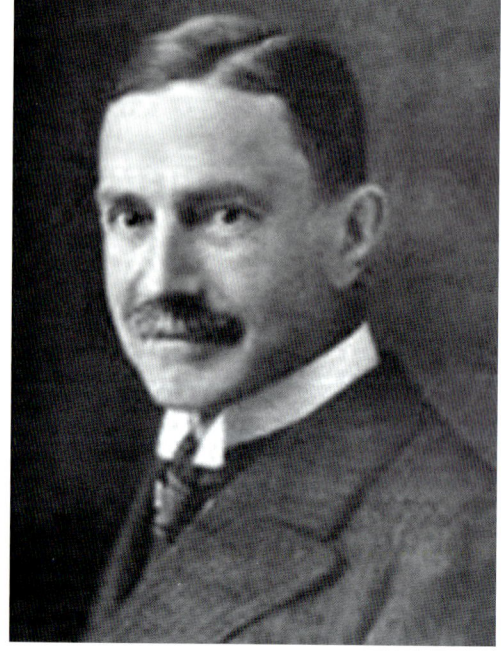

Karl Ludloff

worked as assistant at the physiological institute in Königsberg, and the surgical clinics in Königsberg and Breslau. He began his surgical career in 1900, became the chief surgeon in 1906, and director of the university clinic for orthopaedic surgery in Frankfurt, where he was appointed professor in 1919.

On February 10, 1916, The New York Times (via London) reported from the convention of the German Orthopaedic Society, then in session in Berlin. (At the time, the United States was still not at war with Germany). The headline was "CUT NERVES UNITED IN LIFELESS LIMBS. False Hand Controlled by Upper Arm Muscles. Another German War Invention."

Obviously impressed by the achievements of the surgeons gathered in Berlin, The New York Times reported:

Dr. Ferdinand Sauerbruch, Professor of Surgery at Zürich University, showed the delegates an artificial hand which was able to grasp objects of all forms and to lift weights up to twenty-two pounds. The hand and all the fingers are controlled by muscular action in the upper arm, which is prepared for such work by two operations. The muscular power afterward is transmitted to the hands through a system of wires and pulleys.

Dr. Karl Ludloff, Professor of Surgery at Breslau University, described a method for uniting severed nerves and receiving the muscular action of nerveless limbs. He pointed out that the natural tendency of severed ends of nerves to reunite was hindered by the fact that the cicatrized new flesh between them was impervious to growing nerve fibres.

Professor Ludloff said he restored the connection by a piece of an artery of an ox filled with gelatine, through which nerves readily grew, even bridging gaps of several inches. After several weeks crippled limbs regained their motor activity. The Professor said that many cases had been successfully treated where permanent lameness would have followed.

He was a brilliant scientist, innovator, engineer, designer of instrumentation, and also an imaginative surgeon who invented many techniques. He first described the adductor approach in 1908. His classical publication in 1939 in The American Journal of Orthopaedic Surgery on his medial incision is a classic that needs to be read in its original form to be appreciated.

It is indeed unfortunate that I couldn't find a picture of this great man and so his description will have to do!!

Access

Medial hip capsule
Lesser trochanter
Medial and inferior acetabular border.

Dislocation

Anterior

Position

Supine
Leg draped free
   Hip is abducted and externally rotated to make adductors taut
   Perineum is well prepared. Scrotum is taped back in a male.

Plane

Between adductor longus and brevis straight to hip joint. Division of iliopsoas facilitates exposure.

Incision

From pubic tubercle downwards over adductor longus for about 10 to 12.5 cm.

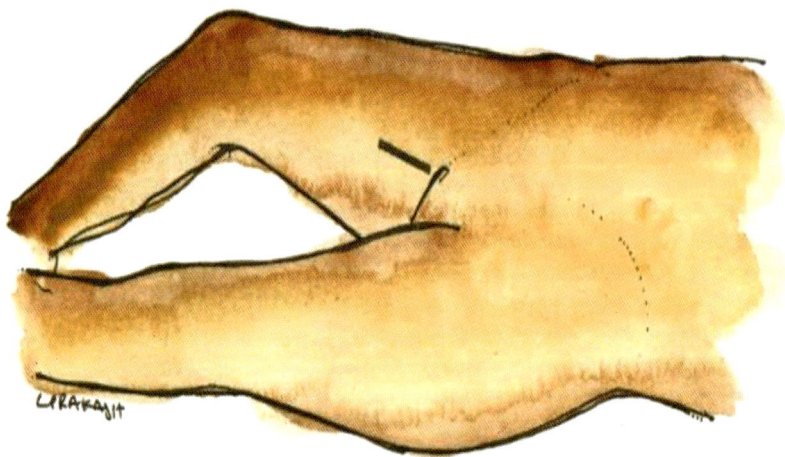

Dissections

Deep Fascia is incised over adductor longus.

This muscle is detached from its insertion if tight.

The plane between Adductor longus and brevis is developed.

The obturator nerve is identified and protected. It lies in front of adductor brevis.

Flexion, abduction, external rotation of the hip (by keeping the heel on the opposite knee) will stretch the capsule for incision or excision.

Indications

Approach of lesser trochanter, e.g. osteoid osteoma.

Hip exposures accompanied with psoas tenotomies and adductor releases.

Pathology of inferior acetabulum.

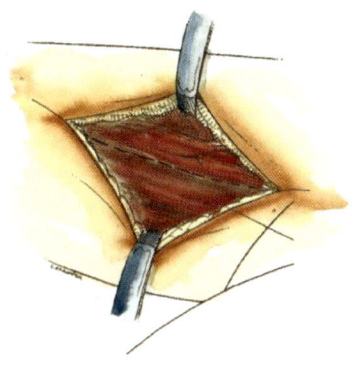 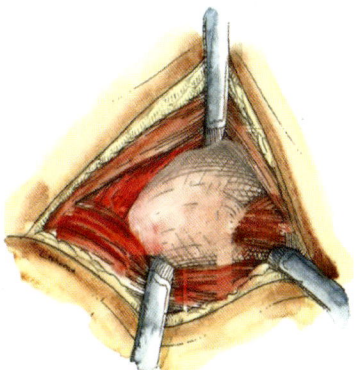

Advantages

Short bloodless exposure

Direct access to lesser trochanter.

Early quick post-operative recovery.

Disadvantages

Extremely limited exposure to medial hip joint.

Being close to perineum, the area is relatively unclean.

Unsuitable for CDH due to limited blood supply. In addition, anteriomedial dislocation places the head at risk of avascular necrosis.

3

Evolution of
Total Hip Arthroplasty

Irregular joint surfaces cause pain when they are moved against each other and there are only three logical methods of relieving this pain. An *excision* would no doubt take away the joint surfaces, but at the cost of stability. An *arthrodesis* on the other hand gives an excellent and long lasting pain relief, but robs one of the much desired movements. *Replacement* arthroplasty would logically be thus an ideal choice.

A little insight into the history and the struggle to develop the artificial hip joint may well be an insight into the development of modern orthopaedics itself.

The earliest recorded case of attempts to perform hip replacement procedures date back to as early as 1891 when Themistocles Gluck tried to use ivory implants to replace the femoral head.

The innovative and brilliant German surgeon **Themistocles Gluck** was born in Iasi, Moldovia (now in Romania) in 1853. His well-known father was an attending physician for the royal family.

Gluck began his university studies in Leipzig in 1873, studying under the Swiss anatomist, Wilhelm. He continued his medical studies in Berlin in 1875. His professors in Berlin included Bernhard von Langenbeck and the eminent pathologist Rudolf Virchow.

Gluck was an excellent student and won a prize for research on nerve regeneration conducted under the supervision of Virchow. He completed his degree in 1882, but, was unable to continue a university career because von Langenbeck retired

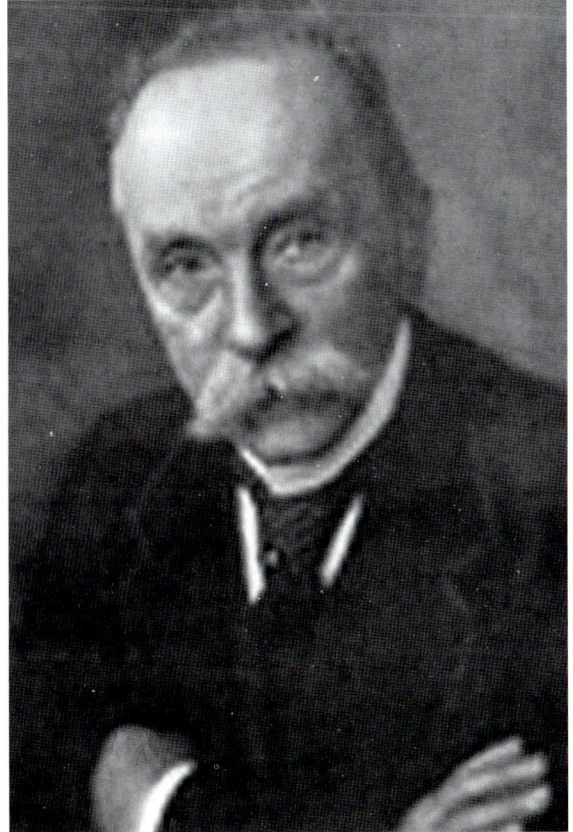

Themistocles Gluck

and his replacement, von Bergmann, evidently found no position for Gluck.

He returned to his homeland and worked for a short time in Bucharest, then practised industrial medicine in Berlin until 1890, when he was appointed as head of surgery at the Emperor and Empress Friederich Paediatric Hospital.

Gluck had a remarkable career and was probably one of the most brilliant surgeons and scientists of his time. He was the first to implant artificial joints in the 1880s. He was also responsible for many other remarkable concepts and developments: stress shielding, joint allografts (although he reportedly never performed any such transplants), intramedullary fixation (with ivory cylinders), biocompatibility (again, with ivory, a material he considered better than others). His interest in bone defects was almost certainly encouraged by his work as a wartime surgeon in the Balkans in 1877 and 1885, during which he first successfully used steel plates to fix a broken femur and replace part of a mandible.

He also experimented with bone cements, including copper amalgam, plaster of Paris, and a stone putty (resin with pumice or gypsum).

He described a number of surgical procedures for the larynx, trachea, lung, and inguinal hernias. It is interesting to note that he performed vessel sutures and venous grafts in the 1880s which predated by many years the work of the American surgeon Alexis Carrel who received the Nobel prize for vascular repair in 1912.

Gluck anticipated Küntscher's popularization of intramedullary fixation of fractures by 50 years. Gluck's pioneering work was often dismissed, but later in life he was honoured for his accomplishments, being listed on the honour roll of the German Surgical Society. Gluck died at age 88 in Berlin in April 1942.

The earliest dates of his implantations of artificial joints are variously reported as the mid 1880s to 1890. Gluck believed that preliminary animal experiments were essential, and implanted his ivory devices in animals before attempting them in humans.

Remarkably, he designed and implanted artificial wrists, elbows, shoulders, hips, knees, and ankles. In May 1890, Gluck inserted a hinged ivory joint in the knee of a 17-year-old girl; this design was not dissimilar from those of the early constrained total knee arthroplasty prostheses introduced in the second half of the 20th century. He reported performing 14 arthroplasties in that year, including a hip, but only provided details on five cases: three knees, a wrist, and an elbow.

The procedures appeared successful over the short term; however, all the five patients in the report suffered from tuberculosis, and all developed complications because of the chronic infection. Three of the five prostheses were removed (the wrist and one of the knees were left in situ). He later realized that prior joint infection was a contraindication to joint arthroplasty.

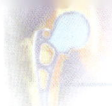

The first recorded total hip replacement should be certainly credited to Philip Wyles in Middlesex hospital and he published the results of replacing both femoral and acetabular components in 1958.

He described animal experimentation, and later the insertion of six of these prostheses into patients. He also noted that he had no adequate followup, as the war intervened and of the six patients, he only knew of one later.

That patient had a painful, stiff, but slightly mobile hip, which was removed and now finds a pride of place in the archives of the British Orthopaedic Association (B.O.A.), on loan to the Hunterian Museum at the Royal College of Surgeons. This first attempt at total hip replacement had some similarity to the present-day, so-called 'surface' replacements.

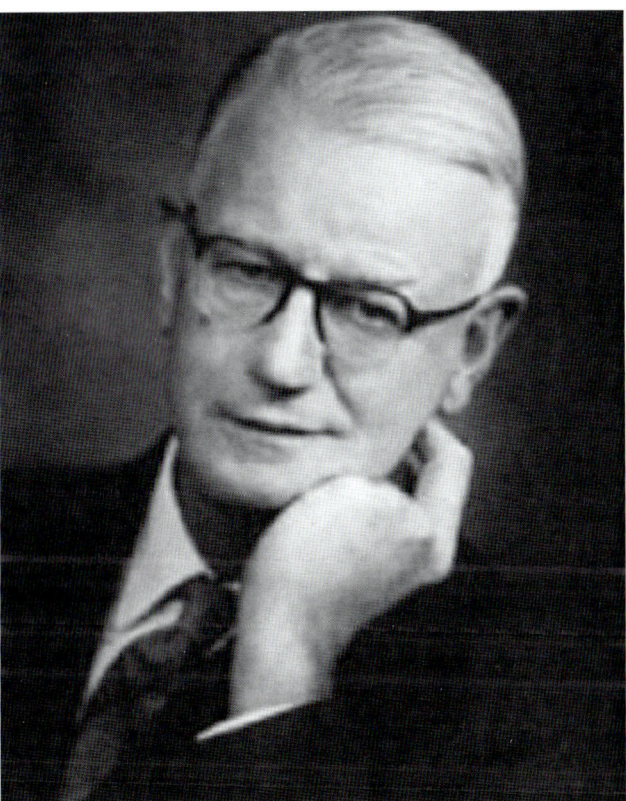

Philip Wyles, the inventor of modern total hip

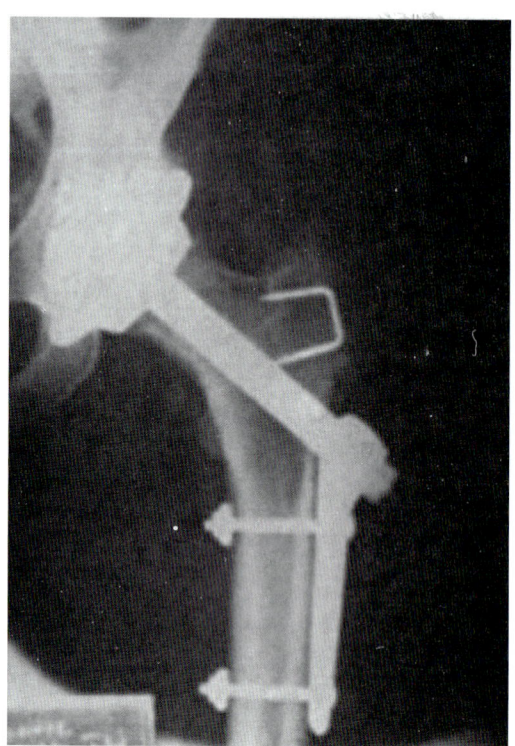

Xray of Wyles hip published in JBJS in 1950

There is still a controversy as to who is the father of the modern hip replacements, and between Wyles and Gluck, I would choose the latter for his documentation, radiographs and records. Gluck however was a far greater genius, way ahead of his times.

Marius Nygaard Smith-Petersen was among the most prominent and innovative orthopaedic surgeons of the first half of the 20th century. He described a new approach to treating fractures of the neck of the femur, mould arthroplasty, osteotomy of the spine, and continuous irrigation for Osteomyelitis, all innovations far ahead of his time.

Dr. Marius Nygaard Smith-Petersen, son of Morten Smith-Petersen, was born on November 14th, 1886 in the coastal town of Grimstad in Aust-Agder County, Norway.

After the death of his father, the family immigrated to the U.S. and settled in Milwaukee, Wisconsin. There he graduated from the University of Wisconsin, receiving a B.S. in 1910. He worked as a laboratory assistant to Nobel Prize winner physiologist Dr. Joseph Erlanger while attending the Medical School at the University of Wisconsin. Marius Smith-Petersen then transferred to Harvard Medical School in Cambridge, Massachusetts, earning his degree in 1914.

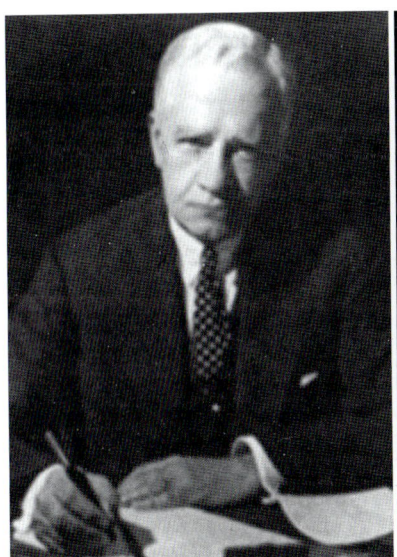 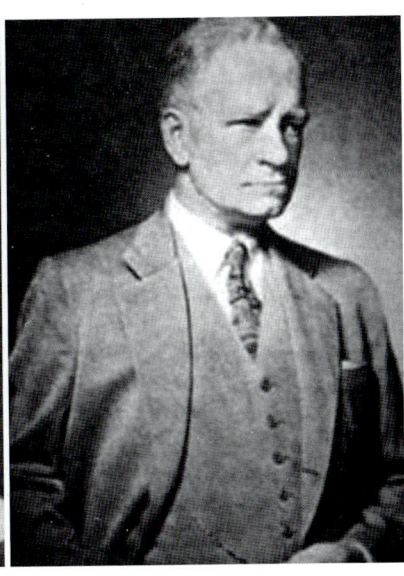

Marius Nygaard Smith-Petersen (November 14, 1886–May 1953)   *Marius Nygaard Smith-Petersen (November 14, 1986–May 1953)*

He went into private practice in Boston, Massachusetts in 1923. He served as Assistant Instructor, Instructor, and then Clinical Professor. He was then appointed as Chief of Orthopaedic Service at Massachusetts General Hospital from 1929–1946 and as consultant to The Surgeon General from 1942 1945.

He is internationally known for the development of the Smith-Petersen nail and hip nailing techniques and for hip-mould arthroplasty, an original model of which sold by Down brothers London has been shown here.

As early as 1952, **Judet brothers** of France designed a heat cured acrylic prosthesis. This was further improved using a metal core. Sterilization was by formalin followed by a wash in boiling water. There was no stem, just a stub projecting from the head ball. However the head sizes differed and thus one could use a

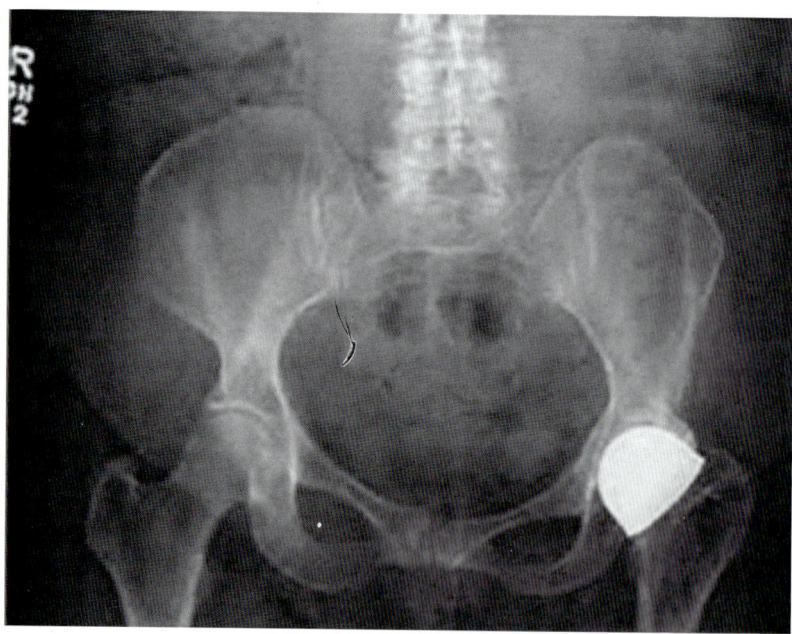

Smith Peterson's mould arthroplasty

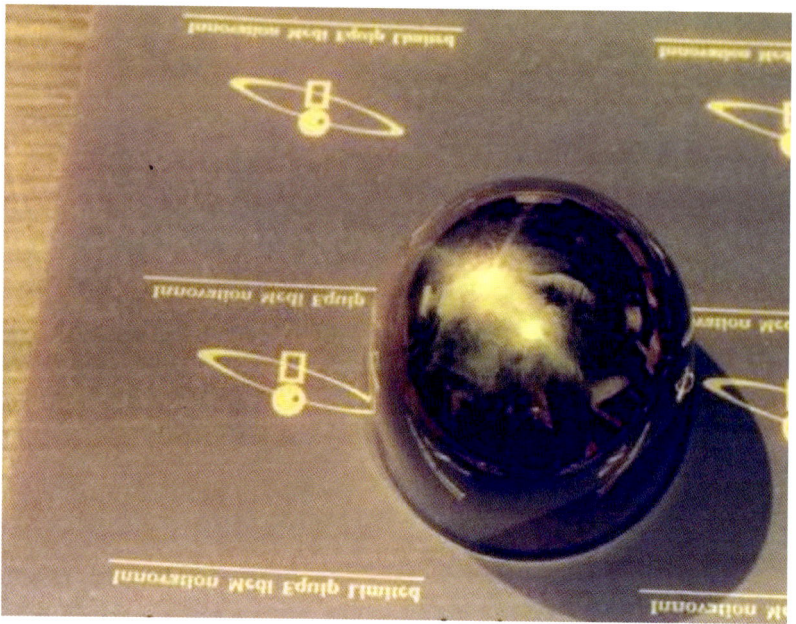

Smith Peterson's hip cap

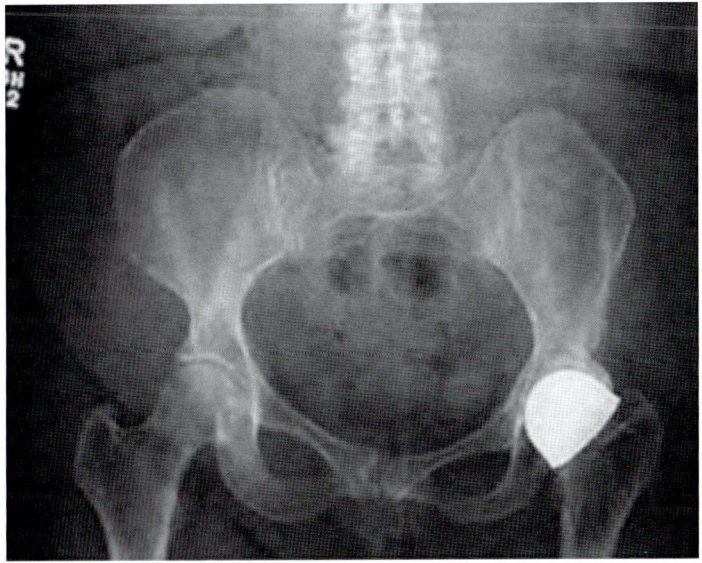

Smith Peterson's mould arthroplasty

reasonable size of the prosthesis. The acrylic was very highly polished and articulated direct with the cartilage. Despite the early use in osteoarthritis with a less than normal acetabulum, the immediate results were spectacular. At an international meeting Judet is quoted as to have said that the operation was so good that he would even do it on his mother.

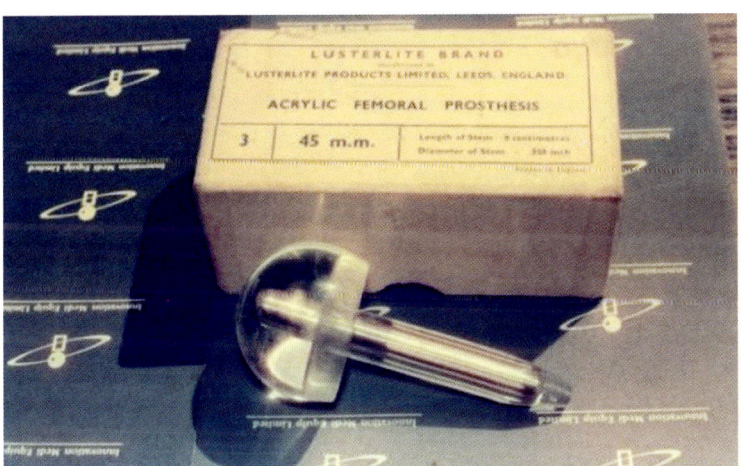

Judet Acrylic femoral head

A large number of cases were done far too quickly without waiting long enough for results, and once they started failing, the failures snowballed leading to so many disasters that it put back the development of arthroplasty by some years.

What went wrong was wear. The acrylic developed scratches during articulation against the hard acetabular wall. These furrowed and expanded. Small particles of debris were released and increased the wear to such an extent that fragmentation resulted in most cases. The wear particles caused a massive tissue reaction, granulation tissue formation and fibrosis, and severe bone destruction. But the pattern of implant failure was not consistent, and some hips lasted longer than others.

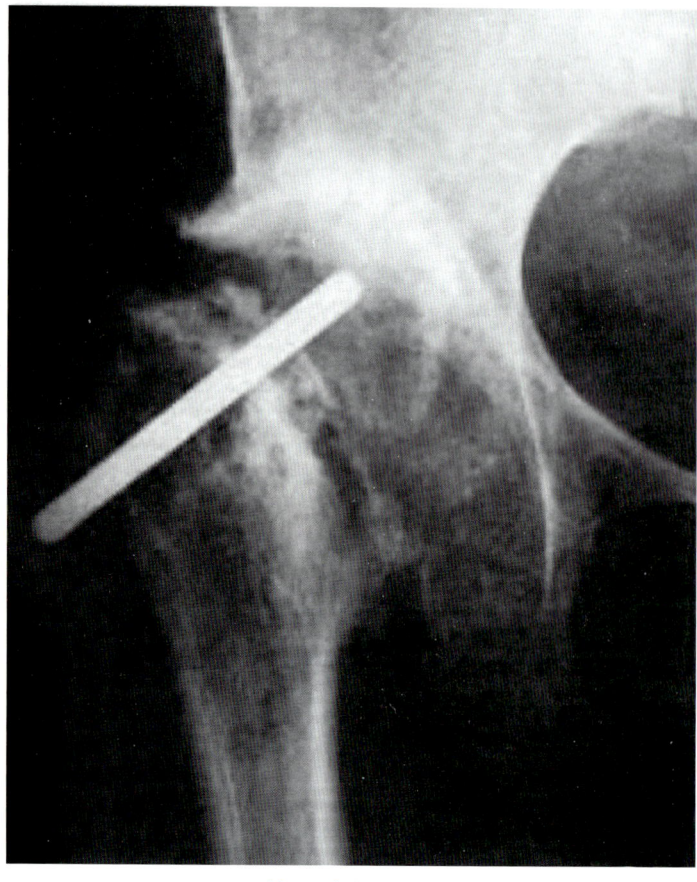

Xray of Judet hip

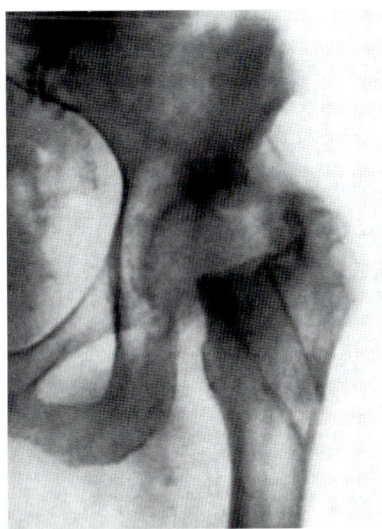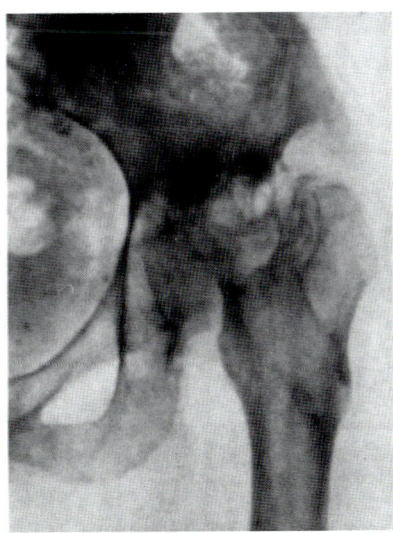

Dramatic wear in a Judet hip in less than a year

However, the Judet hip laid the foundation on which other hips were subsequently developed.

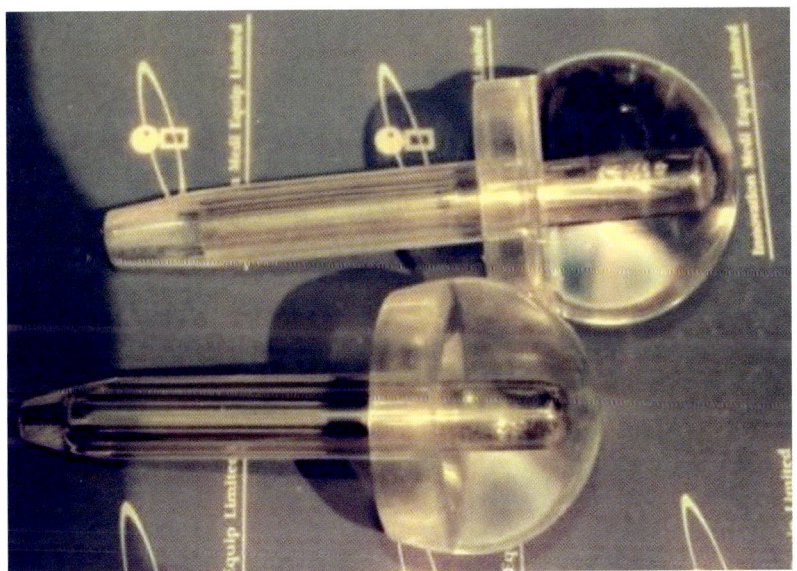

Judet acrylic prosthesis

Above is the original Judet Hip marketed by Down Brothers London and below are pictures of Judet Brothers.

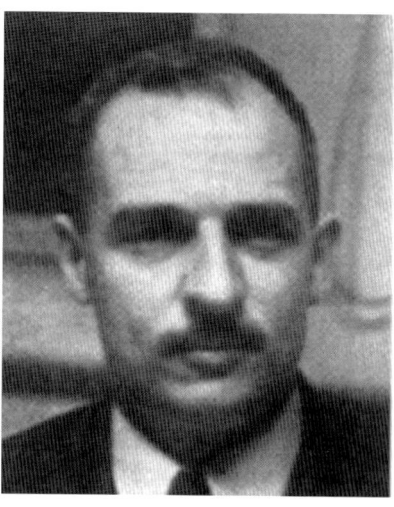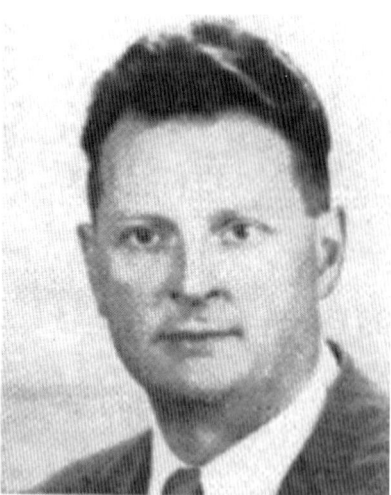

The use of metallic endoprosthesis was then tried by Moore and Thompson. Both had a stem for medullary purchase and the highly polished metal head was far less likely to wear than the acrylic one. The acetabular problems were not addressed, and the press fit stems produced a varying amount of bone resorption. Though in practice these worked reasonably for normal acetabulum (and are even now regularly in use for fresh sub capital fractures in the elderly), the erosion on the acetabular side was unacceptably marked, especially in more active patients.

In 1940, an American surgeon **Dr. Austin Moore** (1899–1963) performed the first metallic hip replacement at Columbia Hospital, South Carolina. Moore had designed a proximal femoral prosthesis with a large head. The implant was around 30cm in length and attached with bolts to the end of the femoral shaft, offering an early form of hemiarthroplasty or partial hip replacement.

Dr. Moore's prosthetic implant gained popularity and he later developed an improved version—the Austin Moore prosthesis – which is still in use today.

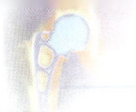
However, today, the implant is inserted within the medullary canal of the femur, where bone growth eventually leads to its more permanent attachment.

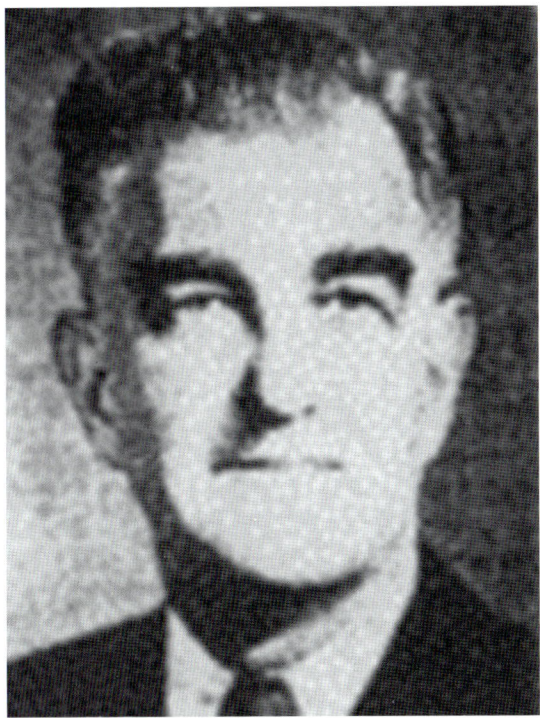

Dr. Austin Tally Moore

Even today, this is the treatment of choice in many hospitals for displaced subcapital fractures in the very elderly.

The need for a polished cup led to the development of metal-on-metal hips from Phillip Wyles, Urist, Peter Ring, Mckee Farar and others. As with their predecessors, the initial results were very satisfactory, but the high friction between the bearing surfaces led to an unacceptable amount of loosening and pain.

Ken McKee was born on 5 January 1906 and educated at Chigwell School before winning a scholarship to the Medical School at St. Bartholomew's Hospital. After qualifying, he held house surgeon appointments at Bart's and also at Chailey

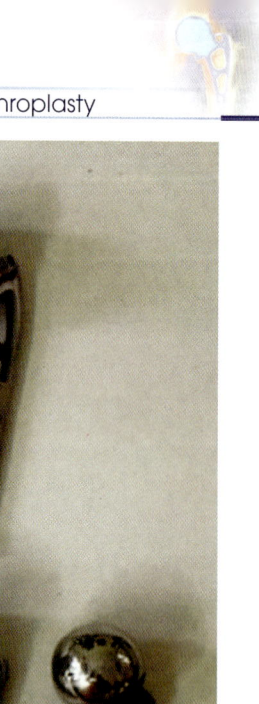

Implants are from Dr L.Prakash's personal collection

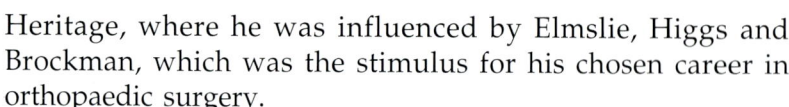

Many versions and makes of Austin Moore's prosthesis are available in the market

Heritage, where he was influenced by Elmslie, Higgs and Brockman, which was the stimulus for his chosen career in orthopaedic surgery.

His subsequent training included registrar posts in Sheffield and the Norfolk and Norwich Hospital. He obtained his F.R.C.S. in 1934 and joined H. A. Brittain on the staff as a consultant at the Norfolk and Norwich Hospital in 1939. Orthopaedic surgery proved to be a fertile field for a man who was fascinated by all things mechanical. His early interest in taking motorcycles and cars to pieces prepared him for an outstandingly inventive

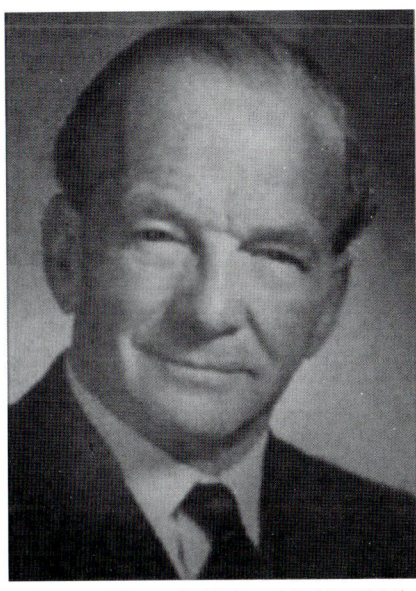
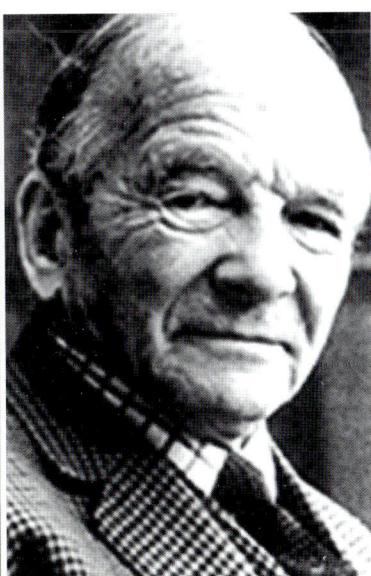

George Kenneth Mckee (1906–1991)   *George Kenneth Mckee*

career. The following photos from my implant collection show the design and details of the McKee-Farar cemented metal-on-metal hips.

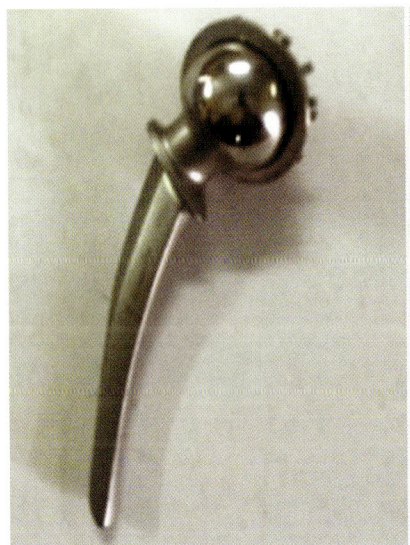
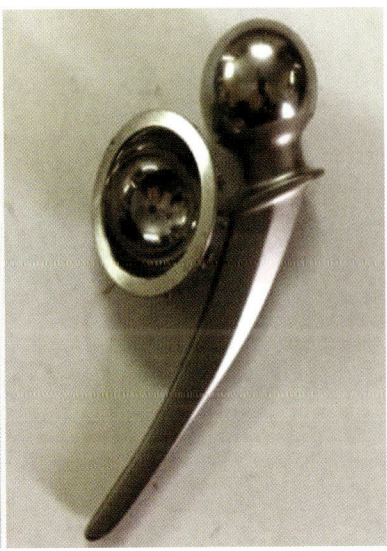

The original Mckee hip, the father of MOM   *See the polished cup interior*

Though these are no longer used, the surprising fact that quite a few of these hips lasted for 25 years plus, leads to the re-emergence of interest in metal-on-metal hips with larger heads.

He himself admitted that "replacing worn joints was a fairly obvious treatment to me." Throughout the 1940s and 1950s he pursued his goal of hip replacement with little encouragement from his more conservative and sceptical peers. Their comments of the time were recorded by McKee: "£200 is very expensive for an operation that is doomed to failure" and "Prosthetic arthroplasty should be reserved for the over 90s."

In later years he would often recall, with a twinkle in his eye, the eminent questioner at a Royal Society of Medicine meeting of 1957, who asked "Where do you put the grease nipple?"

McKee noted but disregarded the hoots of laughter that followed. His first models had been made of brass in 1940, but he delayed putting his ideas into practice until chrome–cobalt alloys became available. He presented his first cases of total hip replacement in a clinical demonstration at the British Orthopaedic Association meeting in Cambridge in 1951. At this time, the management of unilateral hip arthritis was highly controversial.

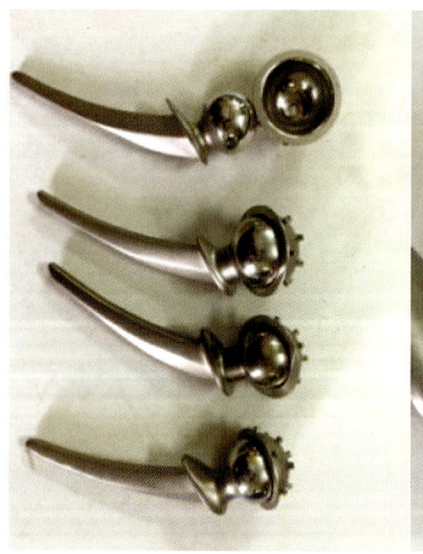

The head sizes changed with the cup dimensions in Mckee Frar hips

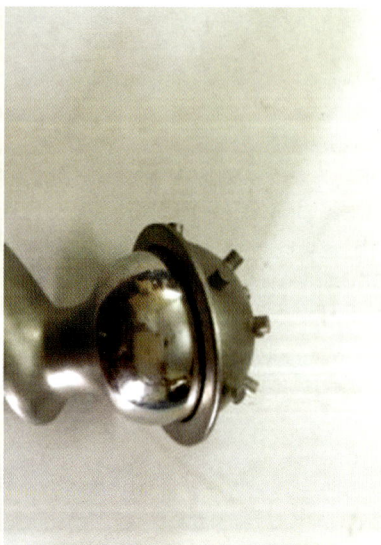

The acetabular spikes give a good cement anchor surface

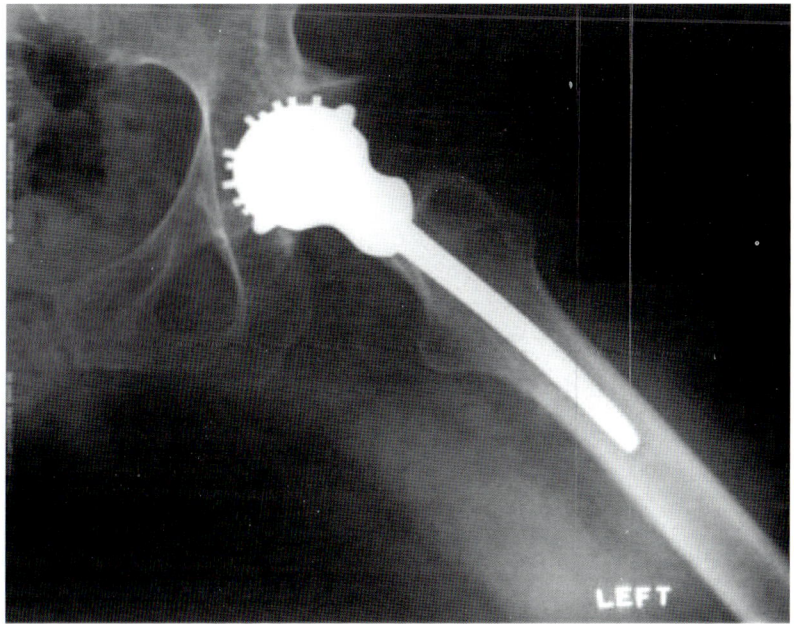

A cemented Mckee Farar hip at 24 years

H. A. Brittain, from whom McKee had remained distant, had published two editions of his book 'The Architectural Principles of Arthrodesis' and Watson-Jones was another proponent of hip fusion. Indeed, in 1948, McKee had invented his own variant of hip fusion using a lag screw and was pleased that the fixation eliminated the need for plaster of Paris. He continued to be committed to total replacement and in 1953 he visited F. R. Thompson in the USA and adopted the Thompson stem for his femoral component, using this in articulation with his chrome–cobalt cloverleaf socket until 1960. He reported a 50% failure rate of this combination in the short term. McKee's confidence in total joint replacement was not shared by others; even John Charnley was uncertain as late as 1957 and still advocated hip fusion.

John Charnley first used acrylic cement to fix a femoral prosthesis in 1958. In 1960, he published his findings in The Journal of Bone and Joint Surgery. This was recognized by McKee as the breakthrough he was looking for. With his registrar John Watson-Farrar, McKee conceived the metal-on-metal cemented hip joint, but unlike Charnley, McKee did not restrict the use of his invention. Metal debris and impingement were major problems and these were addressed by redesign of the Thompson component and by making the femoral head slightly smaller than the socket to diminish equatorial wear. McKee recognized Charnley's brilliant scientific and engineering skills, but was always concerned about wear of high-density polyethylene and unimpressed by Charnley's laboratory studies of friction. Ken McKee was pleased to know that orthopaedic surgeons and engineers were, in 1991, taking a second look at metal-on-metal articulations. McKee's mechanical aptitude was not limited to total hip replacement.

His interventionist approach to fracture treatment led to the use of his own intramedullary nail for femoral fractures in 1941; A. R. Hodgson was his registrar at the time. A trifin nail and plate was developed for trochanteric fractures, and an external fixator incorporated in a Thomas splint was his novel way of treating tibial fractures. McKee also favored plate fixation for closed tibial fractures and even some open ones. He reported the use of moulded plastic corsets for spinal pain and, in the wake of his hip replacement, he designed hinged prostheses for

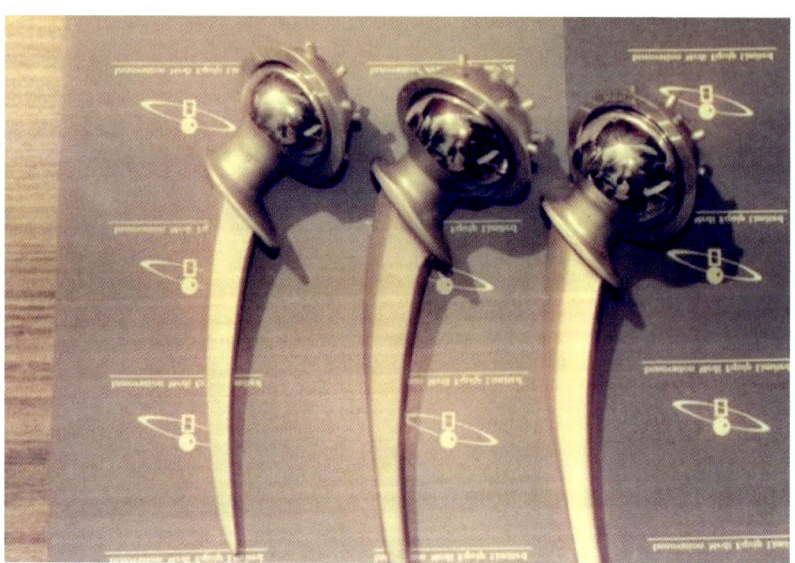

The McKee Farar MOM hip

the elbow and the knee. He even experimented with acrylic cement as a replacement for intervertebral discs.

Though a bold and adventurous surgeon, Ken McKee was a quiet and discreet man, who found public speaking neither easy nor agreeable. His conversation was of cars, golf, skiing and sailing rather than orthopaedics. Ken was not an inspiring orator, and did not readily enjoy the challenge. He was a quiet man, full of brilliant ideas, some of which were before their time.

At this stage a short history of bone cement and its uses would have been appropriate, but I will come to that later as we are studying the history in chronological order.

Peter Ring from Redhill, Surrey, provided the next development in hip arthroplasty. He disliked cement all his life, distrusted it rather. He was also not too happy about polyethylene , as he had been cautioned by Charnley's initial Teflon failures. He was impressed by Sir John Charnley's spectacular results and decided to make his own self-locking total hip replacement for uncemented fixation.

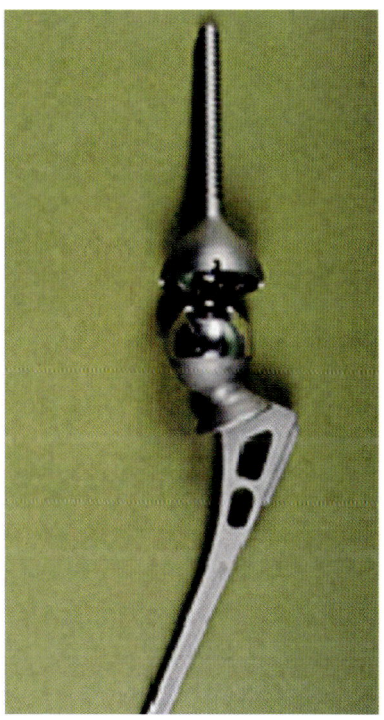

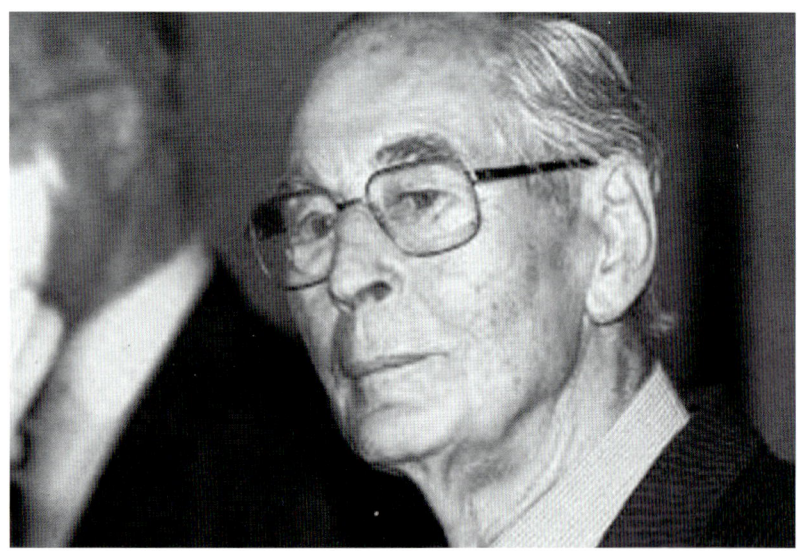

Mr. Peter Ring

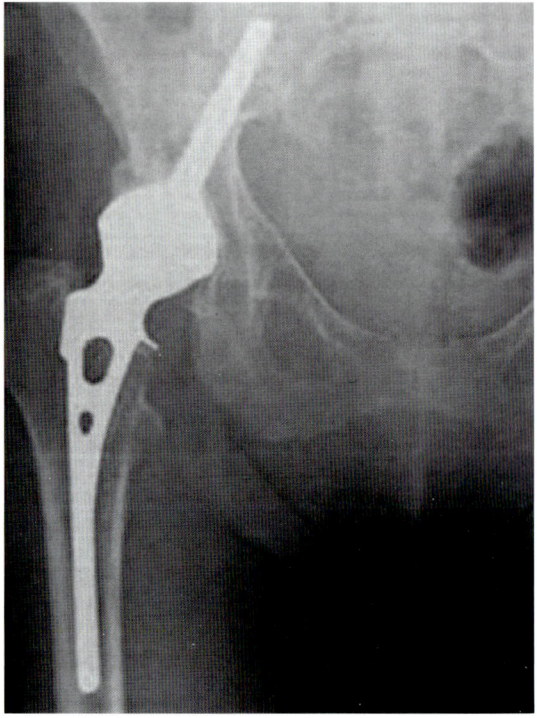

Survival of a Ring cementless metal on metal hip at 25 years

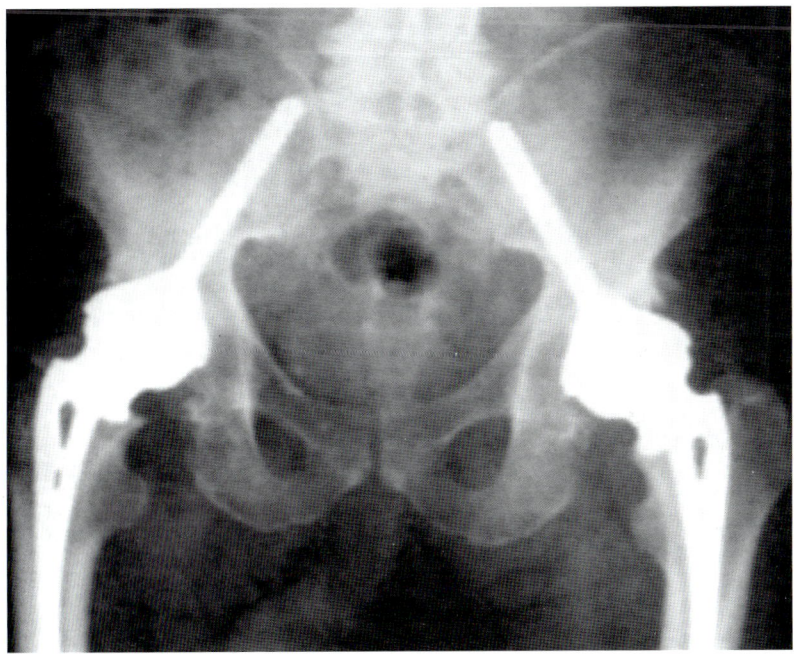

Survival of a Ring cementless metal on metal hip at 25 years

Mr. Peter Ring is considered by many as the father of modern cementless pressfit hips. His firm belief in the metal-on-metal (MOM) articulation and fixation without cement laid the

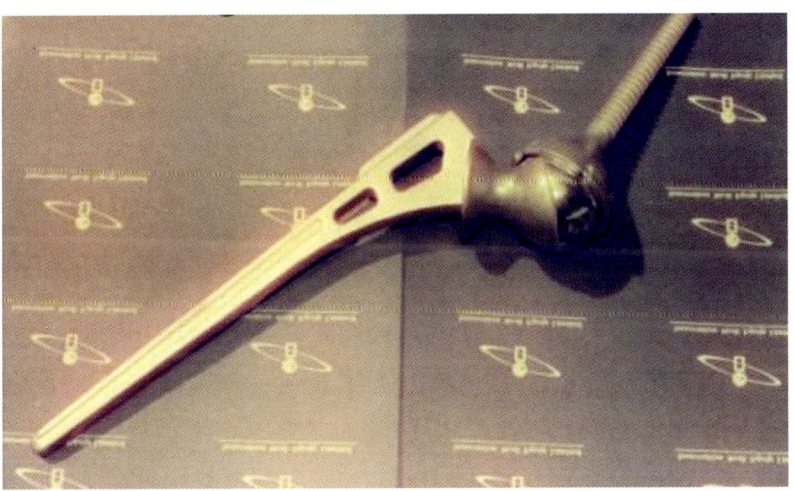

Peter Ring's cementless MOM hip

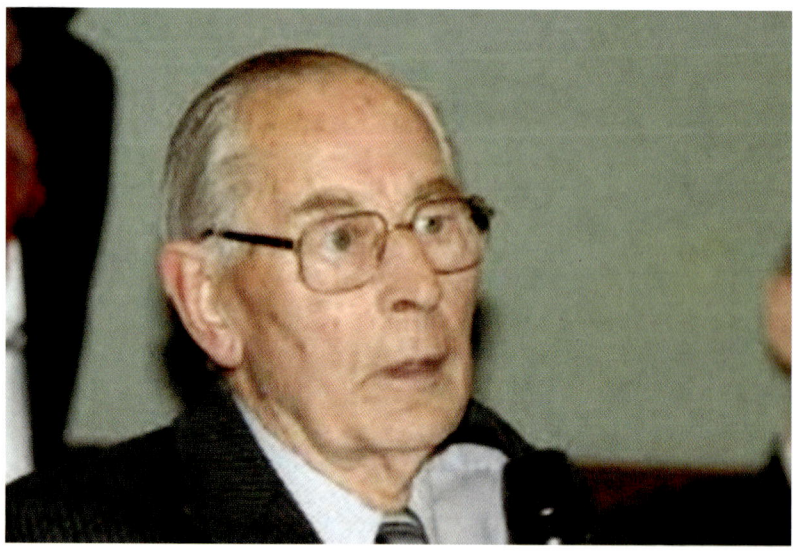

Mr Peter Ring

foundations on which modern hip arthroplasty designs are made. After Sir John Charnley, he is considered the greatest contributor to the science of arthroplasty by many orthopaedicians.

Thus, by the 1970s, three types of total hip replacement were in common use: the McKee, Charnley and Ring types.

Surgeons across the world experienced initial success with all varieties; then attention was focused on which would be more durable. Charnley's intervention at this stage proved decisive. He returned to his favourite theme of frictional torque. He built a pendulum comparator to test the frictional torque of the McKee metal-on-metal joint versus the Charnley metal-on-polyethylene joint. Under test the McKee metal-on-metal came to a juddering halt and the Charnley joint kept on swinging.

Thousands of visiting surgeons to Wrightington were immediately convinced of the superiority of the Charnley joint and the metal-on-metal joint finally ended in the late 1970s when McKee and Ring themselves switched to metal-on-polyethylene articulations for their own hip replacement designs.

Chamley died believing that his metal polyethylene joint had been totally vindicated. McKee died believing that his metal-on-metal joint had been rightly superseded by the metal-on-

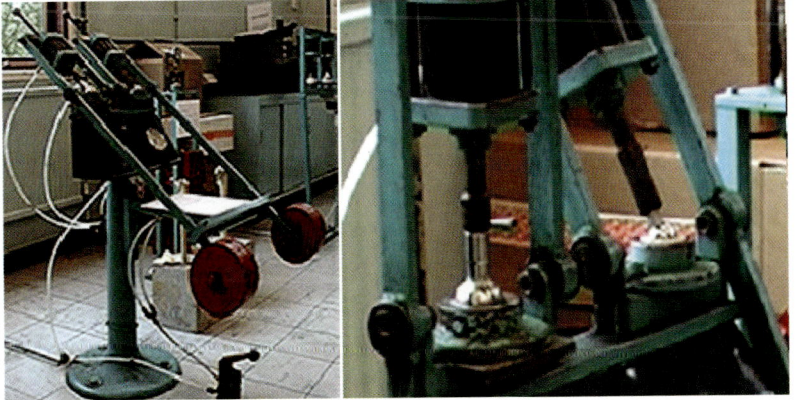

polyethylene articulation. Peter Ring, the last surviving of the triumvirate, was initially optimistic about his new polyethylene joint, but with the passage of time, he saw the results ruined by osteolysis from polyethylene debris, a complication unheard of in his earlier metal-on-metal joint. Ring finally deeply regretted moving away from the metal-on-metal articulation. Satisfactory results have been published for the McKee metal-on-metal, the Charnley and the best for the Ring Metal-on-metal with 5% revision at 17 years. It is now accepted that a Charnley type total hip replacement can give perfectly satisfactory results for 20 years or longer. One man's dedicated scientific studies resulted in this revolution in orthopaedics.

And this brings us to **Sir John Charnley**, the scientist, surgeon, mechanist, biomechanist, obsessively meticulous surgeon, and a genius who will always be the father of joint replacements. I offer no apologies for adding four of his photos. I would have added more if I could find them!

Sir John Charnley, surgeon, inventor, scientist and biomechanical genius

All credit for laying down the foundation of the modern principles of total joint replacements should go to **Sir John Charnley** of Manchester England. He discovered two things: the low friction principle and the cement fixation of the artificial joints. Understanding the principle that however well-polished, steel-on-steel will cause gradual wear and tear as ball bearings do in machinery, he designed a joint in which metal articulated

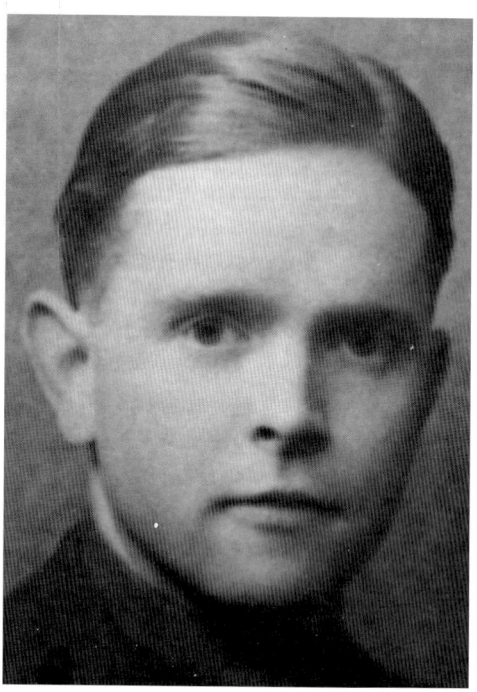

with plastic. Borrowing from the industry where oil free movements were between teflon and steel, he made teflon cups which articulated with steel balls. Eureka!

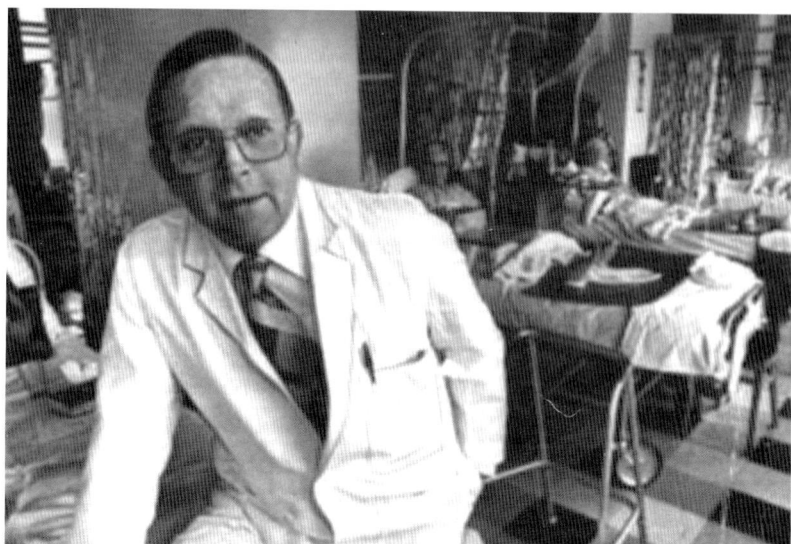

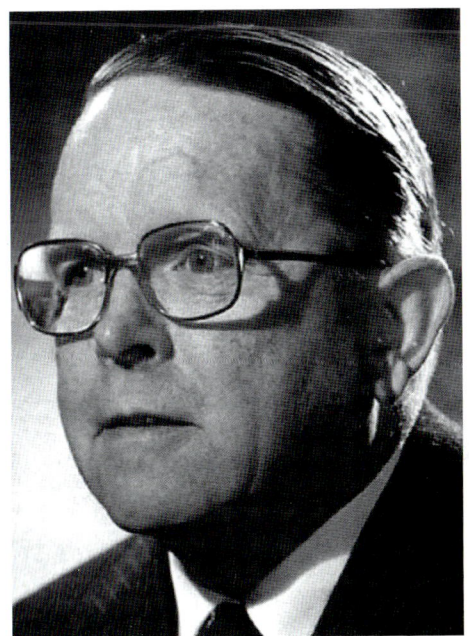

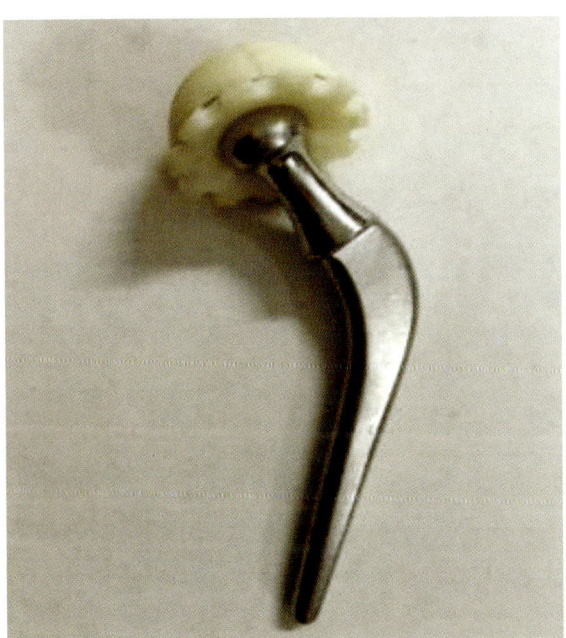

The original Charnley roundback 40, stainless steel stem, HDPE cup, fabricated in Charnley's own laboratory

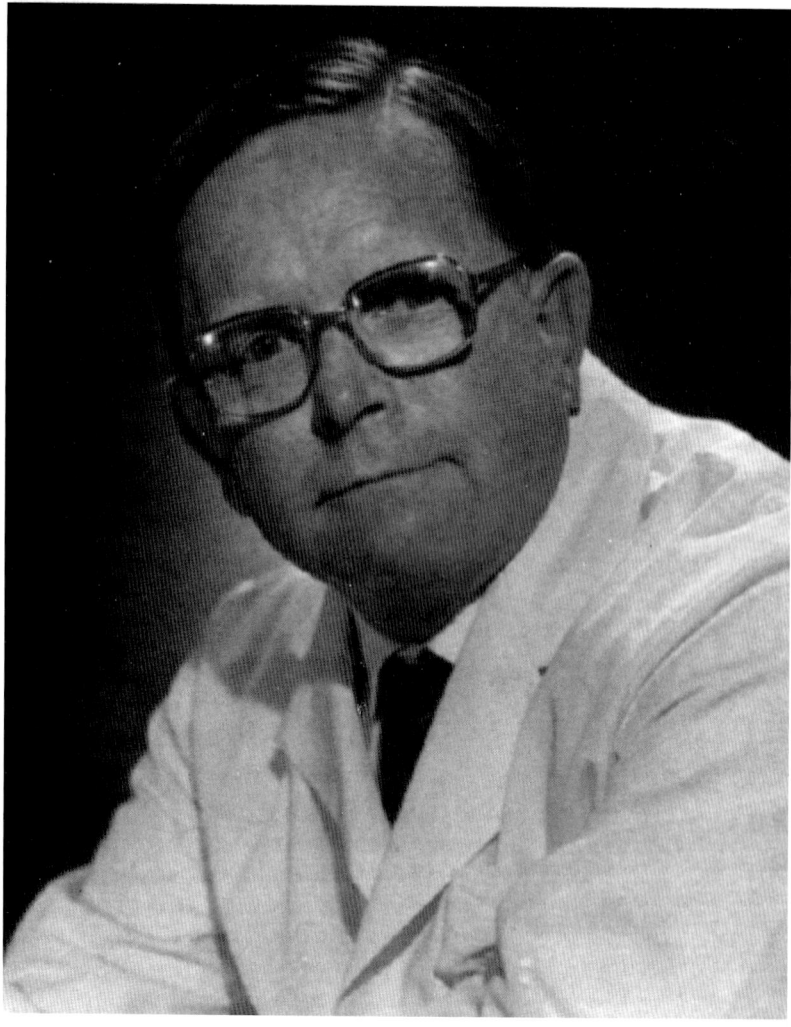

Charnley, an engineer and surgeon, devised a prosthesis made of stainless steel which he machined himself on a lathe and implanted it into a patient. The cup surface was replaced with one of teflon. The initial results were so good that his patients were pain-free immediately after the operation. People who had not walked for years started running. Charnley was thrilled. He went before the orthopaedic surgeons of England and announced that he had discovered an operation he would happily do on his own mother. So spectacular were the results!

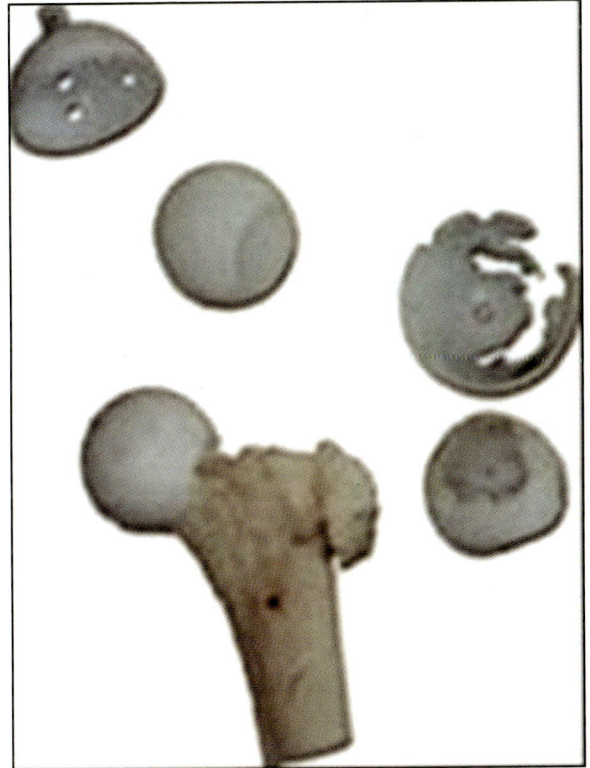

Charnley's Teflon hip showing rapid wear and fragmentation

Alas, the results were shortlived. In his initial enthusiasm, Charnley miscalculated wear and tear. So engrossed was he with friction that he did not anticipate the possibility that teflon can rub out after constant movement against metal. In a human body, the hip is put through vigorous movements with sufficient load over prolonged periods, which causes significant teflon wear. The teflon material just cheesed away in a year's time and Charnley was left with 100 failed hip joints!

Way back in 1963, you could get away with 100 failed operations without a consumer protection council above your head. Charnley was shattered. He went back before the same British orthopaedic surgeons and told them that the operation was no good and that he would not even do it on his own mother-in-law!

Then Charnley was given a piece of HDPE (High Density Polyethylene). He saw another plastic and was not impressed. A hundred failures had disillusioned him. But he did make a trial cup and put it on a machine which he used to test the wear. Someone forgot to switch off the machine that weekend and what was found on Monday was a spinning system which would have been in the human body after two years. Charnley was amazed when he measured the wear and found none! He put it through further tests and the results were the same. HDPE did not wear. At least in experimental situations its wear was not even a fraction of teflon. Further research was conducted and the final UHMUHDPE was invented. UHMUHDPE? Ultra high density, ultra high molecular weight polyethylene to be precise. After considering dentist's cement and modified acrylic compounds, he used polymerised methyl methacralate to fix the components into the human body. Working alone, constantly researching, improvising and improving, he invented what we can call the first modern total joint replacement.

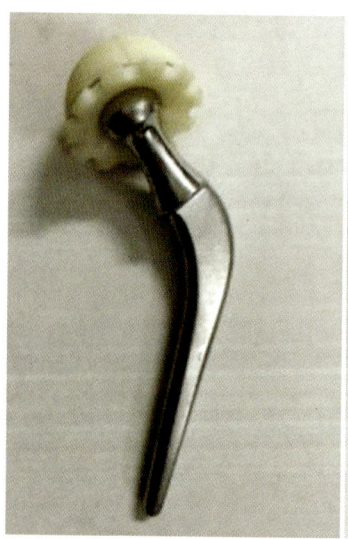 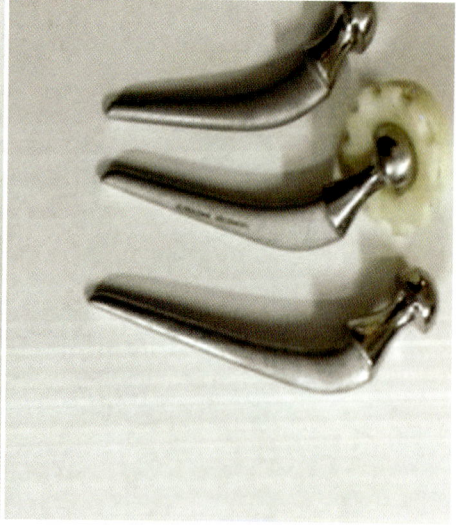

The original Charnley roundback 40, stainless steel stem, HDPE cup, fabricated in Charnley's own laboratory

Narrow, small and CDH stems were added later

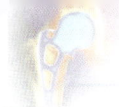

The early results were spectacular. And the results remained spectacular. Hundreds upon hundreds were relieved of pain and crippling. They remained pain-free for a long period, so joint replacements had come to stay. Once the principles were established, replacement of other joints began to follow.

But this was not enough for a dedicated perfectionist like Charnley. Charnley, the meticulous and obsessive scientist, continued to work very hard on all aspects of this specialty.

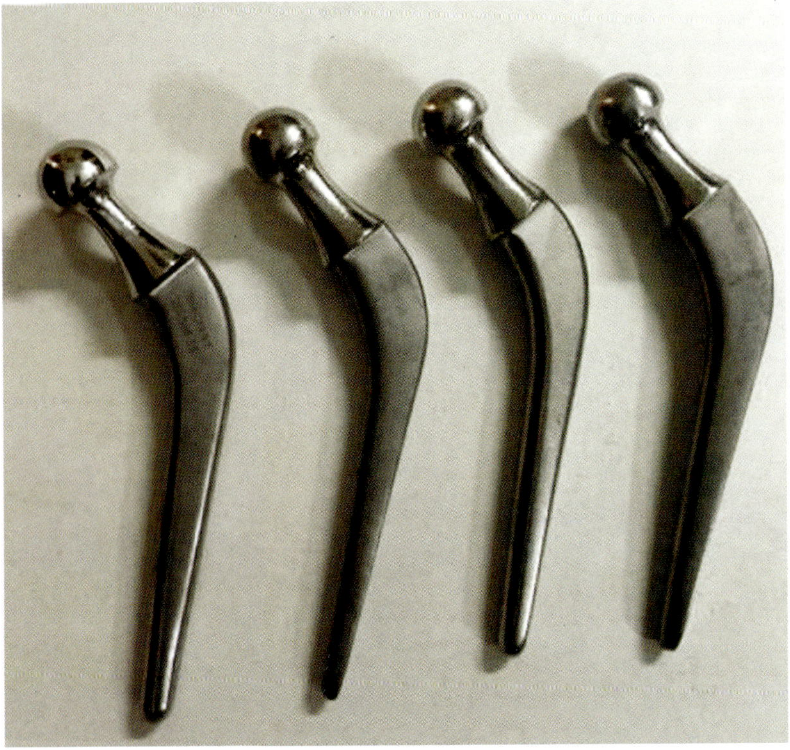

Stems with different neck shaft angels. Round back 35, 40, 45, etc.

The next step was changing the neck shaft angle in different components to match the hip anatomy of individual patients. These were the second generation roundback series.

He continuously improved on the design by adding flanges to both cup and stem. The cobra design pressurized the liquid cement far better than the roundback designs.

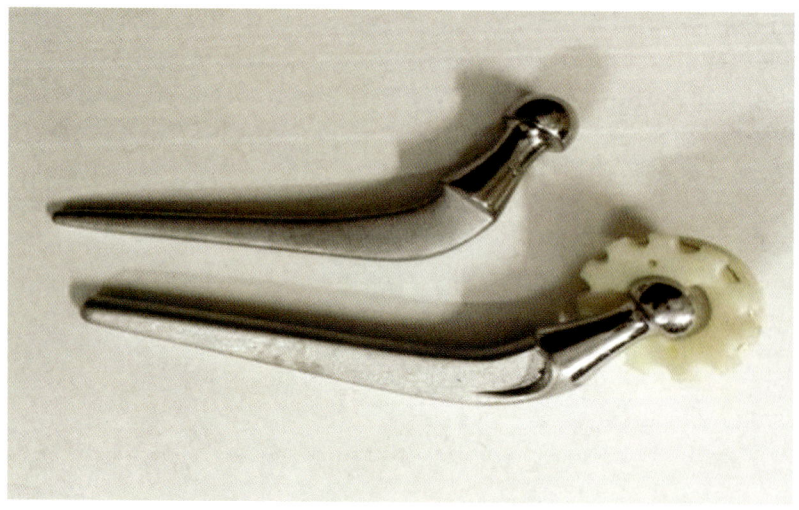

A flanged stem for better cement pressurisation

At this stage, Charnley had done a lot of studies and follow-up, and understood the importance of the abductor lever arm mechanism and its length. Always a proponent of trochanteric osteotomy, he had a magic weapon in his hand to control the

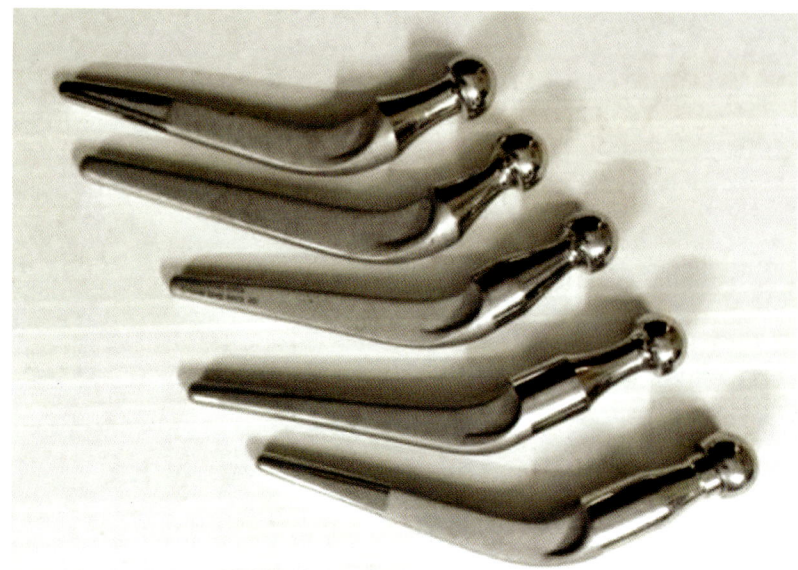

Long neck series, long neck one, two and three

tightness of the hip (distalizing the greater trochanter), but a perfectionist like him was not satisfied. He wanted a better control over neck length and needed designs to work in patients with absent or deformed necks.

Thus came the long neck series, some of which can be used even in intertrochanteric fractures with neck absent up to lesser trochanter, or even when the lesser trochanter is missing.

The next logical step was modularity, which of course did not come in Charnley's time. Later additions were varying head sizes, different inside depths to further fine-tune the neck length and also different sized heads for those who did not like the small 22 mm Charnley heads.

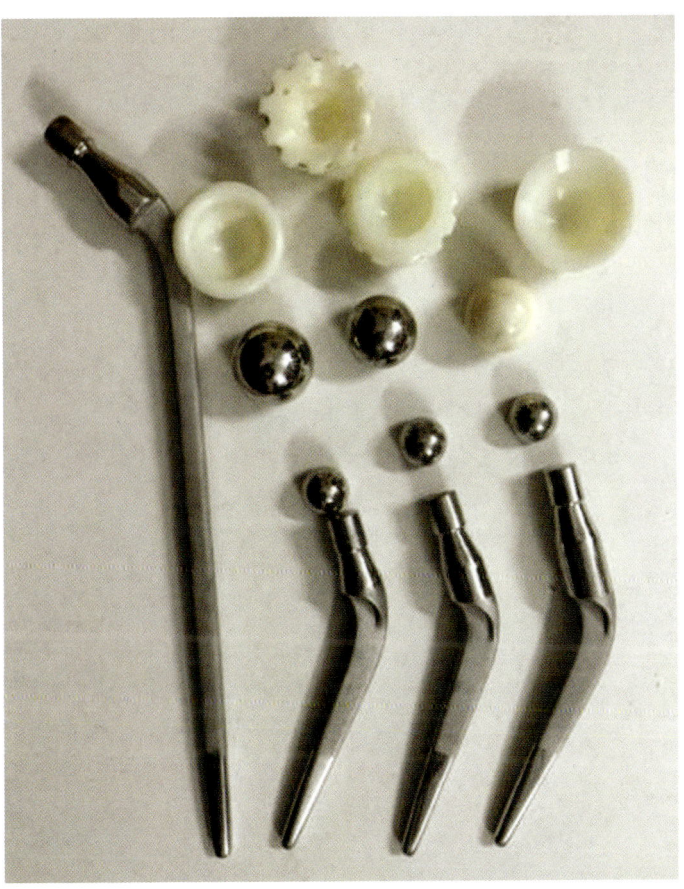

Long stem and modular heads of 22, 26, 28 and 32 mm

Charnley, the first to draft the principles of low friction arthroplasty, laid the foundations of friction and wear in the hip joint. Having burnt his fingers once with Teflon, wear was such an important issue with him that till his last days he insisted on using a small 22 mm head to reduce both the surface area and friction in the joint. The small head of course offers additional mechanical advantages, but at the cost of reduced stability.

Theatre asepsis, laminar air flows, antibiotic prophylaxis, deep vein thrombosis, cement polymerization, cement bone interaction—all these were subjects on which Sir John did a lot of work.

The American surgeons at this time were keen to try out hip replacement for themselves. A number of US surgeons visited Charnley and Wrightington, trained under him and returned with his box of instruments, implants and bone cement.

And as is the custom in America, bone cement was sent to the FDA (the agency that monitors quality and standards of consumables in the U.S.) and they tested it. They tested it on mice and found that cement was carcinogenic for mice!

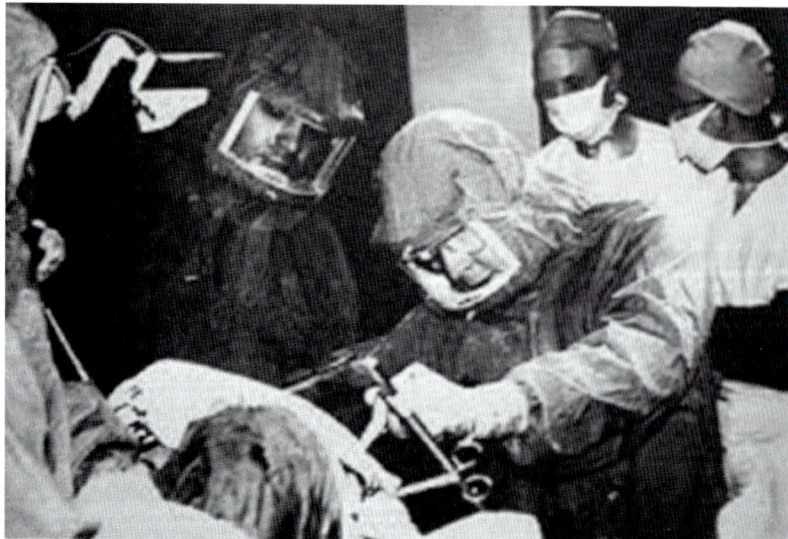

Charnley was also the inventor of space suits and clean air operating rooms

Approval for use of bone cement was withheld and the American surgeons could not use bone cement or do hip replacements. This was in the early 1960s. Plane loads of patients flew into England and got their hips replaced. This state of affairs persisted for a decade. Indignant surgeons from the U.S. demanded a re-evaluation of the facts. And it was found that the mice on which the cement was tested and found carcinogenic were actually carcinogen susceptible in the first place. The experiments were repeated; this time the cement was found to be reasonably safe, and only in the early 1970s cement was permitted for use in the U.S. This gave a ten year lead to the British in the field of hip surgery.

In a way this book is a tribute to Sir John Charnley was an unusual man, and a brilliant scientist on a constant quest for

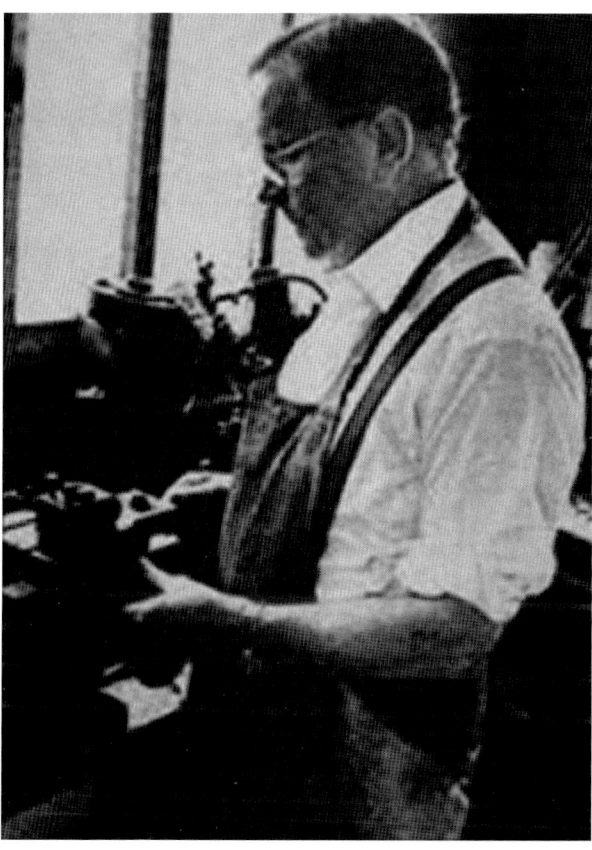

Charnley, working on his lathe

truth. Deviating from hips, I am narrating an event from Sir Charnley's life which would certainly be a great inspiration to most orthopaedic surgeons.

Sir John Charnley was probably one of the greatest minds in orthopaedics. A very keen scientist, he is well known for his total hip, arthrodesis clamps, bone cement, HDPE, book on closed fracture management, antibiotic prophylaxis, clean air, etc.

However, a few incidents of his life are not well known, especially to the younger orthopaedic surgeons, so I am sharing information which is probably not found in Wikepedia.

During his training, Sir John Charnley became interested in the role of periosteum in bone grafts. Wanting to know if supra periosteal grafts would incorporate with the bone, he decided to experiment on his own body.

Against the advice of his senior surgeons, he convinced a colleague to remove a piece of bone from his tibia and reimplant one portion beneath the periosteum and one portion superficial to the periosteum. Unfortunately, Charnley never got an answer to this question as the wound became infected within a few days, and he had to undergo a lot of ordeal and suffering. Finally Charnley required surgery to eradicate the infection. Undaunted, Charnley performed a second self-experiment several years later that revolutionized hip arthroplasty. In the 1950s, Charnley devoted himself to the creation of a low friction hip arthroplasty. He began performing hip replacements that used polytetrafluoroethylene (PTFE, aka Teflon) as a bearing surface, and published his early results in Lancet in 1961. In his article entitled "Arthroplasty of the hip: A new operation", he described how "most patients can execute a straight-leg raise and have no pain or spasm on passive movement." Unfortunately, such promising results were not long lasting. After only a few years, patients returned with failed prostheses and extensive bone loss. Although PTFE had performed well as a bearing surface in the lab and was chemically inert, Charnley suspected that PTFE wear particles were to blame for the osteolysis. To prove this, Charnley placed small particles of PTFE under his own skin in one thigh, and particles of his new proposed bearing surface, High Molecular Weight Polyethylene (HMWP)* under the skin in his other thigh. As he suspected, the PTFE elicited an inflammatory response.

Fortunately, the HMWP did not. To boldly experiment on a patient, conducting untried surgical procedures is one thing, but to get experimental surgery done on one's own body needs not only courage, but also ceaseless undaunted dedication to science. It is because of great dedicated minds like Charnley that a successful procedure like arthroplasty has been able to relieve the miseries of millions of crippled patients.

The next great surgeon in this series is **Maurice Müller**, a great man and personal friend. The year was 1988. I had an opportunity of spending a few precious weeks with Professor Maurice Müller (who even invited me home for dinner!). I had completed a spell in the revision unit of Wrightington Hospital, the Mecca of hip replacements and Charnley's area of operation. I was passionate about orthopaedics, mad about biomechanics and keen on learning.

Müller and I hit it off well and he personally showed me his biomechanical laboratory, his experiments and took me on a conducted tour of Protek factory. (This later helped me to build India's first joint replacement manufacturing factory in 1992, but that's incidental.)

He told me a lot of things that you would probably not find either in J.B.J.S. or Wikepedia. I asked a thousand stupid questions, which he patiently answered, though he was a short tempered surgeon. I assisted him in his private hip operations in a fancy clinic and found his technique a striking contrast from the Wrightington methods. He was a quick surgeon, made large incisions, never bothered about bleeding and did things by eye balling, rather than by instruments.

And here is the story of his hips and their evolution. Impressed by Charnley's work, Müller visited him in 1960. In those times, Chas F. Thackray Ltd. (which made Charnley hips) were allowed to sell them only to those surgeons who trained in Wrightington and learned the technique. If you bought 50 hips and cups, the instrumentation was free. Müller got his sets, began operating and got spectacular success, except for a small problem. 3 of his first 20 hips dislocated and because of component malposition, had to be revised.

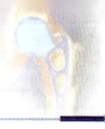

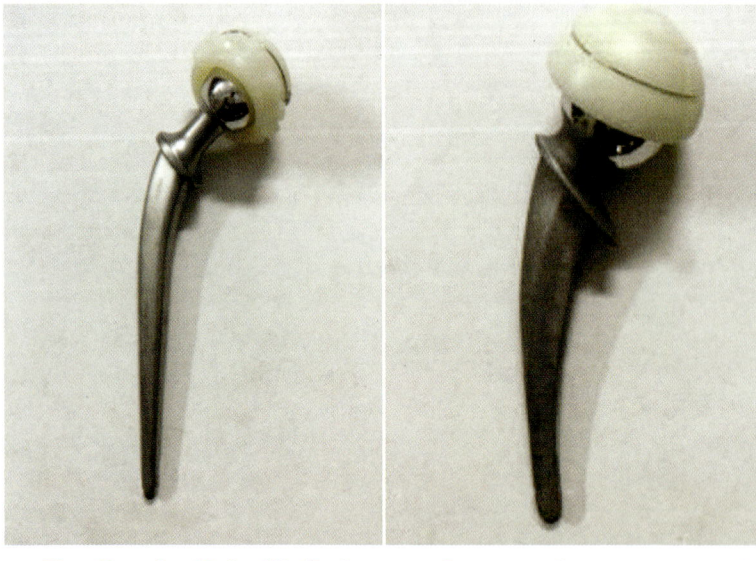

First Charnley Muller Hip Dr. L.
Prakash's collection

Stage two, banana stem, and
35 mm head

Müller wanted a more forgiving system, and tried to analyze the reasons for dislocation. He finally narrowed it to three factors. The small head size, incorrect stem version, and a varus

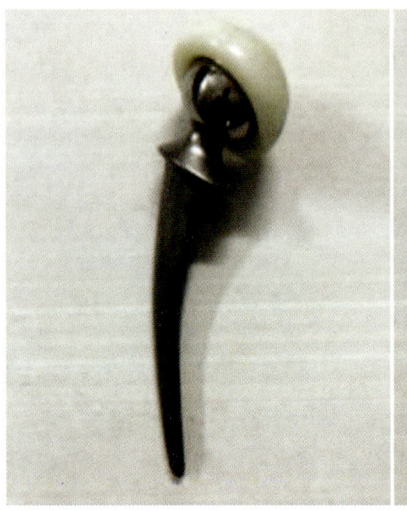

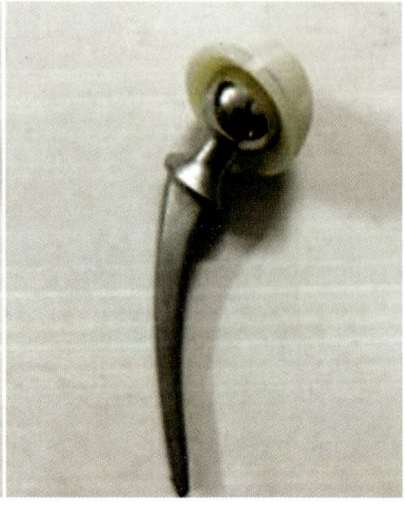

Banana stem for valgus, 32 mm
head standardize, and calcar for
version orientation

Fourth version, valgus banana stem,
small calcar, 34 mm head

position of stem. He thus devised a Charnley Müller Hip, with a head size 30 mm and a banana stem. Being the scientist he was, he constantly improved and modified his designs till he got to the straight stem (later copied as CORAIL) and now the most popular design in the world. I'm lucky to have original implants of the whole series, which I'm posting below. You will see a Charnley copy becoming a banana stem for valgus position, an addition of calcar for better version orientation, head sizes moving from 26, 30 and finally to 32 mm. Material moving from stainless steel to cobalt chrome to titanium. You will also see that he had already made ceramic heads in 1988.

Maurice Edmond Müller, a pioneering hip surgeon, was named surgeon of the century by SICOT in 2002.

Maurice Edmond Müller, born on 28 March 1918, was a surgeon, inventor, scientist, designer, biomechanical engineer, and a very skilled magician. I have had the pleasure of watching him do startling magic tricks.

He was born and had his early schooling in Biel, Switzerland. He had his medical studies in various universities of Switzerland,

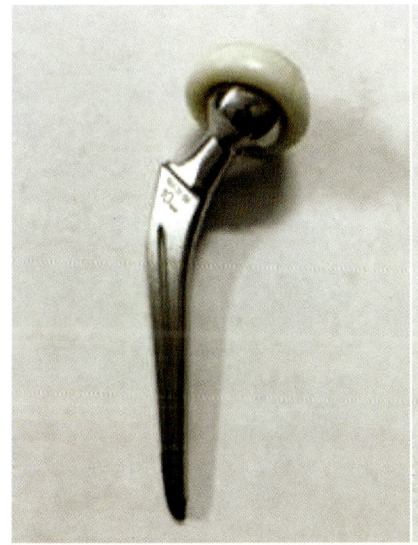

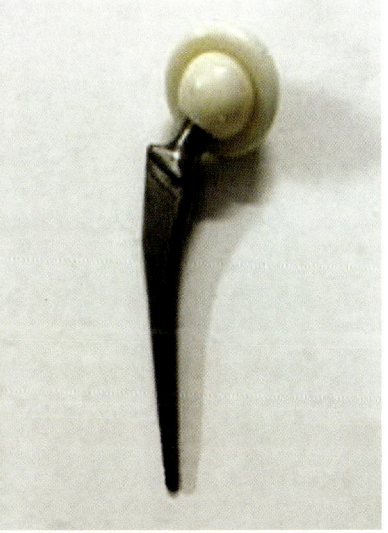

The first stainless steel Muller Hip, straight stem, 32 mm head, no calcar

Titanium straight stem, ceramic head 32 mm, all poly dip

and finally received his M.D. from university of Zurich in 1946.

After spending his initial years serving the poor in Ethopia, he returned to Switzerland to work in its various hospitals. He was professor at University of Berne, and chief orthopaedic surgeon at Inselspital in Berne.

His interest in internal fixation of fractures stemmed from observing results of Gerhad Kuntchner and Robert Danis, the pioneers of intramedullary and plate fixation. After developing his own instrumentation and implant designs, he founded the AO Foundation in 1958 with three other Swiss colleagues.

In the early sixties he developed a strong interest in hip replacements and visited Sir John Charnley in Wrightington U.K. After spending some time there, he returned with a set of instruments and began performing his hip replacements in Berne. Though he was extremely pleased by the results of hip replacements per se, he was a tad dissatisfied with a high post-operative dislocation rate, which he attributed to a small head size used in Charnley hips and the lateral transtrochanteric approach, which in his opinion considerably weakened the abductor mechanism.

In 1963, he modified the Charnley system to produce hips with 28 mm head diameter and began using them by the anteriolateral Watson Jones approach. This was named the Charnley–Müller hip. By 1964, when Charnley expressed dissatisfaction with the use of his name for a design and approach which were not essentially his, Müller modified the hip further, straightening the stem, and using a head diameter of 32 mm.

In 1967, he founded another company Protek AG to market his Müller hips. He was a rich man by his retirement and became a great patron of arts, donating close to eighty million Swiss francs for the cause of building an art museum dedicated to a Swiss painter.

One of the lesser known facts about Müller is that apart from his medical writings, he also published a few articles in magic magazines, explaining certain card trick secrets that he had conceived.

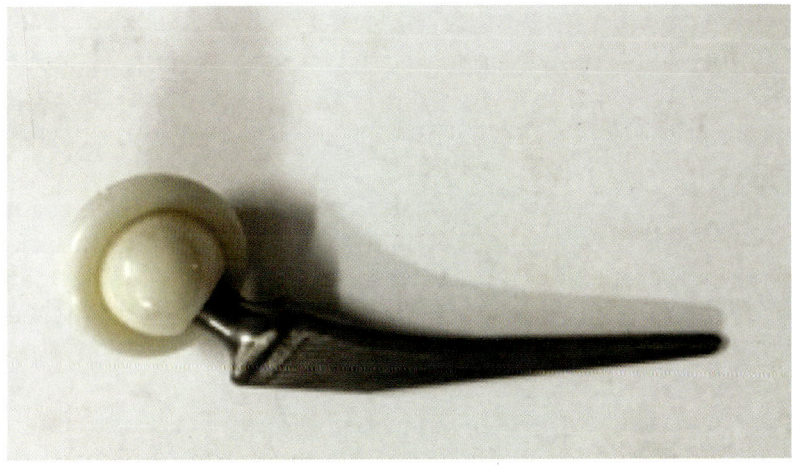

Muller straight stem design, on which Corail, Exedtor, and most other current cemented and cementless hips are based. (Implants from Dr. Prakash's collection)

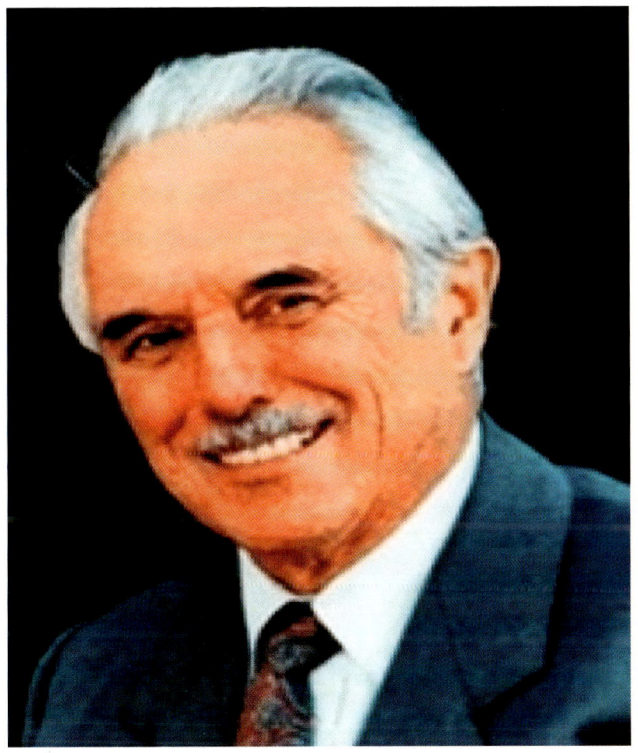

Maurice Muller The Magician Surgeon

BONE CEMENT

PMMA or acrylic cement or acrylic glass is well known to all of us outside the operating room also. The Plexiglas shield for your motorcycle helmet, the plastic fish tank, the fancy transparent door knobs, pseudo crystal plasticky Chinese artifacts, and even an occasional window pane are all made up of acrylic. It is a plastic type polymer, heat curable and was in use for a long time, before researchers found a way to produce room temperature catalytic setting combination, and then as we say, the rest is history!!

See what Wikipedia says about this cement: *Poly methyl methacrylate (PMMA), also known as acrylic or acrylic glass as well as by the trade names Plexiglas, Acrylite, Lucite, and Perspex among several others. PMMA is a transparent thermoplastic often used in sheet form as a lightweight or shatter-resistant alternative to glass. The same material can be utilized as a casting resin, in inks and coatings, and has many other uses.*

Although not a type of familiar silica-based glass, the substance, like many thermoplastics, is often technically classified as a type of glass (in that it is a non¬crystalline vitreous substance), hence its occasional historic designation as acrylic "glass". Chemically, it is the synthetic polymer of methyl methacrylate. Developed in 1928 in several different laboratories by many chemists such as William Chalmers, Otto Röhm and Walter Bauer, it was first marketed in 1933 by the Rohm and Haas Company under the trademark Plexiglas.

PMMA is an economical alternative to polycarbonate (PC) when extreme strength is not necessary. Additionally, PMMA does not contain the potentially harmful bisphenol-A sub-units found in polycarbonate. It is often preferred because of its moderate properties, easy handling and processing, and low cost. Non-modified PMMA behaves in a brittle manner when under load, especially under an impact force, and is more prone to scratching than conventional inorganic glass, but modified PMMA is sometimes able to achieve high scratch and impact resistance.

The era of modern PMMA bone cements comes from the patent by Degussa and Kulzer (1943), who had described the mechanism of polymerization of methyl methacrylate (MMA) at room temperature if a co-initiator, such as a tertiary aromatic amine, is added.

The first bone cement use in Orthopaedics as we all know was by Sir John Charnley, who in 1958, used it for total hip arthroplasty. He had used cold-cured PMMA to attach a PTFE cup to the acetabulum, articulating with a stainless steel femoral head. Sir John was the first to realize that PMMA could be easily used to fill the medullary canal and is easy to blend with the bone morphology.

Charnley's initial success with Teflon, his dramatic failures, discovery of HDPE, and his later spectacular results; make a fascinating story, and bone cement is an essential participant in this saga.

Cement was in widespread use in England from 1958. From 1962 onwards, when PTFE was replaced by HPPE, now the gold standard, cemented hips produced such revolutionary results that it shocked the orthopaedic world, hitherto churning out papers about hip fusions and Girdlestones excision. Charnley however was cautious, insisting that only those trained in his centre, and those buying his instrumentation and implants were allowed to do this surgery. Plane loads of American surgeons came to Wrightington to learn this magical revolutionary operation. But where they able to perform surgeries on their crippled patients back home in USA?? Certainly not!! The stumbling block was FDA.

The USFDA is a bureaucratic body controlled by gigantic commercial interests. It is besides the point that this mindless bureaucracy steals the patients of the latest developments in medicine. FDA tested bone cement in 1963 and rejected its use in humans, as they stated that it was too dangerous, carcinogenic, and fatal in animals. Few surgeons from USA had the courage to defy and replace their hips with cement, and a photo below shows a black market Argentinian bone cement from 1967, which was used by the courageous and daring orthopaedic surgeons thumbing their noses at USFDA.

But the bigger thumb in the nose was given to the FDA by plane loads of American patients with crippling arthritis, who

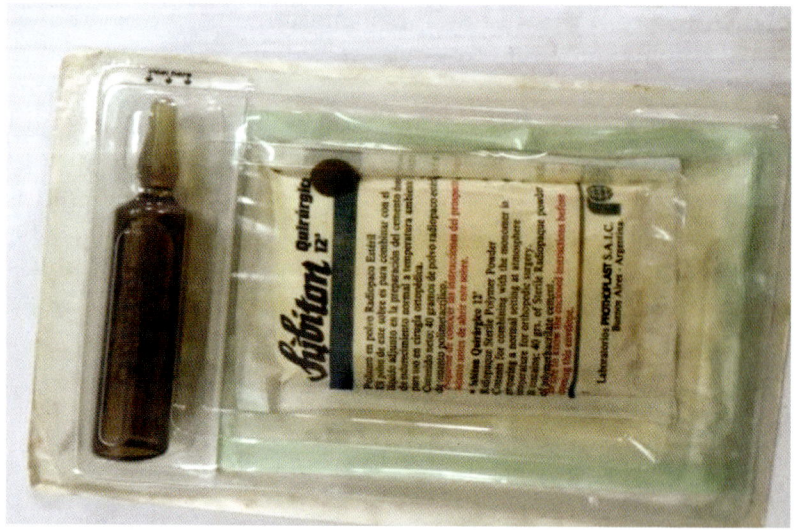

came to Wrightington, England, got their hips replaced and went to Switzerland for a holiday!!

THIS IS THE REASON WHY CEMENTLESS HIPS EVOLVED IN USA. Such are the brilliant laws in USA that the FDA did not distinguish between plates and total joints. Metal inside the body was ok, but not cement to fix it. Try screws, porous coats, beads, whatever you like, but no cement please!!

In 1971, a group of American surgeons, who coincidentally had commercial interests with both Thackeray and Stryker, prevailed on FDA to approve bone cement in human body, because by now there were close to a hundred thousand patients with cement in their body, cancer and complication free. They were painless and mobile as well. This is what the company website says about cement in USA.

"In 1971, Stryker Simplex P Bone Cement revolutionized orthopaedics. Two years later, the product was approved for total knee surgery, and in 1976 for use in pathological fractures and general prosthetic fixation. For more than 50 years, Simplex P Bone Cement, combined with the Stryker cement delivery system, has earned the trust and confidence of tens of thousands of surgeons. Countless articles in respected, peer-reviewed journals confirm its performance."

By now England had not only achieved a ten year lead over USA in hip replacements, but had also bred a new sub speciality of REVISION HIP SURGEONS. The major corporations of USA who had invested billions in cementless technologies would obviously not sit idle and began manufacturing literature to prove the superiority of cementless fixation. David wins against Goliath only in the Bible. In real life, things are a tad different.

1. Chas F Thakery, the company who made Charnley hips was acquired by Depuy, who also acquired Robin Ling's Exeter hips. The latter was a distinctly inferior albeit surgeon friendly model, but more importantly more expensive. Ergo more profits. Charnley hip was killed in favour of Exeter.

2. The profit margins with cement sales were low. Cementless hips produced six times more profit. So began marketing (supported by a lot of pseudo research) into porous coating, beads, titanium, hydroxyappatite coating, etc.

3. Myths and fallacies were spread that cemented hips are extremely difficult to revise. This is certainly not so. I have revised close to four hundred cemented hips and they are routine, if you have the right instrument set. One must read master revisionist Mike Wrobwalaski to appreciate this point. As a matter of fact cementless stems are really difficult to revise!!

4. Though no cementless hip has survived longer than cemented, yet a myth has been created by pseudo literature exactly to the contrary!!

5. Recent animal experiments have shown that you need forty times of the cement we use to actually cause hypotension or cardiac problems. Even reaming femurs or pushing bone wax can cause collapse. You need a proper cementation technique with a tube in the medulla to relieve pressure and a gun to allow liquid cement to ingrain to the bone.

6. No research or papers are being published in the last five years regarding improved cementation techniques. Only antibiotic added inferior cements are making their appearance with regularity.

7. Today you cannot buy a Charnley cobra standard 135 offset hip with an all poly cup in the market, because it is simply unavailable. A product with a 25 year excellent follow-up and it is killed by commerce!

The following points about bone cement may help us to understand and use it better. A lot of this information is gathered from non orthopaedic situations where PMMA acrylic resin is used in large quantities.

1. Acrylic cement is not a glue or adhesive. It is more like a filler or grout. Epoxy resins and Polyester resins bind far better than acrylic.

2. Normally polymer powder to monomer liquid ratio is 2:1 w/v, but by modifying this proportion, setting times can be altered dramatically. A 1:1 mix provides prolonged setting time, as does lower room temperature or chilling before mixing.

3. Additives to powder quicken the setting time and also modify setting behaviour quickening the liquid phase, while hardening time remains more or less the same. Consequently Gentamycin loaded cement is less desirable for cementation.

4. A clean dry porous surface allows cement to "get inside" the cancellous areas and anchor holes, allowing a more uniform distribution of stresses and a better grouting, naturally leading to a longer life of the cementation.

These are the tricks I have followed which has helped my cemented to hips last so long that I find no reason to switch over to uncemented hips.

A, Keep surfaces clean and dry. As clean and as dry as possible.

B, Inject liquid cement under pressure. More liquid, greater the pressure, better.

C, Don't hammer the implant in. Hammering only makes the ductile cement push back the prosthesis. Each blow weakens the grout. Sustained manual pressure is applied on the impactor/positioner, till elbow and shoulder hurts. This is an important trick!

D, A meticulous removal of all overhanging and loose cement debris is essential to prevent particulate debris wear.

The use of bone cement was considered as a weak link in the development process of joint replacement operations and since early days there have been efforts to design and develop a prosthesis that can be anchored without the use of bone cement.

As a matter of fact the Austin Moore endo prosthesis depended on a self locking mechanism as a result of bone in growth to help anchor the prosthesis in the hip. Peter Ring, Chivas, AZmstutz, Müller, and Rob Matheys have all been constantly researching into the possibilities of cementless joint replacements. But to date, cementless joints have not been proved superior to cemented ones in the longest of the long term follow up where the Charnley design reigns supreme. Thus I beg to be pardoned if there is a slant towards cementation and a bias towards the use of the Charnley design throughout this book.

4

Bio-materials of the Artificial Hip

Materials

Metals, Plastic and Acrylic cement form the three common materials used in arthroplasty. Ceramics have now made their appearance on the scene. This chapter will give you enough knowledge not to be fooled by the snake oil salesmen, who are employees of multinational companies, selling those exotic high priced hips at fifty times the manufacturing cost!

In the beginning, when Hemiarthroplasties were done, the implant material varied from heat cured acrylic to resins and then to stainless steel. Stainless steel did not show as much wear as acrylic and soon replaced the latter. The fact that the non replaced acetabulum showed significant wear, prompted research into total joints. Charnley's work laid the foundation of the modern arthroplasty. In spite of the continuing research in implant materials, the time honored combination of metal articulating with ultra high molecular weight polyethylene is yet to be challenged. However the choice of metal has changed from stainless steel of Charnley's time to stronger steel alloys and then to cobalt-chromium and titanium-aluminum-vanadium. Ceramic is also being used because of their excellent frictional and wear characteristics, but has its own disadvantage of brittleness.

There is a lot of confusing terminology whilst describing materials, e.g. yield strength, toughness, ultimate tensile strength, ductility, elasticity, and fatigue strength. This book is not a treatise on material science and hence the reader may have to read more advanced manuals for details about these. I would however teach you enough about biomaterials, and biomechanics, that the next time a high flying scientist from a multinational implant manufacturing company tries to bamboozle you with highly cross linked poly, or plasma coated surfaces, Chiruleen, Gur 10/50, titanium dinitride coatings, or alumina ceramics, you can ask him some questions, the answers to which he would probably not know!!

Metals

Stainless steel: This no doubt the cheapest material, tried and tested for a long period, and has been in use since 1900. 316L stainless steel is popular for implants as it is the most corrosion resistant when in direct contact with biological fluids. What makes 316L ideal as an implant material is the lack of inclusion. Alloys with inclusion will contain sulfur and this is a key ingredient which encourages corrosion of metals.

Stainless steel is an iron alloy. By adding the chromium (16%) to stainless steel, this becomes corrosion resistant. The addition of nickel (7%) helps stabilize the austenite to stainless steel. Type 316L stainless steel selected for the purpose of surgical implants contains approximately 17 to 19% of chromium and 14% nickel. Molybdenum is added to the stainless steel alloy and forms a protective layer sheltering the metal from exposure to an acidic environment. Corrosion resistance can also be achieved with the carbon element but only when the carbon is in a solid solution state.

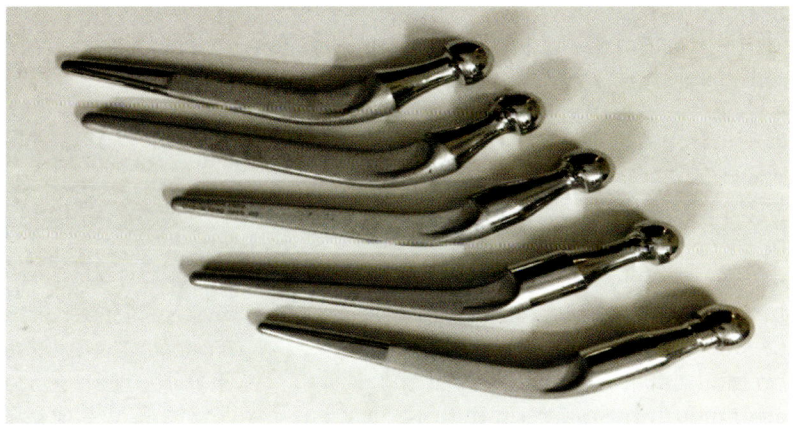

A forged stainless steel implant

Stainless steel can be heat forged, cold worked, machined from blocks or cast into complex shapes. Its final mechanical properties will be entirely dependent on how it is made.

It has to be stressed that the ferrite element should not be incorporated into stainless steel as this gives the metal a magnetic property, which is never used for surgical implants as it could interfere with Magnetic Resonance Imaging (MRI) equipment. One of the most apparent problems with using magnetic implants is their susceptibility to heating which could change its shape or structural composition.

If we evaluate all types of metallic implants that have gone into the human body since nineteen hundreds, roughly 70% would be stainless steel, twenty percent cobalt chrome alloys and ten percent titanium. However a look at the currently available commercial hip implants, will tell us that SS 316L is no longer used. Only the higher priced Cobalt chrome alloys or Titanium form the basic material for most femoral and acetabular components, the purported reason being better strength and biocompatibility of Cobalt and Titanium alloys.

However if the steels of the modern generations are compared with cobalt-chrome alloy, they are only insignificantly weaker than the latter. On the other hand Cobalt-chrome alloys are heavier, and if cast, seldom approach the strength of forged virgin stainless steel. Cobalt chrome molybdenum alloy, which is most commonly used in hip implants, is about three to four times as expensive as stainless steel. Though total joints were initially begun with stainless steel on HDPE constructs, and the initial 100,000 plus hips made by Charnley and Thackeray were stainless steel, and have exhibited excellent mechanical properties and tolerances, surprisingly it is no longer used as an implant material for hip replacements currently.

One would thus like to question the wisdom of generically moving away from stainless steel in implantable joints when this is used extensively in most internal fixation and trauma products. May be commercial considerations outweighs benefits to the patients!!

Cobalt Based Alloys

The material approved for orthopaedic use is ASTM F75. Though these are superior to stainless steel based alloys in corrosion resistance and fatigue failure; there is a tendency for the alloy grains to become non-homogenous and lead to different implant strength in different batches. It is indeed surprising that in the United States, this is the most popular alloy for all endoprosthesis and steel based alloys are almost out.

From the surgeon's point of view this assumption is a little biased, because Charnley's initial experience using simple stainless steel 316L is a definite landmark that is still to be equaled or excelled.

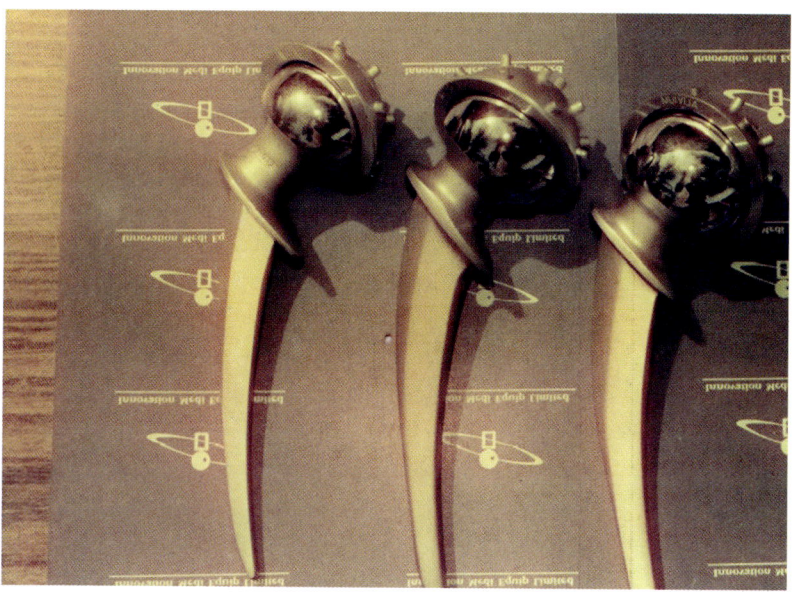

Cast cobalt chrome components of the early Mckee Farar Total hip

The ASTM F75 standard specifies that the alloy should contain cobalt as its principal element, with 27 to 30% chromium, 5 to 7% molybdenum, and limits on other important elements such as manganese and silicon, less than 1% iron, less than 0.75% nickel, less than 0.5%, of nitrogen, phosphorus, sulfur, boron tungsten, etc.

Besides cobalt-chromium-molybdenum (CoCrMo), cobalt-nickel-chromium-molybdenum (CoNiCrMo) is also used for implants. The possible toxicity of released Ni ions from CoNiCr alloys and also their limited frictional properties are a matter of concern in using these alloys as articulating components. Thus, CoCrMo is usually the dominant alloy for total joint arthroplasty.

Titanium Based Alloys

These are the best as far as modulus of elasticity weight and corrosion resistances are concerned, but the adhesive and abrasive wear properties are much less than the above two. In addition, despite the low weight and good strength, Titanium and its alloys suffer from a paradox of excellent bio-compatibility when fixed firmly and a very poor tissue response when they are loose and this leads to particulate debris! Consequently, if a bearing surface is to be made of Titanium, it is indeed imperative that it is either anodized or coated with a non degradable substance to allow for a high quality of abrasive resistant mirror polish. Added to this, the cost of the metal is very high and in many cases especially in our country may be detriment to its selection as a metal of choice in implant manufacture.

Recent studies from the western world do show that the choice of titanium for an implant material is indeed not a wise one! The bio-degradation of the implants fixed not too snugly has not only lead to early loosening, but also to massive osteolysis, migration of the Titanium particles, and even black stained lymph nodes at sites distant from the joint, which does tell us

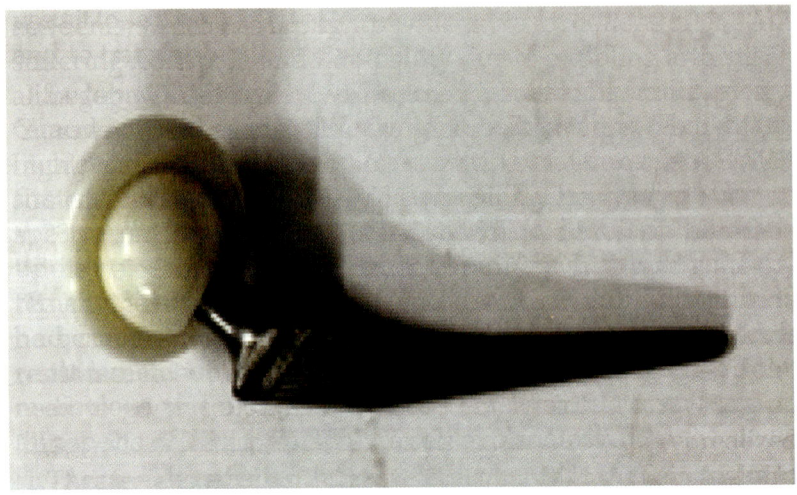

The Muller Straight Stem titanium prosthesis for cemented use

that inertness may be a more important factor that elasticity and weight.

COMPARISON BETWEEN THE THREE COMMONLY USED METALS IN ARTHROPLASTY

1. Modulus of Elasticity

The modulus of elasticity is the ratio of applied stress to the resultant strain in the linear (elastic) portion of the stress-strain curve. This is also referred to as the "Young's modulus, 'E'". This parameter corresponds to the stiffness of a material and thus a high modulus of elasticity would mean a stiffer implant, while a low modulus of elasticity would mean a more elastic implant.

2. Specific Gravity or Density

Weight by volume is density, with water having a density of one. A liter of water will weigh a kilo. Incidentally when Archimedes jumped out of his bath tub and displayed his testicles to the whole of Athens, it was this discovery, his EUREKA moment. Thus materials with high density or specific gravity will be heavier than an identically sized implant of lower SG.

Cortical bone has a Young's modulus varying in the direction of deformation and for a tibia would be about 5 to 10 in transverse axis and 11 to 23 in longitudinal axis. Compared to this 316L SS is 186, Cobalt chrome is 241, and Titanium 5 is 105.

On the other hand, the Density or SG of human bone is between 1.7 to 2.3. Compared to this Titanium is 4.5, Stainless steel 7.9 and Cobalt chrome alloy 8.36.

Other mechanical Properties				
Metal	Ultimate tensile strength MPa	Yield strength MPa	Ellongation %	Area reduction %
SS 316l	480	170	40	0
ASTM F75	890	517	20	20
Titanium 5	900	520	15	25

The four characters which we look for in implantable metals are UTS (ultimate tensile strength), YS (yield strength), Elongation and reduction. This is how the three metals compare

What do these numbers mean? None of the three metals are as light or elastic as human bones. What is the relevance? If you leave aside the commercially motivated research papers, the clear conclusion is that there is no significant difference between cobalt and SS except that the latter is about one fourth the cost. Titanium which is fifteen times as expensive as SS is lighter and more elastic. The latter property may be desirable in implants to avoid stress shielding.

The current trend is shifting towards titanium stems, though cobalt chrome is still widely used and accounts for over two thirds of prosthesis in use currently.

I still believe that Stainless steel 316L is one of the best materials for hip implants. Easily available, manufactured in India, capable of excellent finish, economical to invest cast, easy to machine and with proven 18 to 24 year survivorship! I am working on bringing a commercial model of a sub 200$ hip and knee, and only time will tell if I am able to do something.

ULTRA HIGH MOLECULAR WEIGHT POLYETHYLENE

HDPE was an accident, but probably one of the luckiest accidents, which has brought a wide smile to millions of patients suffering from pain and immobility due to crippling arthritis. It all began with Charnley's experiments in total hip arthroplasty! Charnley first began using the Mckee Farar hips. These were highly polished metal on metal hips fixed with cement. While some failed soon, others lasted surprisingly long, some even up to 23 years. Charnley was a keen observer and excellent clinician. While he examined a few Mckee Farar hips, he heard squeaks. His engineer friends told him that it was a friction squeak, and he became interested to know all about friction. Friction is resistance to two surfaces rubbing against each other. You don't need to go to complex text books of physics to know logical things about friction which are self explanatory.

1. Area—The smaller the area, lesser the friction. It is easier to slide a 25 paisa coin on a table than a dinner plate.

2. Surface—Smoother the surface, lesser the friction. Two sandpapers rubbing against one other will have more friction than two mirrors.

3. Lubrication—A good lubricant naturally reduces friction.

With these points in mind, John Charnley began his experiments with the bearing surface for his hips. Metal was out. He began experimenting with industrial plastics. Teflon or PTFE (poly tetra fluro ethylene), was a new plastic with wonderful properties. Lab tests showed that the friction in stainless steel rubbing against PTFE was practically zero.

Charnley was an engineer and a surgeon. He devised a prosthesis made of stainless steel which he machined himself on a lathe and implanted it into a patient. The cup surface he replaced with one of Teflon. The initial results were very good that his patients were pain free immediately after the operation. People who had not walked for years started running. Charnley was thrilled. He went before the orthopedic surgeons of England and announced that he had discovered an operation he too would do on his mother!! So spectacular were the results!

But unfortunately the results were short lived. Charnley in his initial enthusiasm miscalculated wear and tear. So engrossed was he with friction that he did not anticipate the possibility that Teflon can rub out after constant movement against the metal. In a human body the hip is put through vigorous movements with sufficient load over prolonged periods and this caused a significant Teflon wear.

The Teflon material just cheesed away in a year's time and Charnley was left with a hundred failed hip joints. Way back in 1960s you could get away with a hundred failed operations without a consumer protection council above your head. Charnley was shattered. He went back before the same British orthopedic surgeons and told them that the operation was no good that he would not even do it on his own mother-in-law!

Then Charnley was given a piece of HDPE (High Density Polyethylene). He saw another plastic and was not impressed. A hundred failures had disillusioned him. But he did make a trial cup and put it on a machine which he used to test the wear. Someone forgot to switch off the machine that weekend and what was found on Monday was a spinning system which would

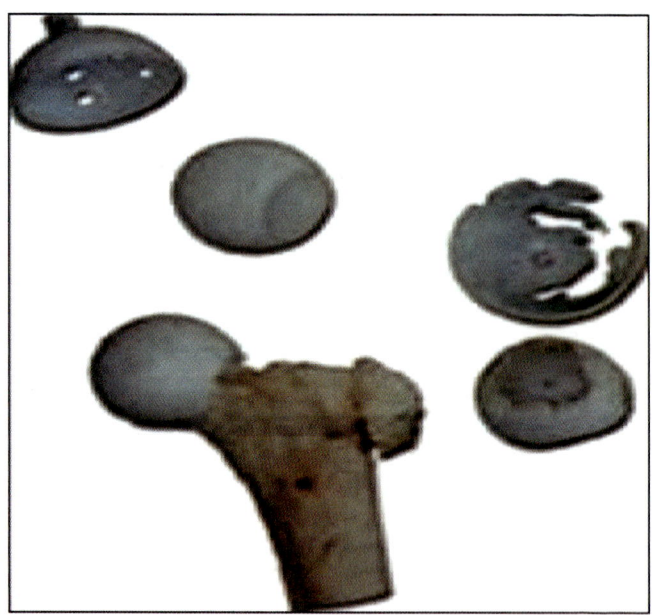

Rapid wear of Teflon cup in Charnley's initial experiments

have been in the human body for two years. Charnley measured the wear and found none! This amazed Charnley. He put it through further tests and the results were the same. Polyethylene did not wear. At least in experiments situations it did not wear even a fraction of that of Teflon. Further researches were made and the final UHMUHDPE was discovered. Ultra high density, ultra high molecular weight polyethylene to be precise.

UHMWPE is a member of the polyethylene family of polymers with the repeat unit $[C_2H_4]_n$, with n denoting the degree of polymerization. The international Standards Organization (ISO 11542) (ISO) defines UHMWPE as having a molecular weight of at least 1 million g/mole, resulting in a minimum degree of polymerization of $n \approx 36{,}000$, while the American Society for Testing and Materials (ASTM D 4020) (ASTM) specifies that UHMWPE has a molecular weight greater than 3.1 million g/mole ($n \approx 110{,}000$). The UHMWPEs used in orthopaedic applications typically have a molecular weight between 2–6 million with a degree of polymerization between 71,000–214,000.

UHMWPE is a linear (non-branching) semi-crystalline polymer which can be described as a two phase composite of crystalline and amorphous phases. The crystalline phase contains chains folded into highly oriented lamellae, with the crystals being orthorhombic in structure. The lamellae are 10–50 nm thick and 10–50 µm long. The lamellae are oriented randomly within the amorphous phase with tie molecules linking individual lamellae to one another.

The two resins of UHMWPE that are currently used in orthopaedics are GUR 1020 (3.5 million g/mole) and GUR 1050 (5.5–6 million g/mole). These resins can either be compression molded into sheets or ram extruded into rods. Both resin and conversion methods are significant predictors of tensile mechanical properties and impact strength. Virgin UHMWHDPE is a non cross linked, non gamma irradiated plastic, which was first used in joint replacements. This is plastic, with slight deformative properties, a reasonable modulus of elasticity and return to shape after deforming forces are removed.

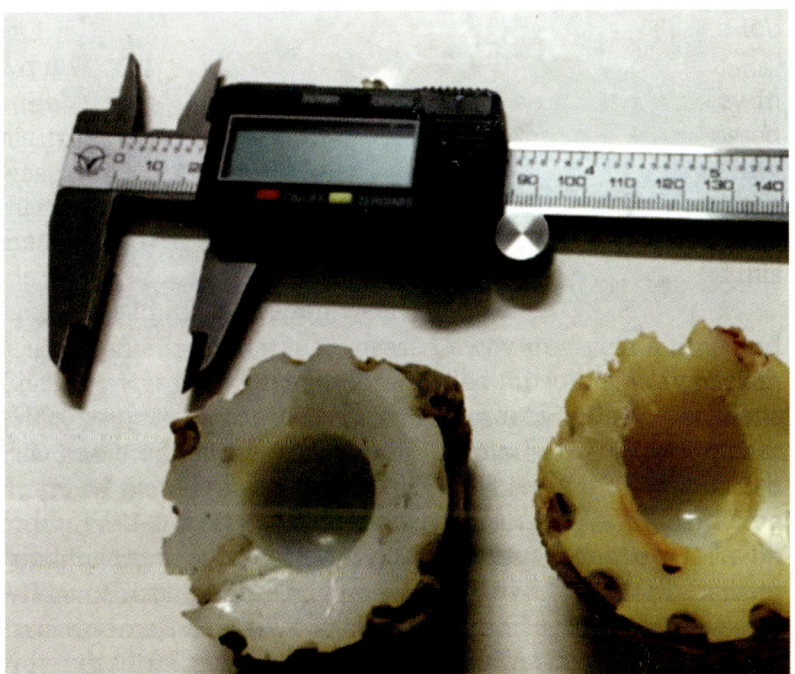

UHMWUHDPE has exceptional wear properties. The cups retrieved by the author show minimal wear at nine years (left) and wear at 19 years. This is non cross linked virgin poly!

Charnley autoclaved his femoral components, but gas sterilized (Ethylene Oxide) the HDPE cups. Around the same time Maurice Muller of Switzerland began doing his larger head (32mm) hips. He gamma radiated both the stems and cups. Initial results of the two systems were similar, but at five years, the wear rate of Muller's radiated cups was extremely high compared to Charnley's non irradiated ones.

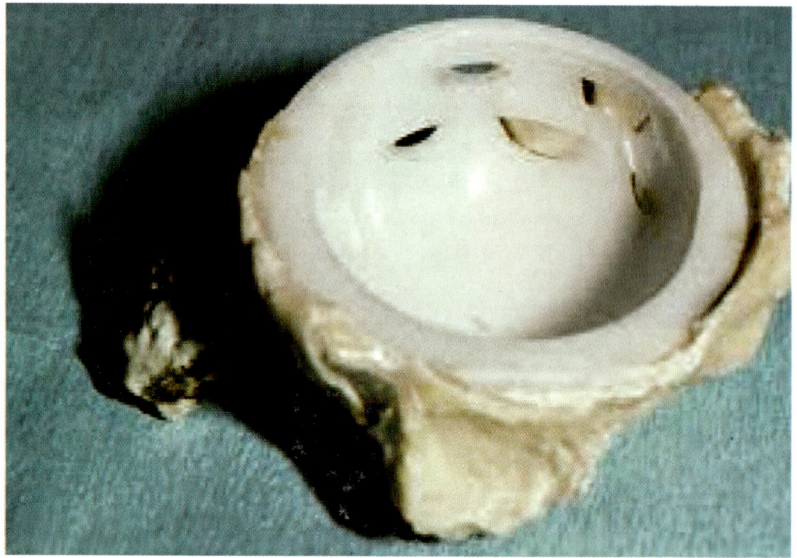

Early Muller cups showed a much greater wear due to two reasons. Thin cup due to large head, and gamma radiation

It was at this time that scientists began to worry about plastic wear. It was found that radiation produced cross-linking of the molecules and when gamma sterilized in presence of air, the cups underwent oxidative degradation, making them brittle over the years leading to progressive wear.

Ruhrchemie AG, the German company first introduced UHDPE for orthopaedic use and it was called RCH 100. (R)uhr (CH)emie 100. This company then became Hoechst and the next gen UHMWHDPE produced by them was named Chirulen. Now the company is called Tikona and the plastics are called GUR or (G)ranular (U)hmwhdpe (R)uhrchemie. The product is designated with a four digit number, example GUR 1050 or GUR

1020, etc. The first digit is the loose density, the second is presence or absence of calcium strerate, the third digit is molecular weight in million and the last digit is the resin grade.

Application of heat and pressure produces sheets or extruded rods, which are then machined to the correct component dimensions. Though some manufacturers directly moulded the granules to the desired component using a die, it was later found that these extra polished components wore out faster. The current concept is to use machined parts from stock blocks of larger size.

Virgin HDPE has stood the test of time so long as it is not irradiated and the components are not too thin. However the principal cause of hip revision was found to be wear. Scientists thus began experimenting with gilding the lilly to produce better variants. Carbon reinforced polymer composite was one such disaster, and Zimmer had to recall its entire stocks and discontinue the product seven years after release. Heat pressing was another disaster.

Cross linking is currently being used in an attempt to improve the wear performance. Normally HDPE is linear linked with long molecular chains. It was assumed that this was the defect of the polymer, causing wear. By adding linking agents like peroxides or silanes, and gamma radiating the plastic to controlled levels, the molecular structure was reorganized to allow linking in both linear and transverse directions, producing what is known as a cross linked polymer.

Though hip cups have shown some degree of wear resistance, due to cross-linking, only commercial publications wax eloquently about cross linking in hip replacements. Some studies have actually shown that cross linking makes the plastic more rigid, brittle and more susceptible to fractures and early failure.

Cross-linking reduces crystalinity, and thereby makes the plastic more brittle, less elastic, stronger in one way but weaker in the other. Whether it is actually beneficial in the long run is a matter to be seen with time.

Ceramics

Ceramics are non-metallic inorganic materials and vary in composition. They are made by mixing the fine powders of the ingredient material with water and adhesive binder. This is then squeezed into a mould to obtain the desired shape, air dried to dry, and the binder is then burned out by thermal treatment. Firing or sintering at this stage at a high temperature (over 100 degrees Celsius) makes the residual material extremely dense.

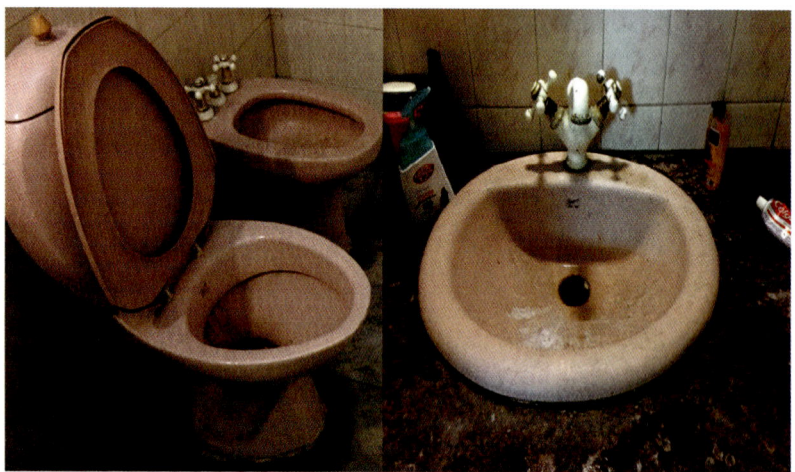

The ceramics used in hips are no different used in our toilets and wash basins. The material and technology are the same

The final microscopic structure of the resultant ceramic is greatly dependent on the thermal process used, the highest temperature reached and the duration of furnace heat treatment.

Five types of ceramics are used in arthroplasty:

1. Glass
2. Plasma-sprayed polycrystalline ceramic
3. Vitrified ceramic
4. Solid state sintered ceramic
5. Polycrystalline glass-ceramic.

Other factors determining the mechanical and biological properties are the purity of the powder, the size and distribution of the grains, and the porosity.

Ceramics used in orthopaedic surgery are classified as *bioactive* or *inert* according to the tissue response when implanted in an osseous environment.

The *bioactivity* of a material can be defined as its ability to bond biologically to bone. An *inert* ceramic merely elicits a minor fibrous reaction. In clinical practice, inert fully-dense ceramics are used as bearings in total joint replacements because of their exceptional resistance to wear and bioactive ceramics are used as coatings to enhance the fixation of the femoral stems or acetabular shells.

Sliding ceramics. The most widely used bearing combination in total joint replacements is metal-on-polyethylene. The long-term survival of the artificial joint however, is dependent on the wear of its components. It is the poly wear, which ultimately leads to osteolysis around the implant leading to an inflammatory response induced by wear debris occurring from both the articulating and non-articulating surfaces.

Pierre Boutin first introduced ceramics in orthopaedics in the early 1970s in order to tackle complications related to polyethylene wear.

They are mainly used in total hip arthroplasty as femoral heads articulating against polyethylene, and as cups in the alumina-on-alumina combination. Because of their relatively brittle nature, fracture of ceramic femoral heads has been, along with cost, the main limitation to their expanded use world-wide.

The risk of fracture, however, has been virtually eliminated because of a great improvement in the manufacturing process

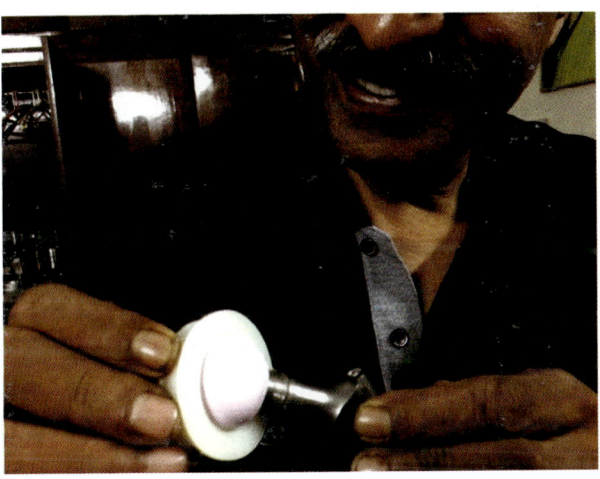

Currently the most popular use of ceramics is as a bearing with HDPE

with increased purity and density, increase in the size and distribution of the grains and better quality control.

Accurate fixation of the ceramic ball to the femoral stem through a well-designed Morse taper avoids undesirable stresses in the head and improved surgical techniques augment the longevity of the implant.

The fracture rate of ceramic heads has been evaluated as 0.02% for alumina heads and 0.03% for those of zirconia indicating that fracture of the ceramic head is no longer an important.

Alumina ceramic. Dense alumina of surgical grade is obtained by sintering alumina powder at temperatures between 1600 and 1800°C. The resultant material is in its highest state of oxidation, allowing thermodynamic stability, chemical inertness and excellent resistance to corrosion.

Improvement in the manufacturing process has lowered the size and distribution of the grains, which are major factors in avoiding cracks and fracture.

Alumina is a brittle material with excellent compression strength but the bending strength is limited. The Young's modulus is 300 times greater than that of cancellous bone, and 190 times higher than polymethylmethacrylate (PMMA).

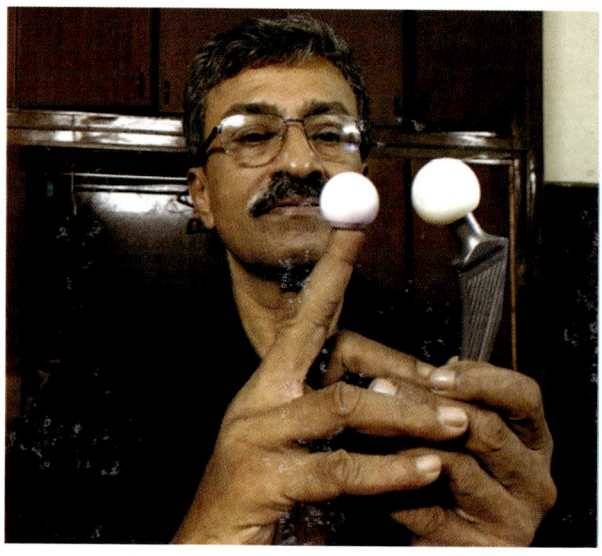

The alumina and Zirconia ceramics are not too differrrent in look and feel on the operating table

Alumina has been a standardised material since 1984 (International Standard Organisation, ISO 6474). The tribological properties of alumina ceramic against itself are outstanding with a linear wear rate 4000 times lower than that of metal-on-polyethylene.

The excellent frictional characteristics are due in part to a high wettability because of the hydrophilic surface and fluid film lubrification which minimises adhesive wear.

These properties, demonstrated both in vitro and on analysis of retrieved implants, are responsible for the limited amount of wear particles produced and the subsequent moderate biological reaction to ceramic wear debris.

The clearance between the two components in the case of the alumina-on-alumina combination should be around 50 nanometers to avoid Hertz stresses at the surface of the alumina which may result in detachment of grains and third-body wear. This Hertz stress is a geometrically progressive wear, as the particles produced exponentially.

Wroblewski, Siney and Fleming recently described the results of 22 mm alumina femoral heads articulating against crosslinked polyethylene in a ten-year follow-up. A running-in rate of penetration was noted which then decreased to 0.022 mm/year after the first 18 months. It is difficult, however, to conclude from this study whether the alumina head, the small diameter of the femoral head, or the crosslinked nature of the polyethylene cups was responsible for the low rate of wear observed.

Comparative physical properties of alumina and zirconia ceramics of surgical grade

Property	Alumina	Zirconia
Purity (%)	>99.8	>97.0
Density (g/cm^3)	3.98	6.05
Bending strength (MPa)	595	1000
Compressive strength (MPa)	4250	2000
Young's modulus (GPa)	380	210
Hardness (Vickers hardness number)	2000	1200
Fracture toughness KIC (MN/m^3/2)	5	7
Grain size (micro m)	3.6	0.2 to 0.4
Surface finish (Ra, micro m)	0.02	

Zirconia ceramic was introduced in the manufacture of femoral heads for total hip replacements because of its higher strength and toughness which would reduce the risk of fracture. Pure zirconia is an unstable material showing three different crystalline phases: monoclinic, tetragonal and cubic.

The phase changes result in a large variation in volume and significantly decrease the mechanical properties of the material due to the production of cracks. Stabilisation of zirconia by adding oxides to maintain the tetragonal phase has therefore been undertaken.

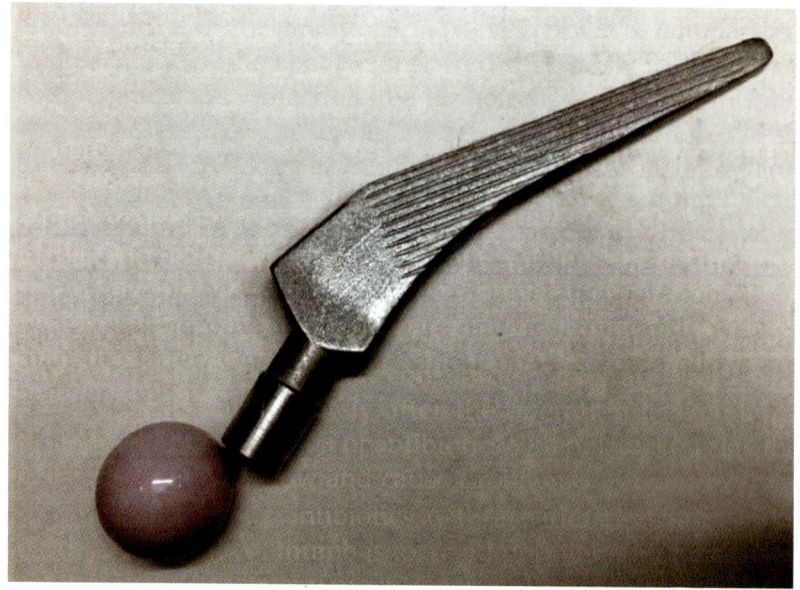

A zirconia ceramic head with a Hydroxyappatite coated stem

Yttrium-stabilised tetragonal polycrystalline zirconia (Y-TZP) has a fine grain size and offers the best mechanical properties (Table I).

This material was standardised in 1997 (International Standard Organisation, ISO 13356). Zirconia femoral heads should articulate only against polyethylene sockets since both zirconia against alumina and zirconia against zirconia20 have been shown to produce catastrophic rates of wear in vitro. Zirconia-on-polyethylene has demonstrated similar rates of wear as alumina-on-polyethylene in vitro, but in vivo the results have not been so favourable.

Allain et al recently described a consecutive series of 78 hips using a zirconia femoral head and a polyethylene cup. Complete radiolucent lines were observed around the cup in 23% of the hips and 17% of the femoral implants had radiolucency greater than 1 mm. Survival at eight years was 63%. These worrying results were confirmed by Hernigou and Babrami in a study comparing wear of the cup and osteolysis in 40 hips over a period of ten years.

Two comparable groups of 20 hips each had either a 32 mm alumina or a 28 mm zirconia femoral head. During the first five years, the zirconia group had a lower rate of wear of 0.04 mm/year compared with 0.08 mm/year, and osteolysis on the calcar measured in square millimetres was similar in both groups.

Between five and ten years, however, the rate of wear increased dramatically in the zirconia group to 0.15 mm/ year at ten years as opposed to 0.07 mm/year in the alumina group. Osteolysis of the calcar was significantly greater in the zirconia group at 135 mm2 compared with 65 mm.

These results are of concern. The long-term performance of zirconia ceramic may well be altered by degradation in vivo with transformation of the material into its monoclinic unstable phase.

Another explanation was suggested by Lu and McKellop who measured the frictional heating of polyethylene cups in a hip joint simulator. The steady-state temperature of the polyethylene reached 99°C with heads of zirconia ceramic compared with 45°C with alumina prostheses.

This may account for the long-term wear because of the consequent structural changes and may also produce precipitation of lubricant proteins. Better results are apparent in current clinical trials.

Mixed-oxide ceramics. A new class of materials has been developed recently to combine the tribological properties of alumina and the mechanical characteristics of yitrium stabilised zirconia.

These mixed-oxide ceramics containing 40% to 80% zirconia have shown rates of wear in vitro comparable to those of alumina ceramic. Preliminary results in hip joint simulators have been promising, but further investigations are needed to assess their long-term performance.

Bioactive ceramics. These are osteoconductive, acting as a scaffold to enhance bone formation on their surface, and are used either as a coating on various substrates or to fill bone defects. An osteoconductive material can only elicit bone formation in an osseous environment, whereas an osteoinductive substance can promote bone formation even in an extraosseous situation.

Calcium phosphate ceramics. Two bioceramics belonging to the calcium phosphate family have had extensive evaluation as orthopaedic implants, namely HA and tricalcium phosphate (TCP). Stochiometric synthetic HA ($Ca_{10}(PO_4)_6(OH)_2$), with a calcium-to-phosphate atomic ratio of 1.67, was introduced as a bone-graft substitute because its formula is similar to that of the inorganic mineral phase of bone.

Biological HA, however, is Ca deficient and a carbonated apatite. The bonding mechanism of HA to bone, although not

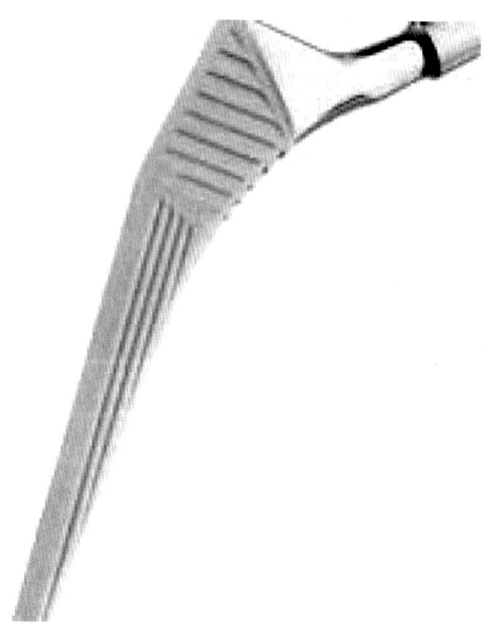

A Hydroxy Appatite coated stem

completely understood, seems to be due to the attachment at the surface of the HA of osteogenically-competent cells which differentiate into osteoblasts.

A cellular bone matrix is then formed at the surface of the HA. An amorphous area is present between the surface and the bone tissue containing thin apatite crystals. As maturation occurs, this bonding zone shrinks and HA becomes attached to bone through a thin epitaxial layer, resulting in a strong interface with no layer of fibrous tisue interposed between the bone and HA.

Bone formation grows from the surface of the HA towards the centre of the pores. HA coating is widely used on femoral prostheses and on sockets as a means of fixation in order to avoid complications related to the use of PMMA. It is usually applied by plasma spray.

An American multicentre study has reported excellent results, with a rate of femoral revision of 0.3% at a mean follow-up of 8.1 years, with one case of loosening out of 324 implants.

However it has not yet been clearly shown that HA offers improved fixation when compared with bone cement. The thickness of the coating, the chemical composition of the material and the roughness and nature of the metal substrate seem to be key factors in ensuring good results.

The main Disadvantages which have limited the clinical application of HA as a bone-graft substitute are related to the brittle nature and poor tensile strength of the material. Consequently, information on the clinical use of ceramic bone-graft substitutes is scarce.

TCP has been evaluated in spinal fusion with results comparable to those with autogenous bone.

Bioactive glasses. Bioactive glasses were first developed by Hench and Wilson and have a vitreous structure. They bond chemically to bone. The model in this class of materials is Bioglass 45S5 of which the composition in weight % is: 45% SiO_2, 24.5% CaO, 6% P_2O_5 and 24.5% Na_2O.

The bonding mechanism of silicate bioactive glasses to bone has been attributed to a series of surface reactions ultimately leading to the formation of a hydroxycarbonate apatite layer at the glass surface.

Greater production of bone has been demonstrated with Bioglass 45S5 when compared with HA, but due to its poor mechanical properties this material has not been used in load-bearing applications.

Recently, in order to improve the reactivity of the material, sol-gel processed glasses, hydrolysed at ambient temperatures, have been developed to obtain bioactive gelglasses in the SiO2-CaO-P2O5 system, with an initial high specific surface area.

These materials have similar osteoconductive properties to melt-derived glasses, but have an improved degradability.

The low temperatures used to produce sol-gel glasses allow them to be used as a coating on alumina substrates. When implanted in an animal model, sol-gel glass-coated alumina has demonstrated the ability to form an interface mainly composed of newly-formed bone by 24 weeks

In this class of material, apatite wollastonite (CaOSiO2) glass ceramic developed by Kokubo et al has osteoconductive properties similar to Bioglass 45S5 but increased mechanical strength. It has been used as a spacer at the iliac crest, for vertebral prostheses and as a shelf in procedures about the shoulder with favourable results.

Bioactive bone cements. Bioactive bone cements have been explored as an alternative to PMMA in order to avoid complications related to PMMA debris and to enhance fixation of the prosthesis. These materials have undergone extensive basic

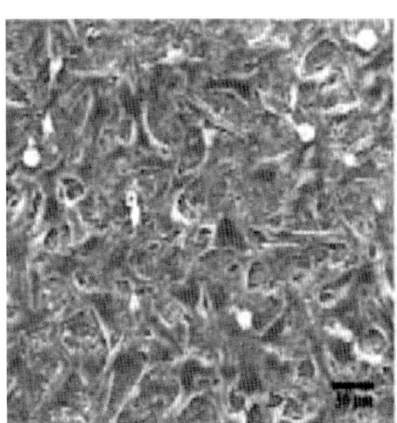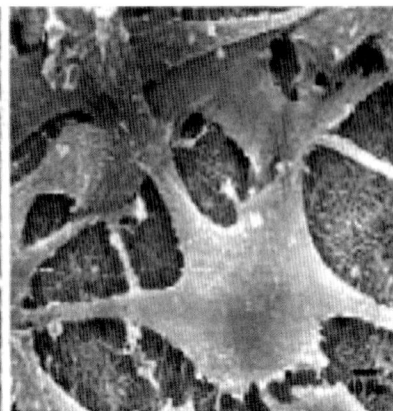

Bone, bioactive glass interface at 26 weeks

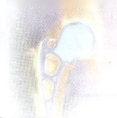

research. They include calcium-phosphate based bone cement and glass-ceramic bone cement. A strong cement-bone interface is obtained by the formation of HA at the surface of the cement. Moreover, calcium phosphate cements are resorbable and are progressively replaced by newly-formed bone.

Ceramic coatings provide an attractive alternative for biological fixation. In the near future, ceramic substitutes for bone grafts will probably be used in association with osteoinductive materials such as bone morphogenetic proteins or mesenchymal stem cells to accelerate bone formation further.

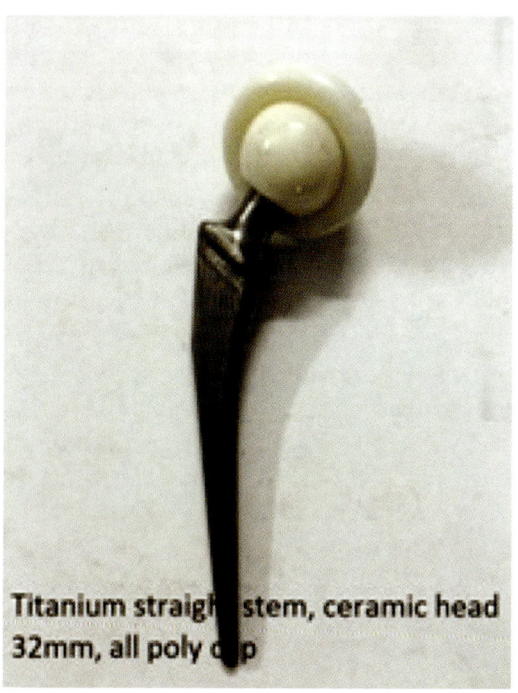

Titanium straight stem, ceramic head 32mm, all poly cup

Ceramic or ceramic coated hips are still being evaluated

POLYMETHYL METHACRALATE

Polymethylmethacrylate remains one of the most enigmatic but enduring materials in orthopaedic surgery. It has a central role in the success of total joint replacement and is also used in newer techniques such as percutaneous vertebroplasty and kyphoplasty.

In reality, "cement" is a misnomer because, the word cement is used to describe a substance that bonds two things together. However, PMMA acts as a space-filler that creates a tight space which holds the implant against the bone and thus acts as a 'grout'. Bone cements have no intrinsic adhesive properties, but they rely instead on close mechanical interlock between the irregular bone surface and the prosthesis.

Polymethylmethacrylate (PMMA) was first employed by orthopaedic surgeons over 60 years ago and remains a key component of modern practice. The understanding of its properties has evolved and progressed alongside the advance of the specialty, and has indirectly helped improve implant design, particle science, cell biology and biomechanics. The use of acrylic by orthopaedic surgeons is likely to continue, and knowledge of the properties and applications of this material remains essential. Polymethylmethacrylate was unveiled by the chemical industry in 1843 and named 'acide acrylique' on account of the acrid smell of the monomer. In 1936 it was noted that mixing ground polymer with monomer produced a dough that could be manipulated and moulded; hence it became one of the early biomaterials.

Early applications were in dentistry. Its use as a grout to improve implant fixation was pioneered in 1953 by Haboush. However, the major breakthrough in the use of PMMA in total hip replacement (THR) was the work of Charnley in 1970 who used it to secure fixation of the acetabular and femoral components and to transfer loads to bone.

Sir John Charnley can well be credited with introducing bone cement in Orthopaedics. Working alone, constantly researching, improvising and improving he invented what we can call as the first modern total joint replacement. The early results were spectacular. And the results remained spectacular. Hundreds upon hundreds were relieved of pain and crippling. They remained pain free for a long period and so joint replacements had come to stay. Once the principles were established, replacement of other joints began to follow. Charnley the meticulous and dedicated scientist was working very hard on all aspects of this specialty.

Theater asepsis, lamellar air flows, antibiotic prophylaxis, deep vein thrombosis, cement polymerization, cement bone

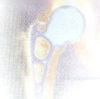

interaction, all these were subjects on which Sir John did a lot of work.

The American surgeons at this time were keen to try out hip replacement for themselves. And as was the custom, bone cement was sent to the FDA (the agency that monitors quality and standards of consumables in the US) and they tested it. They found that cement was carcinogenic in the rats they tested them in! Approval for use of bone cement was withheld and the American Surgeons could not use bone cement or do hip replacements.

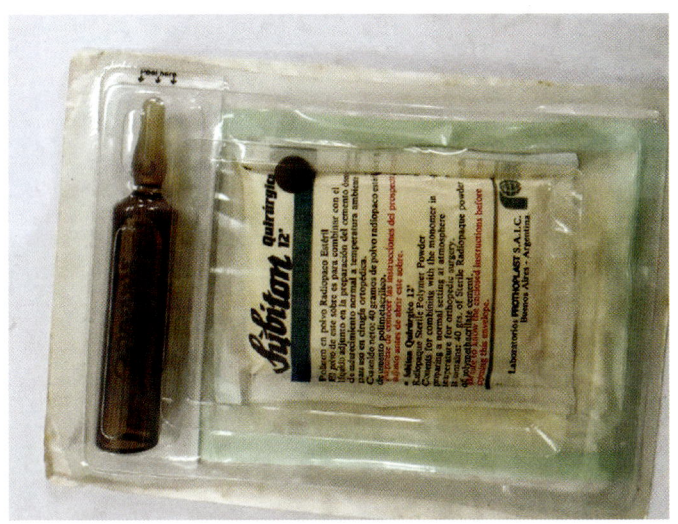

Argentinian black market cement used in USA when FDA had not yet approved the use of bone cement

This was in the early nineteen sixties. Plane load of patients flew into England and got their hips replaced. Back in USA they thumbed their nose at the FDA!!! This state of affairs persisted for a decade. Indignant Surgeons from the states demanded a re-evaluation of the facts. And it was found that the mice on whom cement was tested and found carcinogenic were indeed carcinogen susceptible mice in the first place. The experiments were repeated and this time it was found to be reasonably safe, and only in the early seventies cement was released for the use in America. This gave a ten year lead to the British in the field of hip Surgery.

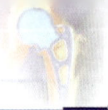

The use of bone cement was considered as a weak link in the development process of joint replacements and since early days there have been efforts to design and develop a prosthesis that can be anchored without the use of bone cement. As a matter of fact that Austin Moore endo prosthesis depended on a self locking mechanism as a result of bone in growth to help anchor the prosthesis in the hip.

Bone cement is available in two components a polymer and a monomer, the polymer is a sachet containing a white powder and most manufacturers conventionally have 40 grams of this powder. This is available in a double or triple packing and sterilized by gamma irradiation. The monomer is a liquid usually available in a 20 ml ampoule and this too is double packed and sterile by gamma irradiation.

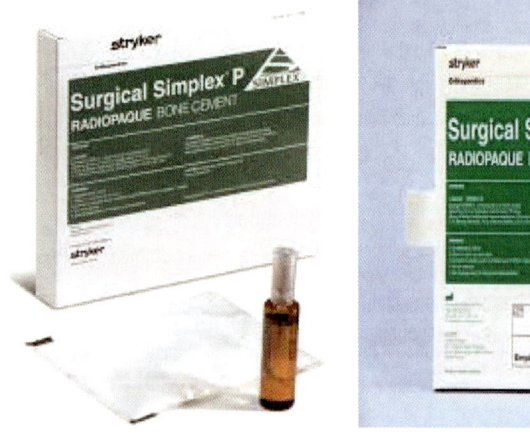
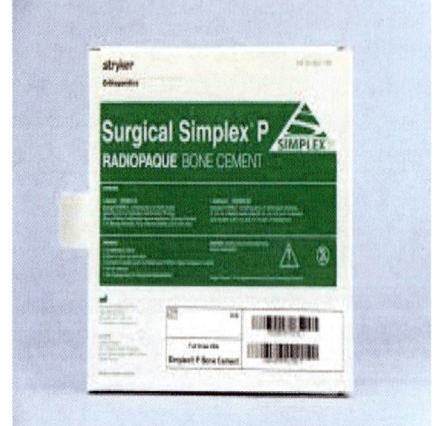

The original low viscosity cement best for injection under pressure

PMMA is a self curing acrylic polymer, rather that a heat cured one as used in the original Judet hips. There is a catalyst in the powder and an accelerator in the liquid. Both these act together in causing a polymerization by which longer chains of the acrylate are formed and the same changes its constituency with the passage of time. The cement is not glue and does not have any adhesive qualities. As a matter of fact it is a grout or a filler to enable a more uniform transmission of forces.

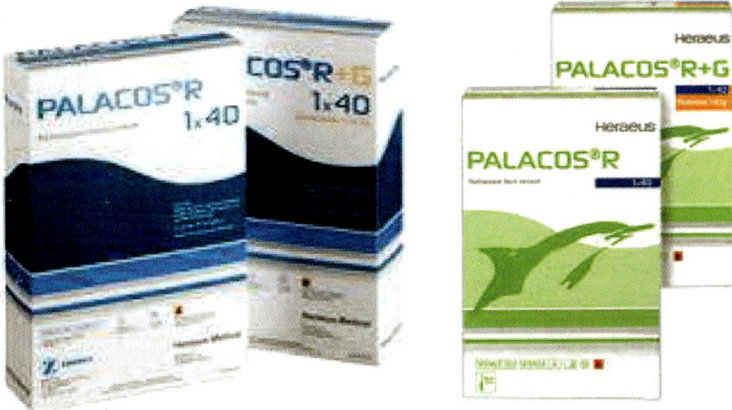

Antibiotic loaded bone cements are slightly less viscous

As it sets and is mouldable this is distributed uniformly all over the surfaces transmitting weight proportionately across all dimensions of the implant. Due to the absence of mechanical bonding properties, the cement does not adhere to the polished surfaces of the prosthesis. However it does slightly bond to the rough metallic surfaces or the plastic tibia. Some manufacturers however precoat the surface of the implant with a thin coat of PMMA to enhance its bonding qualities. However since the time of Sir John cement was never intended to be glue; it was neither intended to bond either the prosthesis or the cup to the body. Especially with the knee replacement it is to be understood that it is, a rigid and brittle structure and only when fully conforms to the outer surface of the implant will it act as a uniform weight transmitter.

Recent studies have shown that bone cement is 3 times stronger in compression rather than with shear forces. Actually a good analogy would be the building cement between bricks. This would stand a strong ceiling and a weight on the ceiling, but would be weaker to a blow from the side as is used to demolish the buildings. Thus in the long run, failure would often be because the cement is not packed tightly enough and the crevices in it would fail due to the rotatory and bending movements rather than compression.

Subsequent studies have shown that the properties of the cement implant bondage not only depend upon the stage at

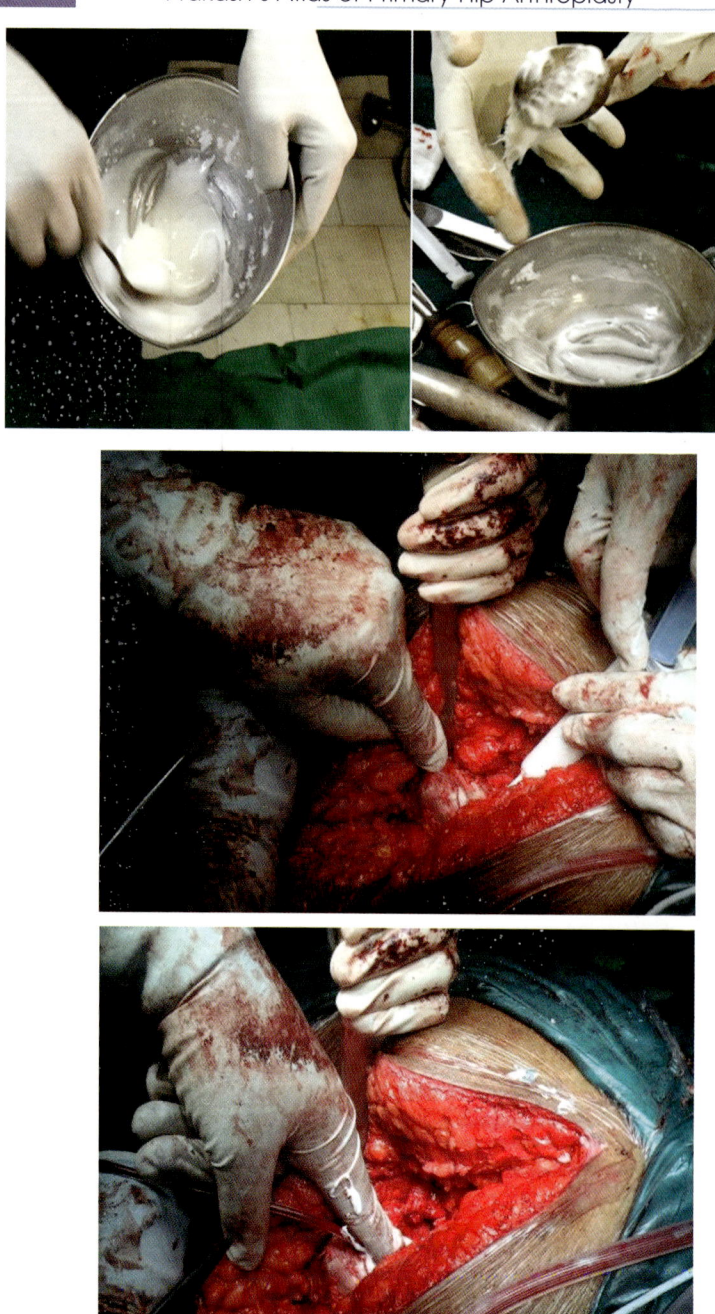

Cement can be hand pressurized or injected with a gun or syringe

which it is introduced, it also depends upon constant pressure exertion at the time of setting and absence or diminution of air bubbles in the mixture leading to porosity of the cement. Newer methods like vacuum stirring and pressure injection address this problem. A closed cavity onto which liquid cement is pushed with pressure will of course enhance the bondage between the walls and the cement and hence the newer techniques of syringe injection are currently being used.

Many surgeons have advocated the use of antibiotics in bone cement and it has been found that less that 2 grams of heat stable antibiotics in a powder form added to 40 grams of the cement powder does not significantly inhibit the tensile and compressive strength. Very recent studies do show that fatigue strength may be compromised by such addition and hence a routine use in primary arthroplasty is not recommended. Further as the chances of infection is much less in a primary replacement arthroplasty than a revision, and as routine antibiotic loaded cement usage in primary arthroplasties may cause the development of resistant strains of organisms, it is not routinely recommended.

Radio-opaque substances like barium sulfate are now being routinely added. These are very important for an accurate correlation in follow up radiographs. The use of cement without this is almost given up. After remaining in the body for a sufficient time the cement tends to attain a light brown shade and in many revision cases it may be difficult to distinguish this from the cortical bone and to help identify cement in revision procedures certain companies have started addition of pigments like methylene blue and chlorophyll.

A word here about hypotension induced by cement. It has been found that after femoral cementation, between three to four minutes a transient hypotension is noticed. This is more marked with liquid preparations rather than doughy masses. The reason for this is the absorption of the monomer into the blood. The monomer absorbed is subsequently metabolized as methacrylic acid and then to carbon dioxide. The anesthetist should be warned and the blood pressure has to be kept a little high to avoid complications.

In our country almost all brands of cement are available. The expiry date of the monomer is earlier than that of the polymer

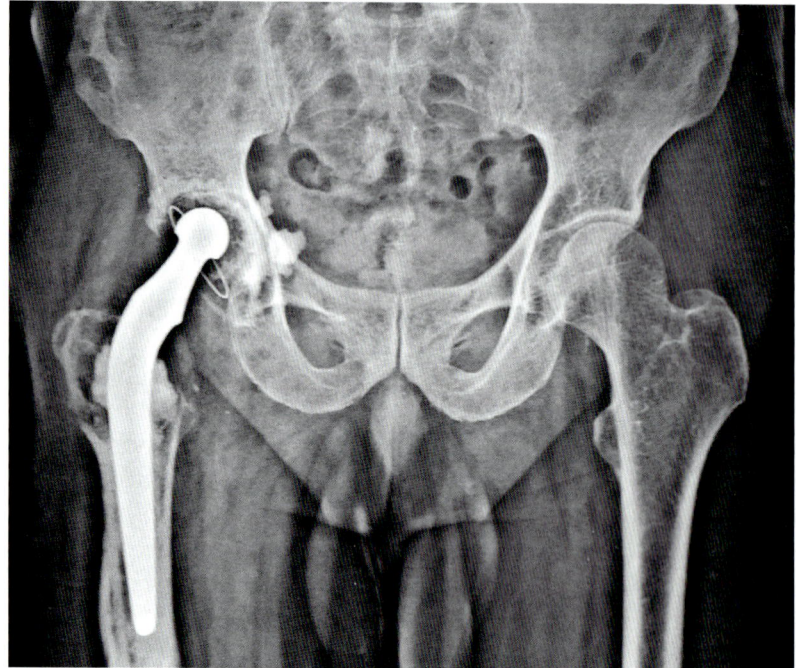

Mixing of radioopague substances with bone cement allows us to radiologically study the cement bone interface

and one must note the date carefully prior to purchase. There is not much to choose between the various forms of cement except when you are using pressurization techniques and the need to use a cement gun. Low viscosity cements available are Surgical Simplex, and CMW. Doughy mixes are Zimmer, Palacos and Sulfix.

In conclusion bone cement is a good thing. But only as long as one understands how to use it properly. Use it well and it will last you for years. Bad cementation will lead to early failures.

Even today, best results of cemented hips are superior to cementless hips both in short and long terms.

5 Indications and Pre-operative Planning of a Total Hip Arthroplasty

It is more important to know when not to do a total hip replacement, than when to do one. Primary indication would be a painful hip. Of lesser importance would be stiffness and instability. To give a pain-free mobile and functional hip is not very difficult. The main problem is to make sure that the improvement lasts. And lasts at least for twenty or more years. With this perspective though some latitude can be given to the indications in those, patients who are over 65 years of age, one must be careful in prescribing this form of management in patients below 50.

An useful method to assess the indication is the Girdlestone test.

When a girdlestone excision arthroplasty will improve the patient's status, irrespective of his age, a total replacement can be considered, because even when the replacement fails and we remove all the implants, the patient is left with a girdle stone pseudoarthrosis.

Even this test should be considered carefully in the very young because results of primary excision are far better than salvage of a failed hip by removal of the implants. Parameters that are of additional importance are whether the disease is unilateral or bilateral, how active the patient is, what is the body weight, and whether sufficient conservative means have been tried to relieve the pain.

The indications for which it is performed routinely in my set up are

1. Rheumatoid arthritis
2. Ankylosing spondylosis

3. Avascular necrosis
4. Old subcapital fractures
5. Old inter trochanteric fractures
6. Secondary osteoarthritis
7. Secondary to Perthes or CDH
8. Quiescent tubercular arthritis
9. Hip fusion and pseudoarthrosis
10. Failed procedures on hip like hemi, internal fixations, etc.
11. Primary Osteoarthrosis.

The contraindications are:
1. Active infection anywhere in the body
2. Neuropathic joint
3. Conditions rapidly destroying the bone mass.

These are absolute contra indications. There are plenty of relative contraindications and these are patient, surgeon and the hospital dependant. A good rule of thumb is that whenever one is in doubt about the indication it is better not to perform the surgery but to wait and review the patient after some time, by then the pain or symptoms would have become sufficiently bad and the indications clearer.

PRE-OPERATIVE EVALUATION

We are treating the patient as a whole and not just replacing a hip. Thus a pre-operative planning and evaluation schedule is very important and should be strictly followed. The following is my personal schedule and has stood me well.

1. History of the present problems, past problems, special mention of diabetes mellitus, hypertension, and bleeding and coagulation disorders. Smokers should be counseled and so should the obese. In addition history of infections or sepsis anywhere in the body, drug allergies and past medication should be known.

2. Clinical examination of the affected hip, opposite hip, both knees and spine. Peripheral vascular status of the same and opposite limb is to be examined.

3. A general examination to assess the heart lungs, exclude systemic diseases and the status of teeth and prostate. On occasions it may be wise to get a physician's opinion as to the fitness of the patient for a major surgical procedure as this.

4. Blood and urine examination, a chest radiograph and ECG are mandatory both from the surgical and anesthetic point of view. Specific investigations not to be missed are bleeding and clotting times, blood urea and sugar, creatinine, Hemoglobin and PCV and a urine culture.

5. One unit of fresh blood is usually required and adequate preparation for the same should be made. In my set up relative donors or autologus transfusion is preferred to avoid transfusion related problems.

Certain special requirements and situations demand special preparations. On occasions with severe bilateral hip disease or with the involvement of one hip and knee when a double arthroplasty is planned, sufficient attention should be paid to the patient's fitness and the surgeon's stamina.

I still do these routinely as the patient benefits by a single procedure, shorter hospital stay and easier physiotherapy and rehabilitation.

PRE-OPERATIVE SURGICAL PLANNING

A complete range of instrumentation is a must for a proper job. Different implants need different instrumentation sets and are supplied by the manufacturer. A full set of retractors, deepening and reaming devices, and drill-saw system is a must. Full set of femoral and acetabular trials are essential and it would be unwise to embark upon the surgical procedure without this.

If there is a pre-existing internal fixation device or prosthesis, instrumentation needed for removal is also necessary. For revision hips one must have the special cement removal chisels. Bone cement of the appropriate type and sufficient quantity of the same is mandatory. Adequate range and sizes of the prosthesis including one size above and below and a longer and shorter neck length must also be kept ready and handy.

PRE-OPERATIVE ANAESTHETIC PLANNING

An anaesthesist reviews the patient a few days before the operation and does all the assessment needed. He reviews the investigations and plans for the type of anaesthesia depending upon the patient's condition. A regional anaesthesia is always preferred and over 97% of our hips are done this way. In simple uncomplicated cases a Sensorcaine spinal anaesthesia is used. If the surgery might take longer than an hour, a continuous epidural anaesthesia administered with a catheter is used. General anaesthesia is rarely used.

The final choice of the anaesthetic agents and mode of administration is left entirely to the anesthetist. An anesthetic chart is maintained in which preoperative intra operative and post-operative parameters are recorded.

PRE-OPERATIVE THEATRE REQUISITES

Much has been written about the operation theatre conditions needed for hip replacements. A lot has been said about the unsuitability of average operating rooms for a hip replacement. A lamellar flow with space suits though ideal is a very expensive proposition for most average operating rooms. Bio occlusive clothing too is not easily available in our country as it is all imported.

If one looks into the literature, the original Charnley series of total hip replacements had an incidence of about 8% infection. He was of the opinion that air borne microbes are the cause and set about to remedy this problem. Whilst working on this problem, he took the help of persons maintaining clean air in breweries and distilleries where a strict abacterial status was essential for proper fermentation of the alcohol. He postulated that the air in the operating room must be changed many times a minute and the fresh air blown into the theatre should be ultra filtered and abacterial and aparticulate.

Further he postulated that the surgeon emits bacteria from his skin and breath, and if the surgeon were encompassed in a space suit like contraption with hoods and if all the air expired by the surgeon is let out through a separate outlet, infection must be reduced.

He was correct! By using these methods he managed to reduce his infection rate from 8% to less than 1%. Simultaneously surgeons found out that prophylactic antibiotics too, reduce the infection rate despite the surgery being performed in a conventional operation theatre. Nelson and Phillips reported a reduction of infection from 5.8% in a conventional theatre to just 1.3% with the use of antibiotics.

It has been postulated that clean air, prophylactic antibiotics, and clothing all act complementary to each other and their use together causes a reduction of infection rate to less than .5%.

Laminar flows are fairly common and easy to install. They have proved their cost effectiveness. In addition prophylactic antibiotics are mandatory. Space suits and body exhaust; if available would certainly give additional protection against infection, but I don't use them.

My protocol is fairly straightforward and easy to implement in most operating rooms.

1. The operating room must not be used for the previous day and must be cleaned thoroughly. It should be properly fumigated and an ultra violet lamp is illuminated all night.

2. One or two air conditioners allow for a flow of clean filtered air into the theatre. This also keeps the temperature of the operating room cool, avoids the surgeon and theatre staff sweating and allows the cement to set slowly.

3. The Boyles machine, theatre furniture, and all loose and bulky machinery and objects in the operating room are cleaned, and wiped with isopropyl alcohol disinfectant the evening before surgery.

4. The patient is prepared in a side room and all ward clothing is discarded and the patient is re-gowned prior to entering the operation theatre.

5. The clothes worn by the operating team are all autoclaved. Two caps and masks are worn and in case of female personnel the hair should be completely covered.

6. The procedure proceeds with a proper planning, minimum time is wasted and a quick, precise job is done with a minimum of the wound being exposed to the outside.

7. In the initial stages entry of too many personnel into the operating room was not allowed. But subsequently as the

number of visitors from outside the town rose, and on many occasions as many as six observers were inside the theatre without any problems, the rule was relaxed so long as all personnel followed the theatre protocol.

8. Special drapes are used. These are thick cotton ones very large in size, completely drape the patient and isolate the operating field from the anesthetist's end.

It has been found that it is easy to enforce this sort of a discipline in an operation theatre where only orthopaedic operations are done routinely. In general nursing homes, and those with a great turnover, it might be sometimes difficult to enforce all the above conditions. However it must be emphasized that each one of the above is followed religiously to avoid any complications. An infection in a hip joint is a disaster. Sir John was all his life working towards a zero percent infection. We all must treat an infection as our own personal responsibility and must take all precautions, and efforts to minimize it.

ANTIBIOTIC PROPHYLAXIS

The current pharmacological literature tells us that air borne bacteria are prone to cause infection only during the actual surgical period. If sufficient concentrations of antibiotics are present at and immediately after the operation it is enough. Prolonged administration of antibiotics will only encourage the resistant strains to grow and cause problems.

Any of the newer antibiotics with a wide spectrum can be used. A good rule of thumb is to avoid popular antibiotics used commonly by the general practitioners as the rarer the antibiotic, lesser the chances of resistant strains.

The current prophylactic antibiotic is: 1.5 grams of cefuroxime iv at induction, 1.5 grams iv at 6 hours and 1.5 grams iv at twelve hours.

6

Hemiarthroplasty of the Hip

The surgery is performed under general or regional anesthesia.

As the average surgical time is a little under thirty minutes, even a spinal anesthetic can be used.

Epidural anesthesia is a safe option, allowing for post-operative analgesia.

First dose of prophylactic antibiotic is administered with the anesthesia.

One unit of blood is usually reserved for use during surgery or during the post-operative period.

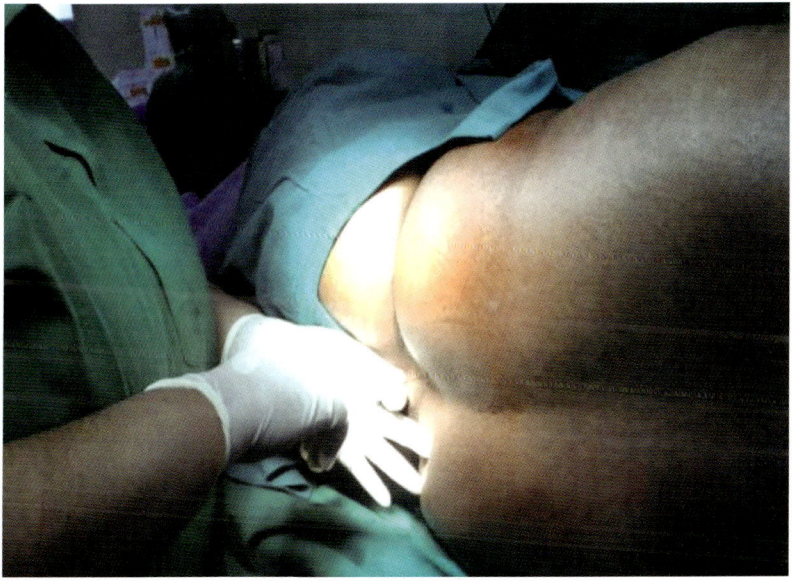

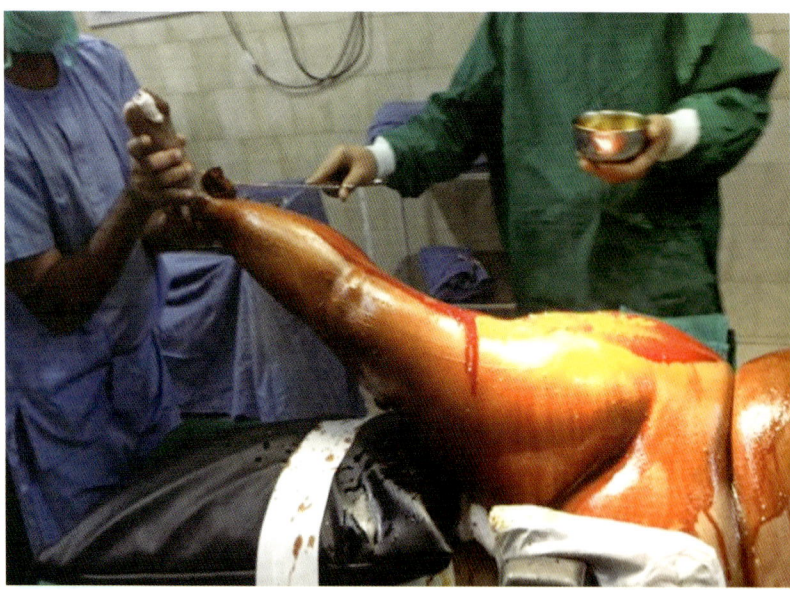

The patient is placed in a lateral position with sand bags and table attachments to keep the pelvis stable. The leg is draped free for manipulations and dislocations.

The opposite limb is strapped to a pillow and the operating table.

The knee is flexed and kept flexed throughout the procedure to ensure that sciatic nerve is kept relaxed during the entire period.

The preparation extends from ankle to iliac crest.

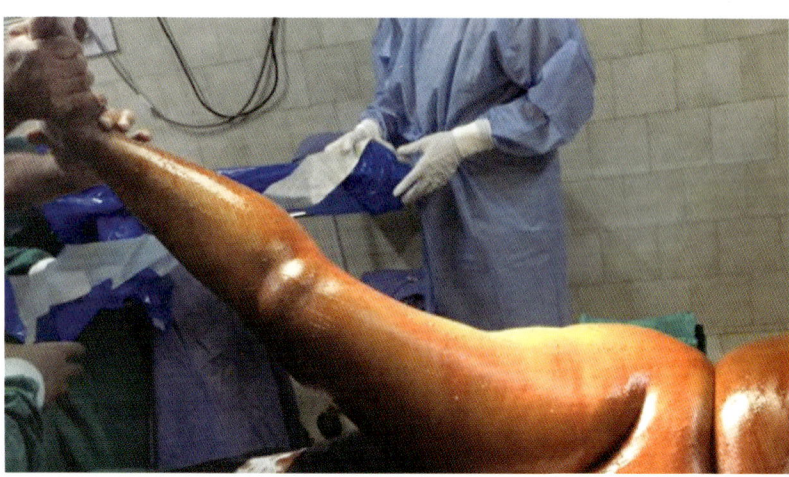

The area from ankle to groin below and iliac crest above are first cleaned with savlon and soap solution.

This is then swabbed with isopropyl alcohol solution.

A generous coat of povidine iodine paint is then applied to the above area.

As the patient has been fixed in lateral position with back supports, she stays in the same position throughout the surgery.

Adequate stability in the lateral position is essential for getting the prosthesis orientation correctly.

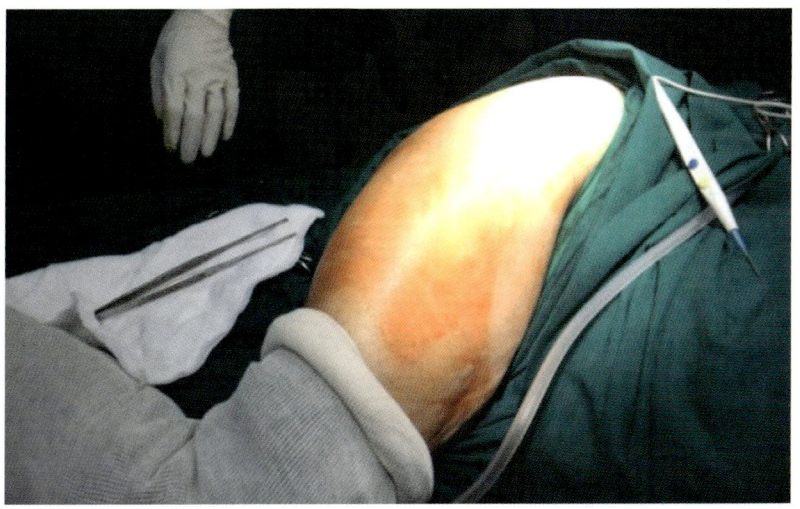

Large drapes are used. The drapes in the author's operating room are twelve feet square and cover the operating table floor to floor.

The area from iliac crest to a little above the knee are left exposed for the procedure.

The knee is draped free to allow intra operative manipulation.

The knee is flexed and kept flexed throughout the surgery to keep the sciatic nerve relaxed.

A straight lateral incision centred on the trochanter extends to equal distances proximally and distally.

The subcutaneous tissue and Fascia is cut in the line of skin incision.

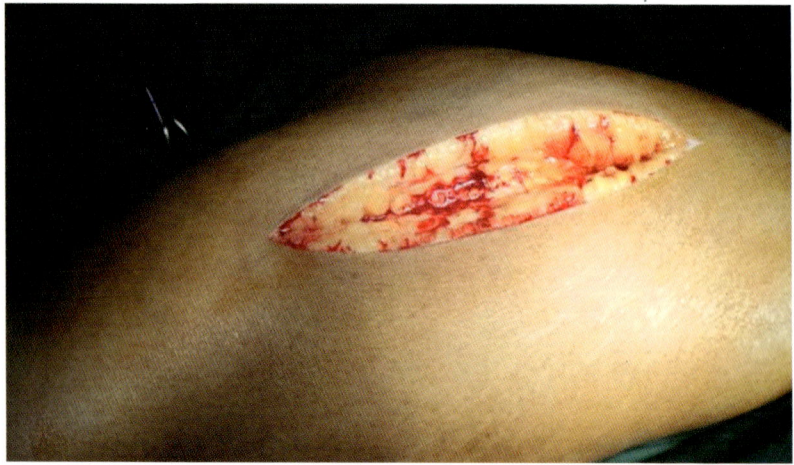

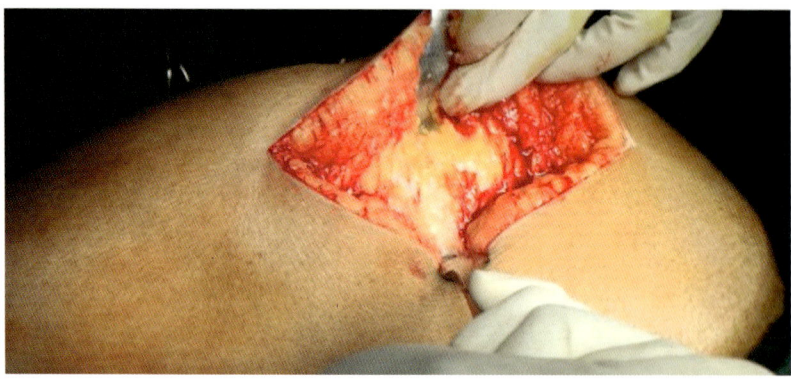

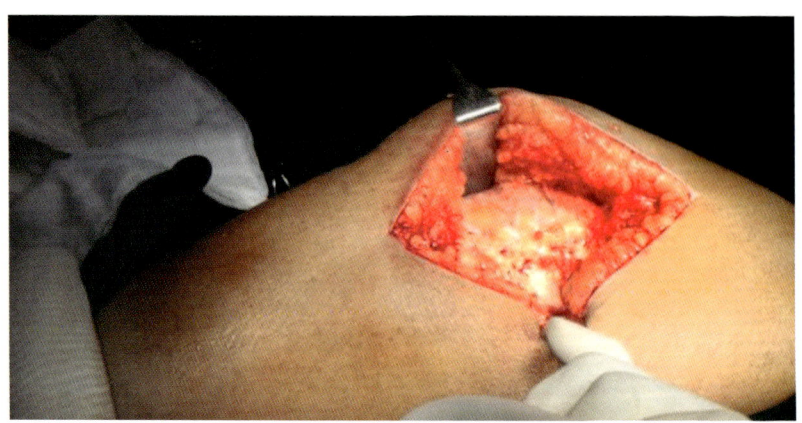

The fat is incised in the line of skin incision, and the fibres of glutei are split to expose the small lateral rotators of the hip.

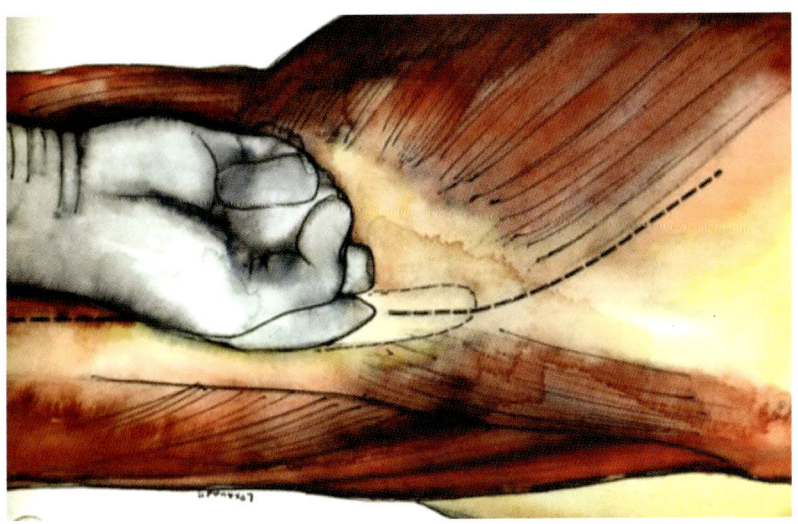

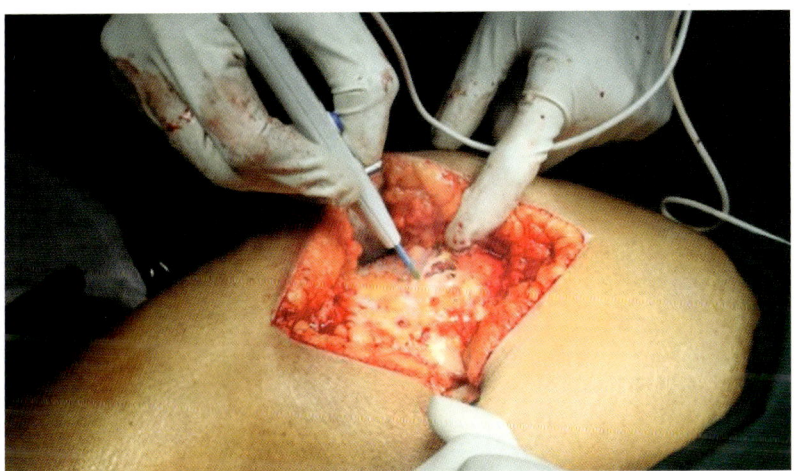

The short lateral rotators are now cut, leaving an attachment to the trochanteric flare for subsequent reattachment.

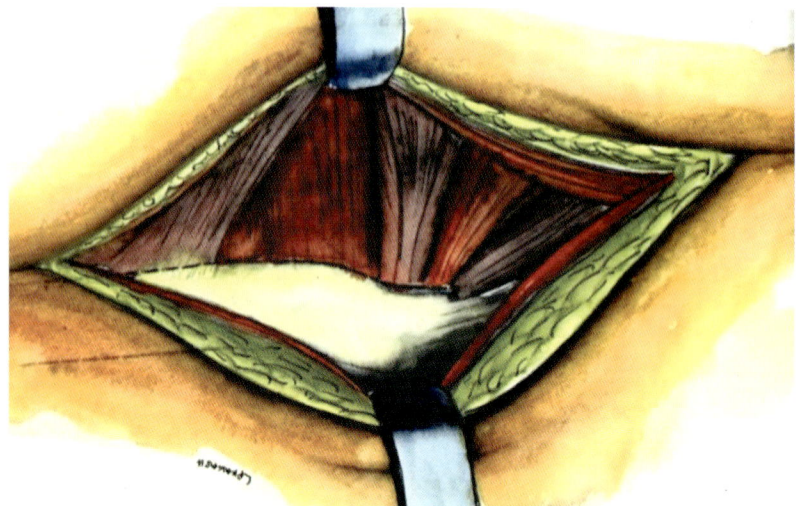

The inferior part of prifiormis is detached as well.

If the hip appears tight, additional soft tissue releases are performed.

The assistant internally rotates the hip, using the flexed knee as a lever, and this maneuver tightens the short rotators, making them prominent.

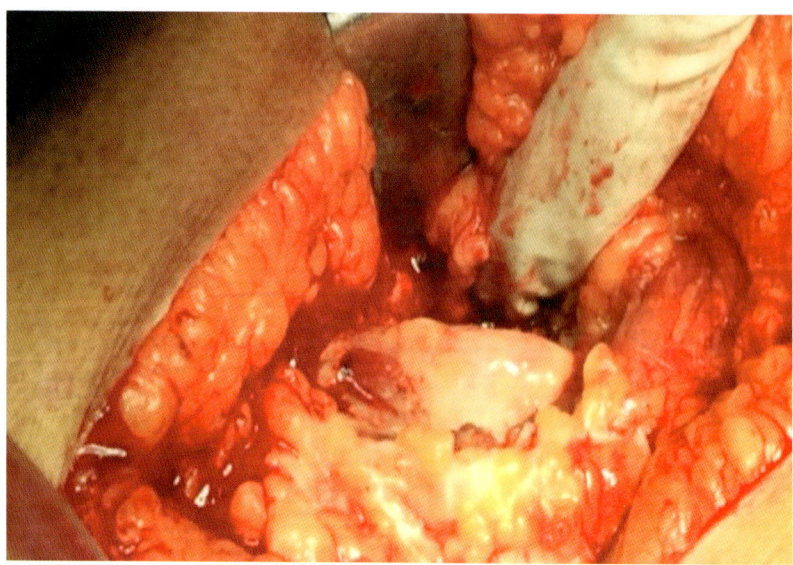

Some surgeons use stay sutures in the rotators to facilitate reattachment.

A precise positioning of Homman retractors allows the head to be visualized.

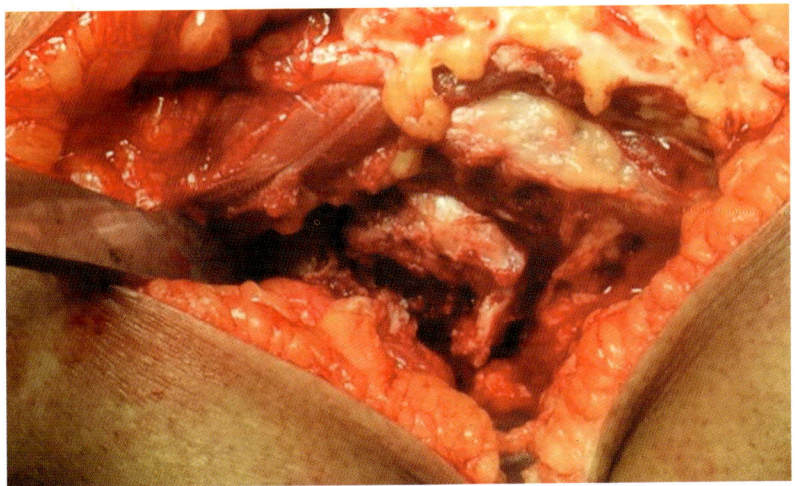

A gentle rocking movement of the flexed knee towards internal rotation, exposes larger areas of the head.

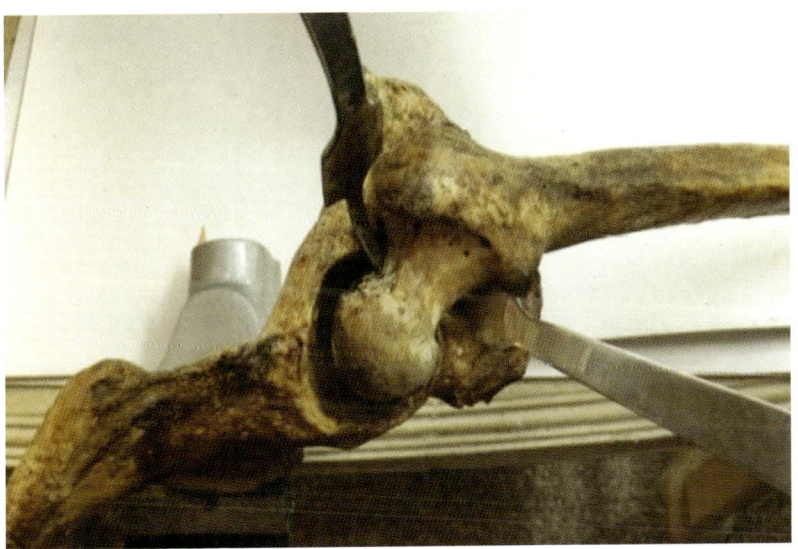

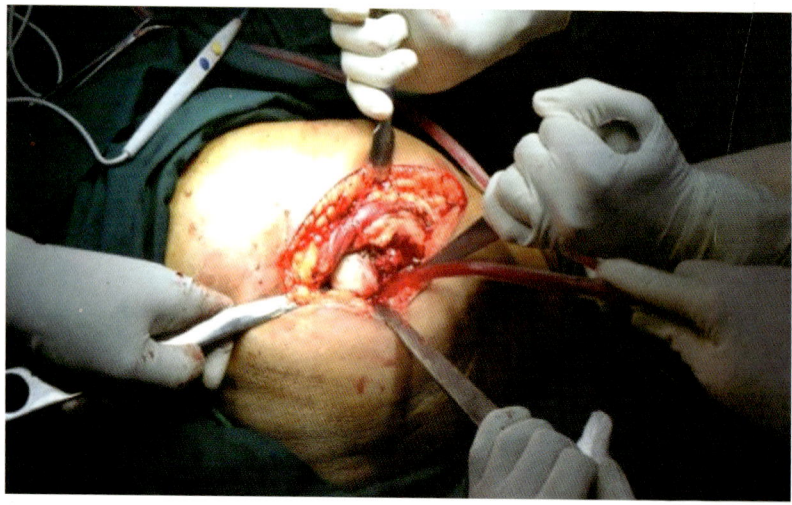

The assistant should not use excessive force during internal rotation, especially in patients with osteoporosis and rheumatoid arthritis, because there is a risk of spiral fracture of the shaft of femur.

As the limb is internally rotated, greater areas of the head become exposed. 2

Adduction and further internal rotation dislocates the hip joint

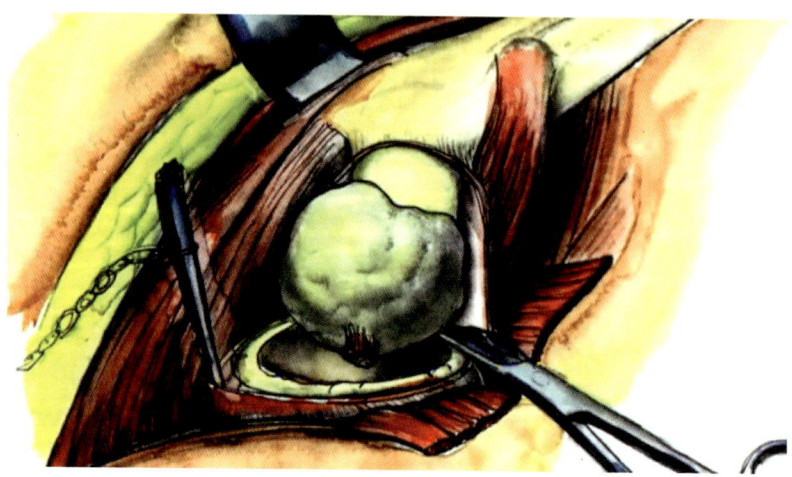

The head is gently levered out using Homman spikes or a cork screw.

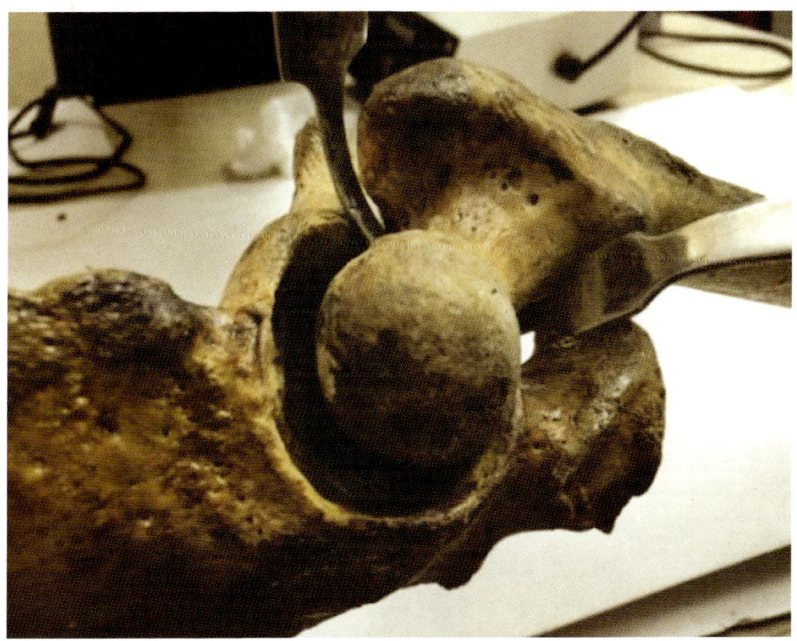

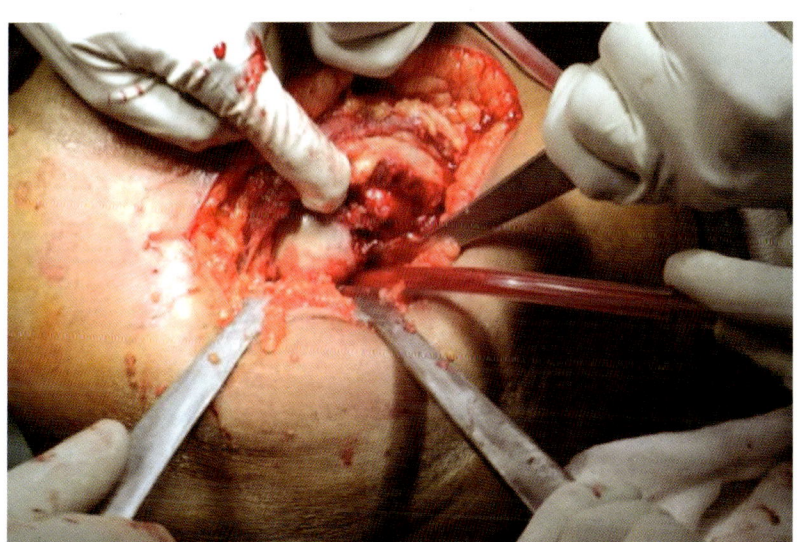

It is essential to ensure that no damage is caused to the acetabular articular cartilage during the process of head extraction.

If need be, the head can be even removed piece meal, but it is absolutely essential to ensure that the acetabulum is left unscratched.

The older method of using a shoe horn to lever out the head is mentioned only to be condemned. This has to be strongly discouraged.

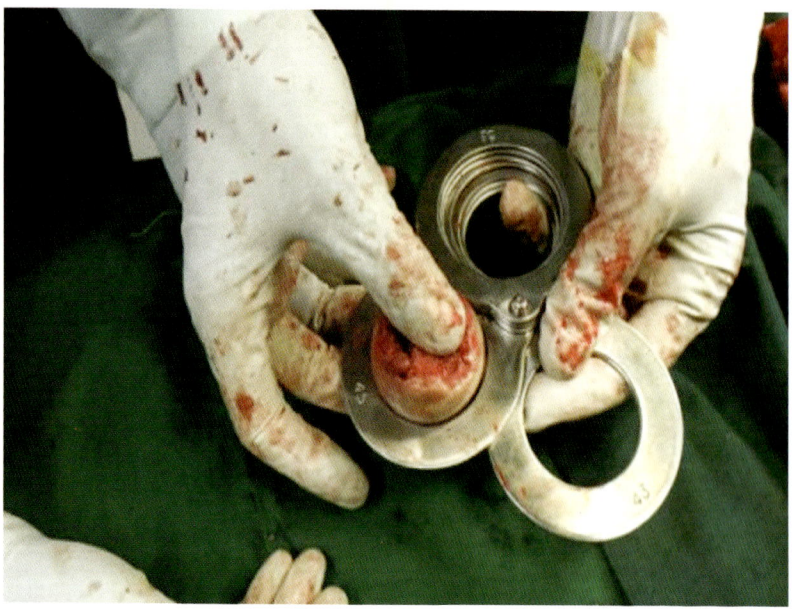

The extracted head is now measured. The head diameter of the actual implant should be the same or one millimeter lesser than the head size.

As bipolar hips are usually performed for otherwise normal hips, the acetabulum is hemispherical and so is the head. If the head is found deformed or irregular or not perfectly hemispherical in its widest extent, it would indicate a preexisting acetabular pathology and would render the patient an unsuitable candidate for a hemi arthroplasty. In such cases a total replacement should be considered.

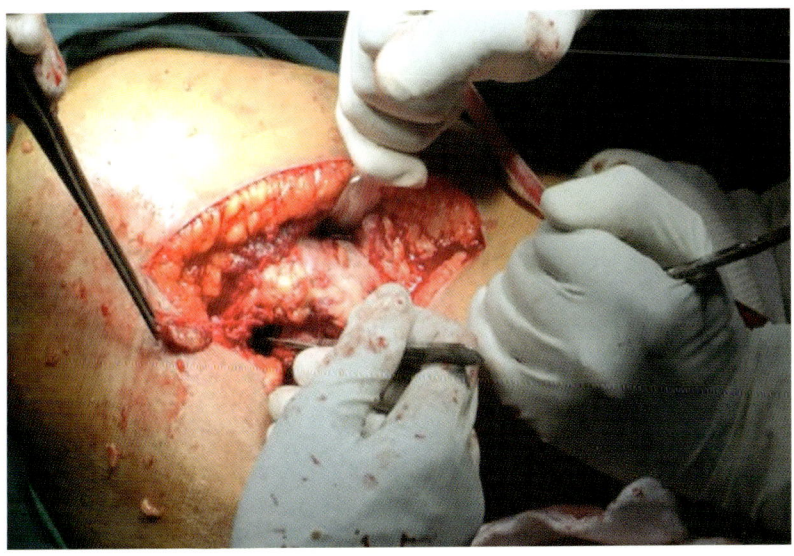

The neck is identified and using a diathermy, a mark is made to define a subsequent cut with an oscillating saw.

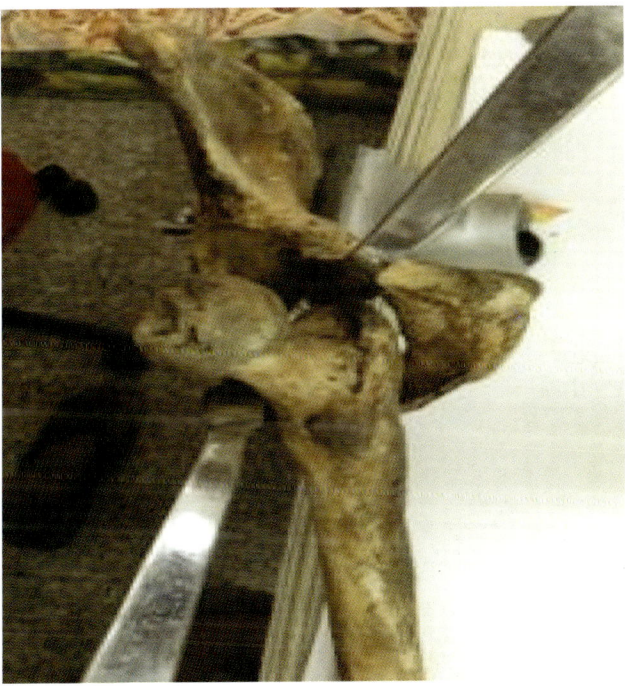

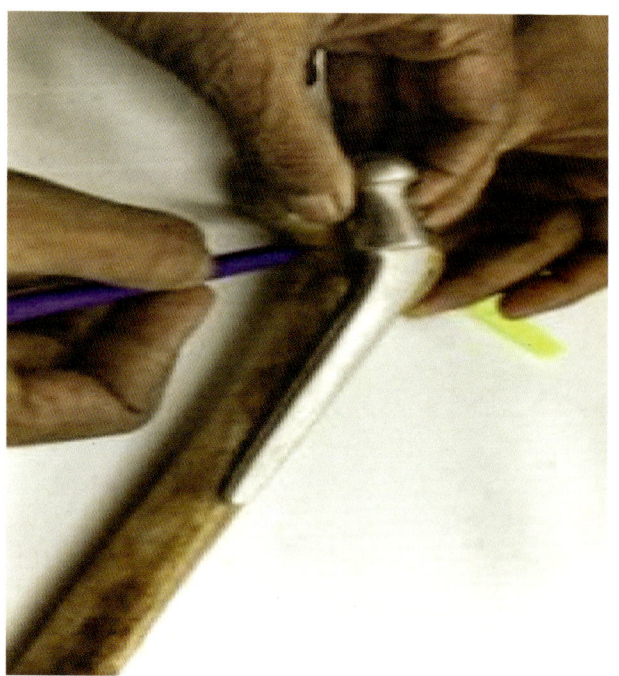

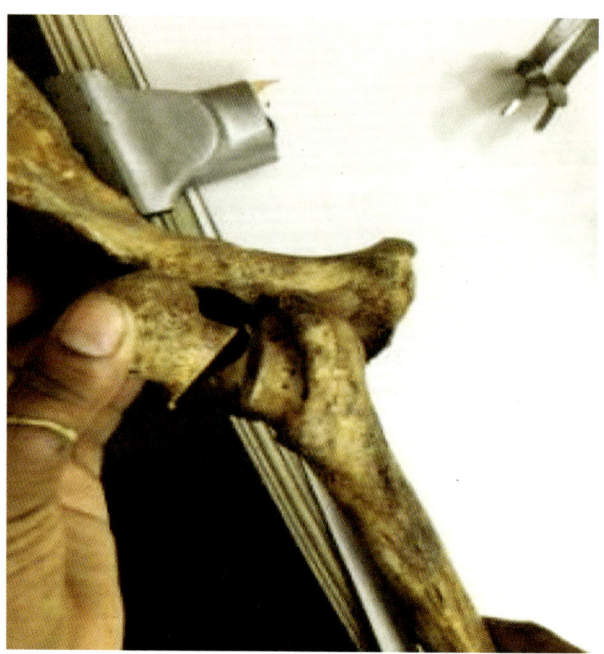

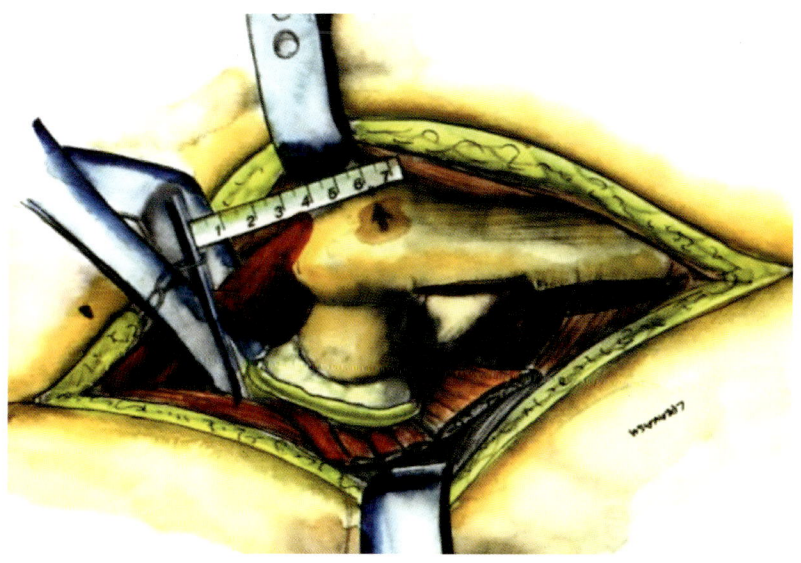

The angle of cut should match the angle of the implant to be used. Many instrument sets have neck cutting guides for this purpose.

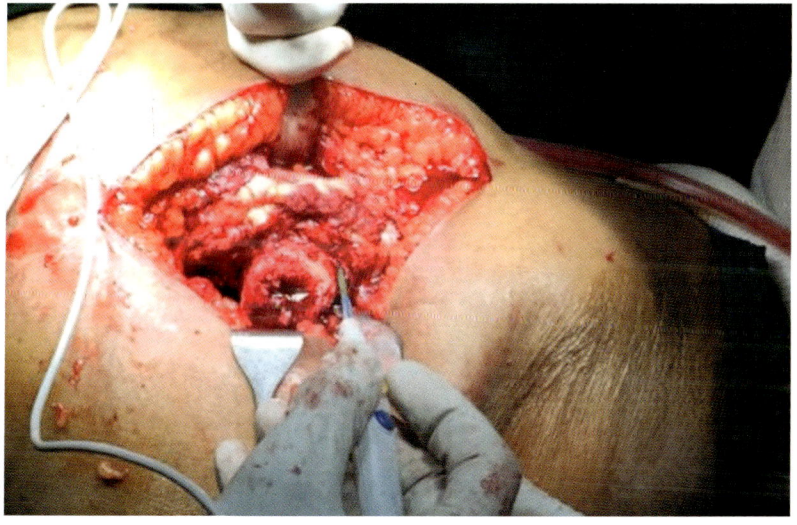

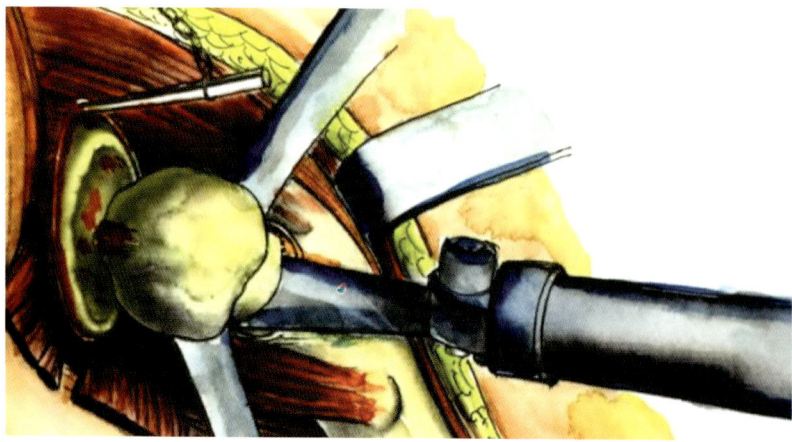

The neck is cut to the appropriate level, and the actual prosthesis can be placed over the neck and shaft to ensure that the cut has been made at the correct level and at a correct angle.

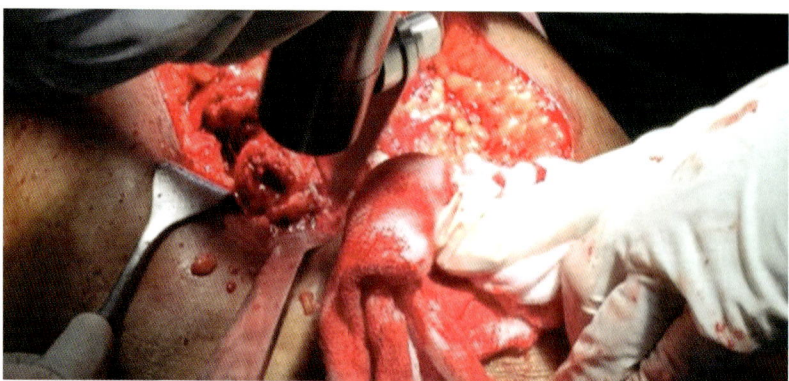

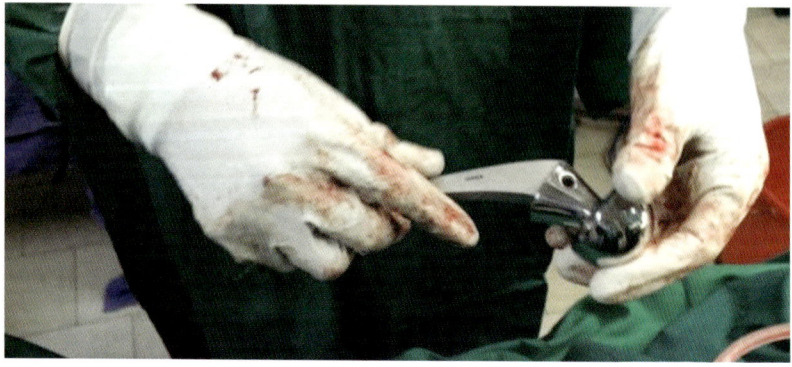

The bone model shows the process of placing the actual prosthesis over the shaft to define the level and angle of neck osteotomy.

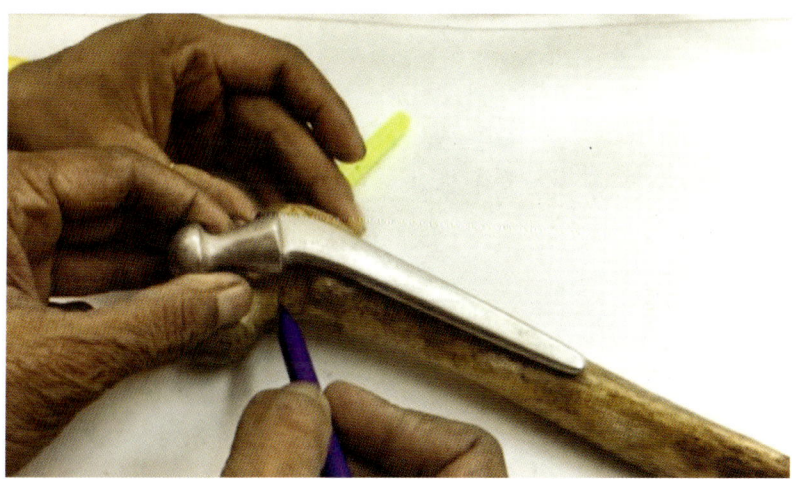

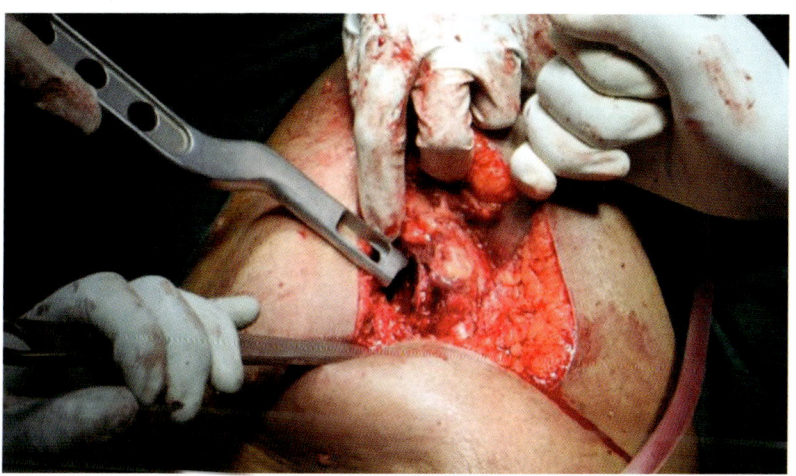

A box chisel is now used to cut a slot in the femur. This slot should reach far back posteriorly to ensure a proper seating of the prosthesis and its final placement in a valgus position.

This is an important step as it defines the version of the prosthesis.

The normal version is about fifteen degrees though it varies from person to person. The chisel cut is precisely aligned to the correct version of that particular neck. The rule of thumb is to stay about fifteen degrees rotated from the lesser trochanter.

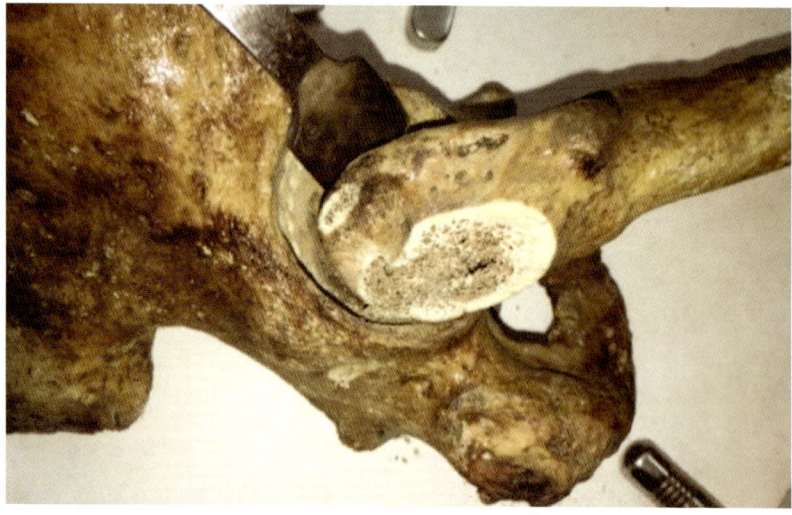

A broach finds the posterior aspect of trochanteric fossa beside the attachment of piriformis to locate the entry point for femoral reaming.

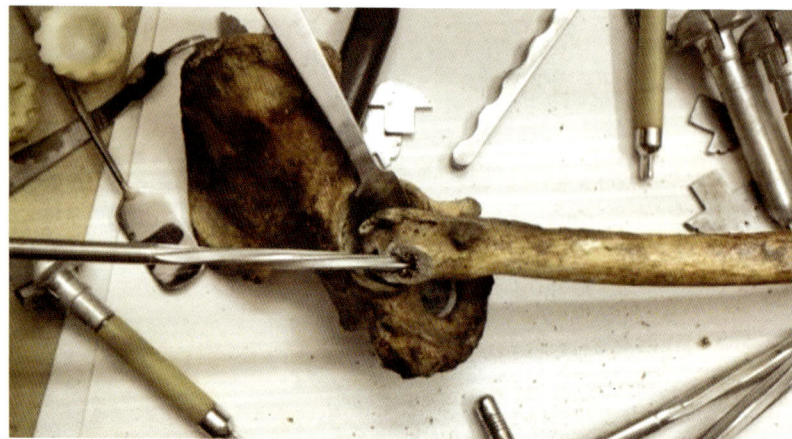

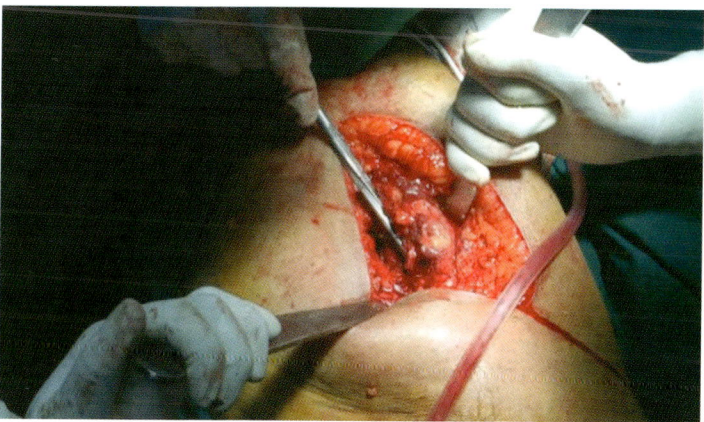

The medulla is widened with successive broaches, especially at the isthumus level to allow an easy passage and uniform cement mantle around the stem.

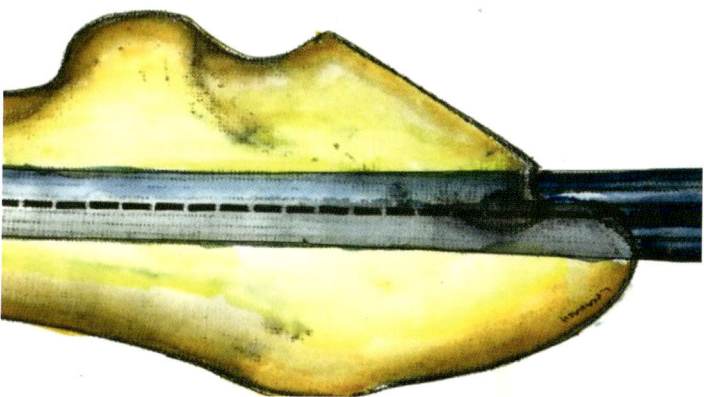

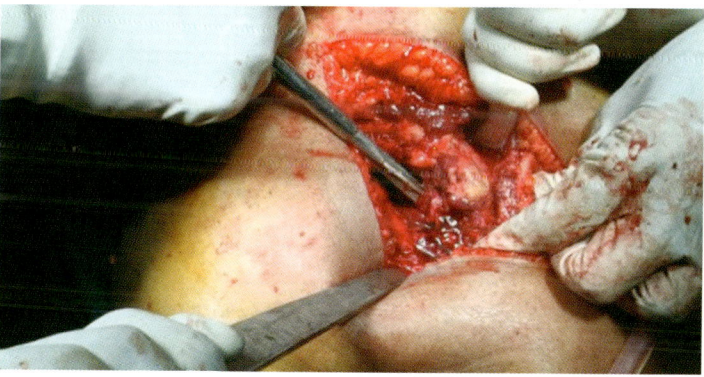

Most bipolar hips available in this country have a fixed stem size. The isthemic diameter in these stems is close to 8 mm.Iin case the femoral medulla is narrower than this, one must use hand reamers to expand the lumen.

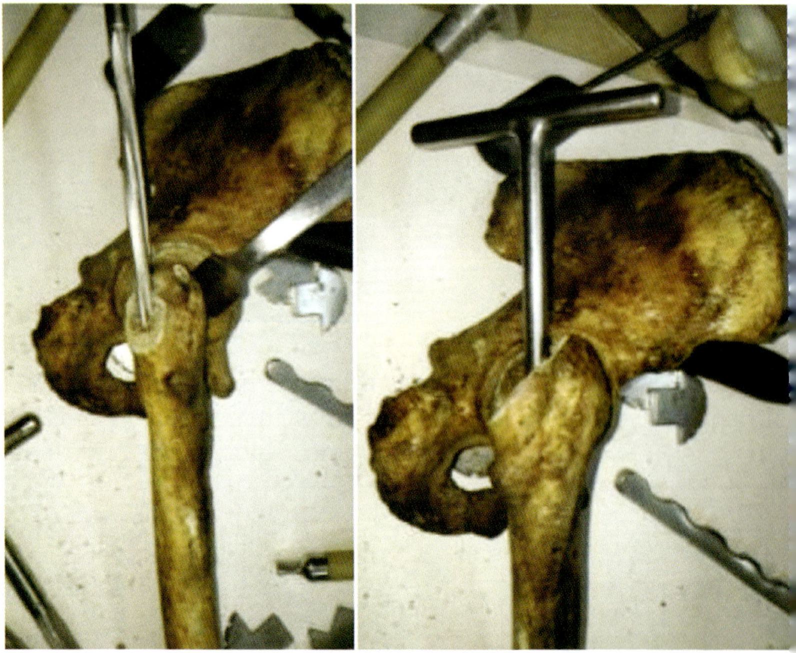

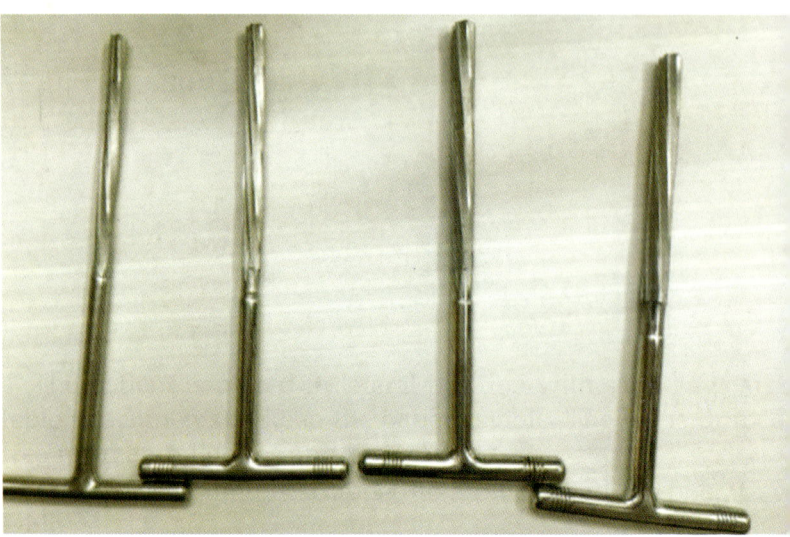

Hand reamers are available from six millimeters upwards and have sharp cutting edges.

Occasionally power reamers may be required, but these are contraindicated in osteoporotic bones.

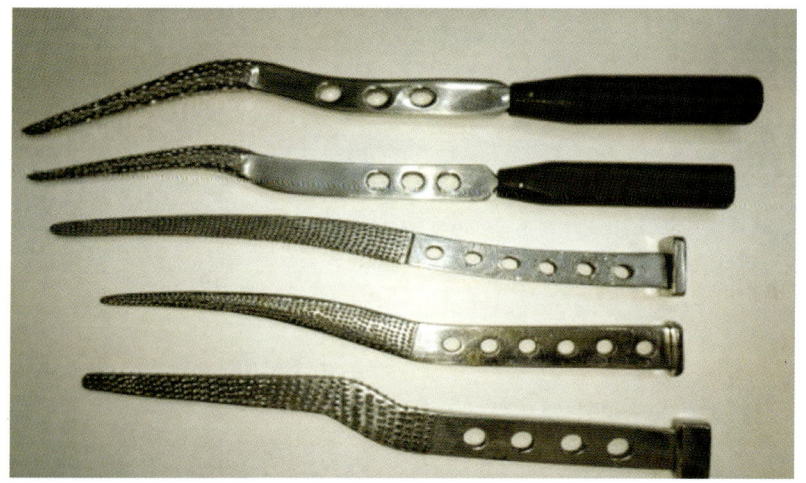

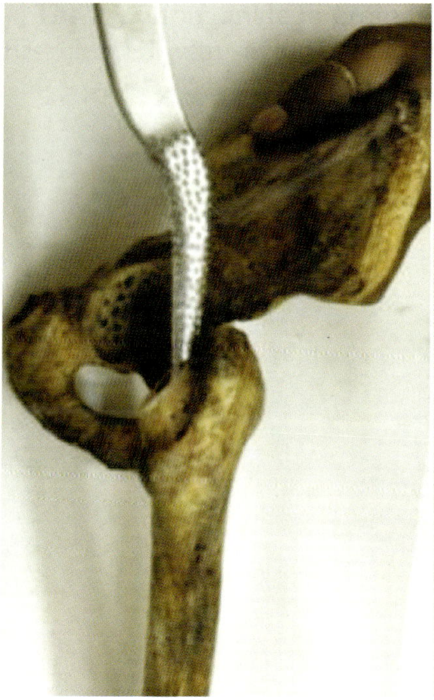

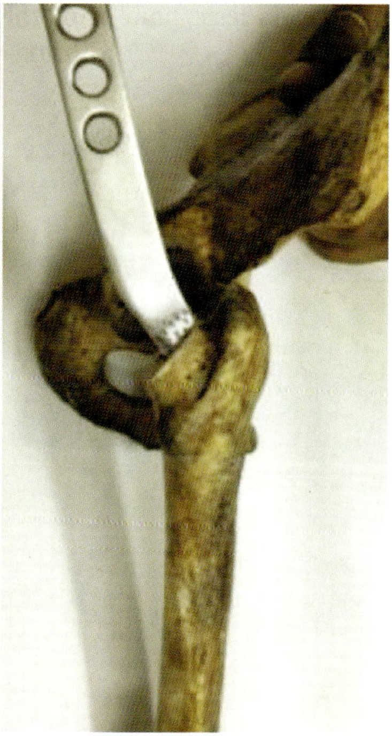

The assistant, who holds the leg, applies counter traction against the knee and keeps a tight hold on the flexed knee. He is thus able to provide a haptic feedback in case the medullary reaming is impinging on the cortex and producing jolts to the knee.

These precautions are necessary to avoid a femoral fracture while broaching, which is a real possibility.

Rasps are available in progressive sizes and the largest rasp that will accommodate the femur should be used.

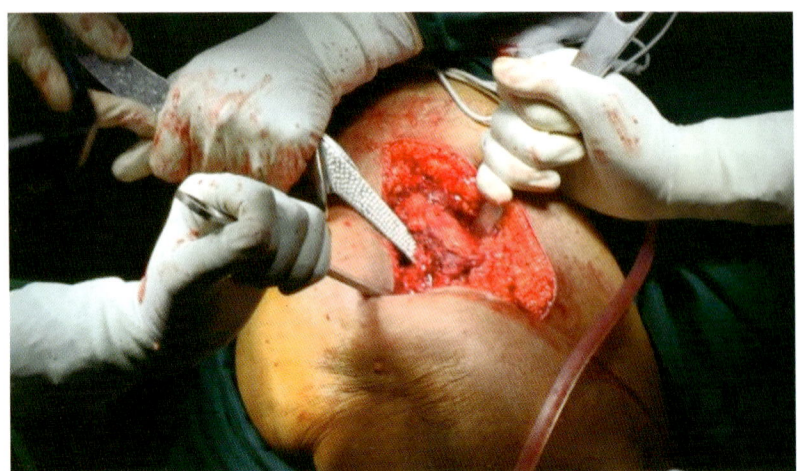

Femoral rasps are used to ream the canal. We must attempt to get a loose fit of the implant with a two to three mm space all around.

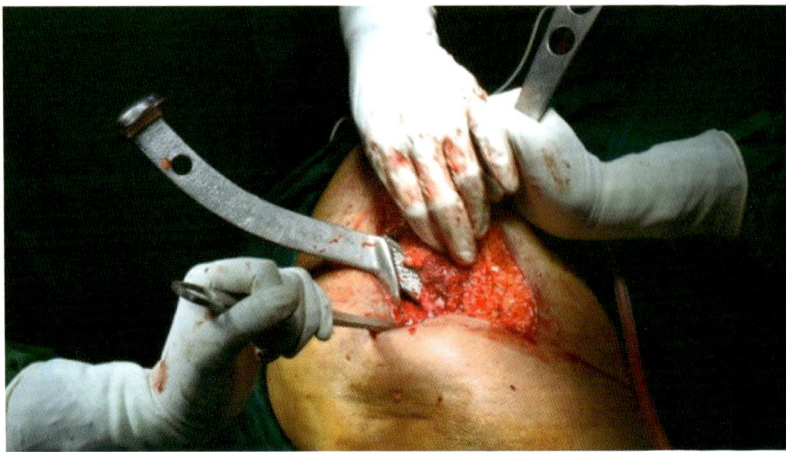

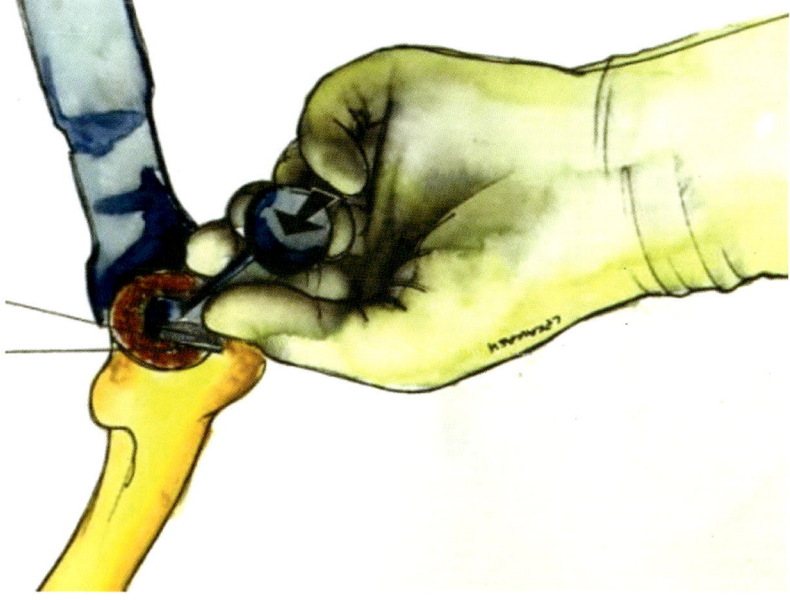

A ten to fifteen degree posterior sway from the lesser trochanter is the axis of version. This can be easily located by following the neck.

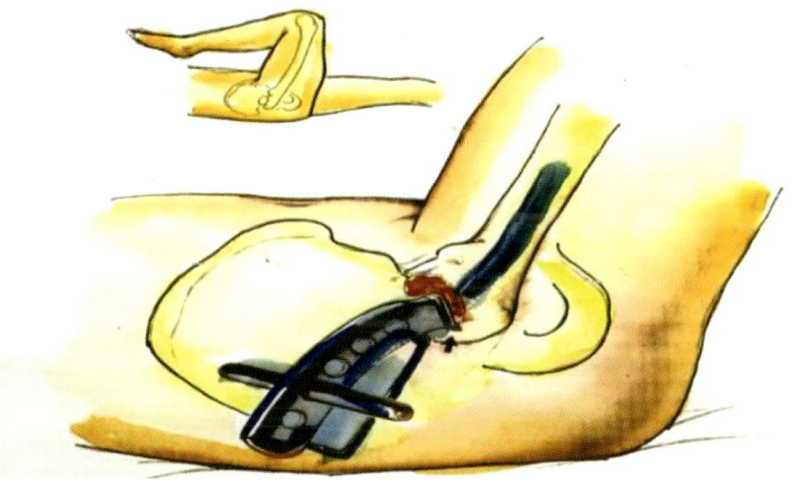

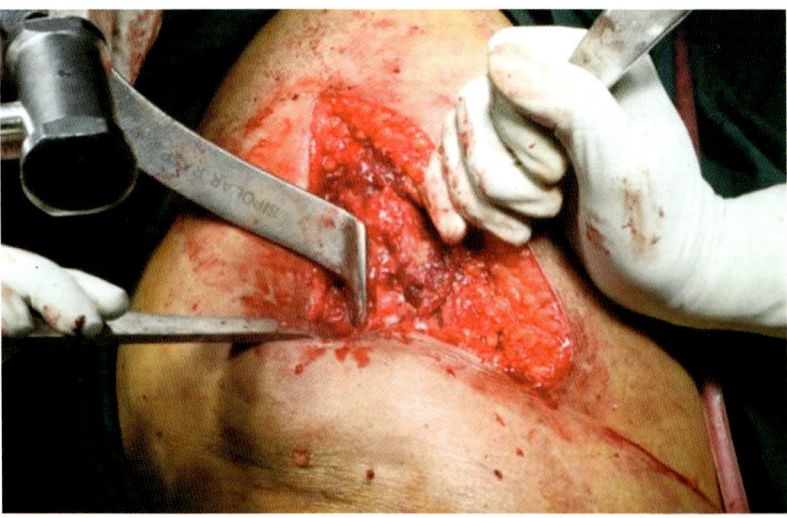

After ensuring that the rasp seats well on the calcar, the prosthesis is inserted and its seating evaluated.

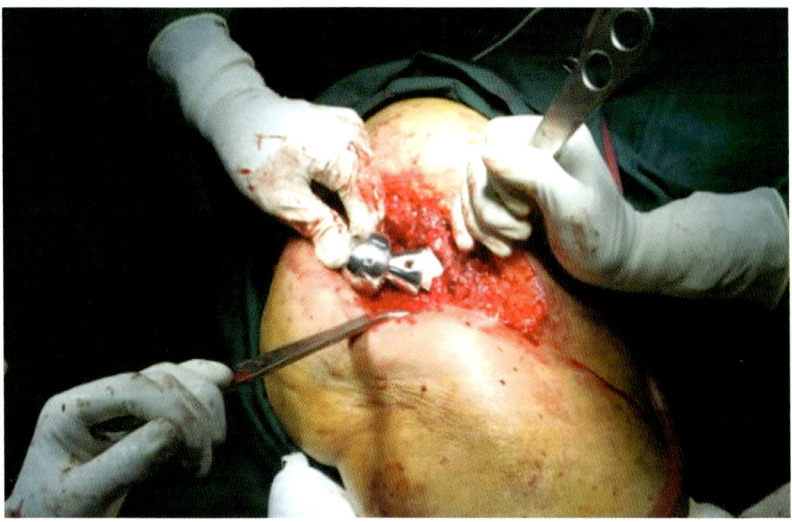

The hip is then reduced and put through the range of movements it allows. A properly placed hip will be stable in 100 degrees flexion and 30 degrees internal rotation.

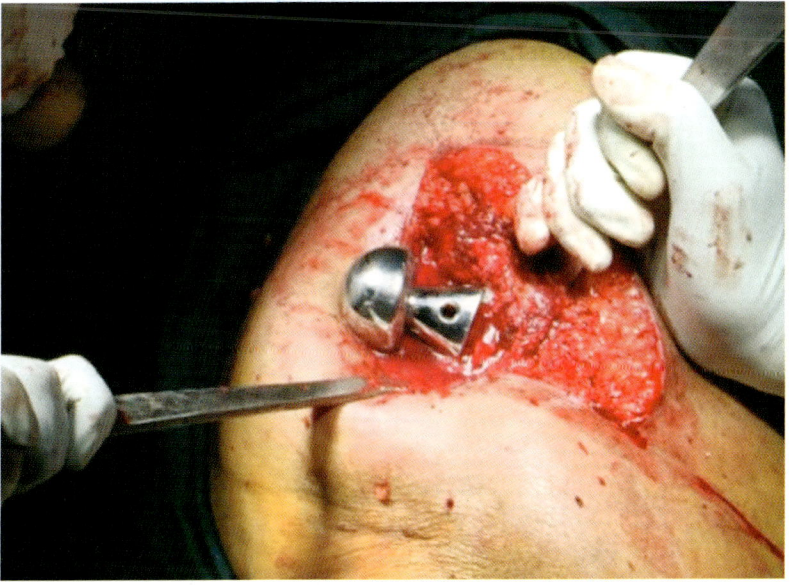

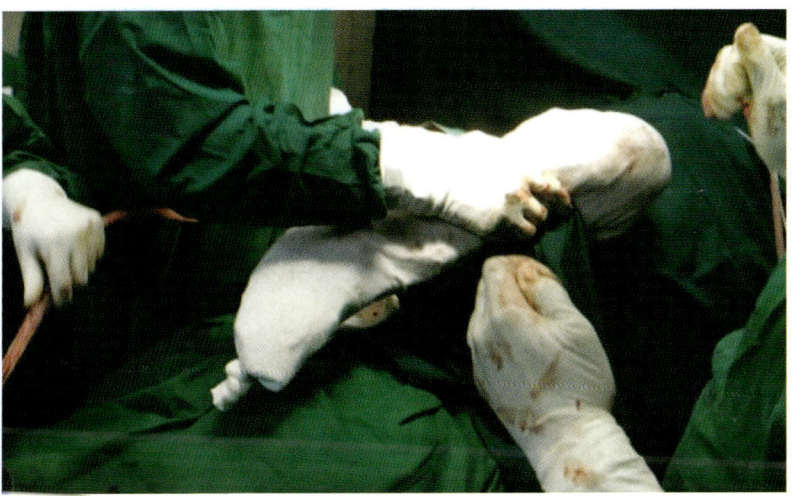

Flexion or internal rotation should not uncover more than twenty percent of the femoral head under any circumstance.

The prosthesis is tapped out, the medulla thoroughly washed and packed with ribbon gauze soaked in adrenaline, to render it dry and bloodless during cementation.

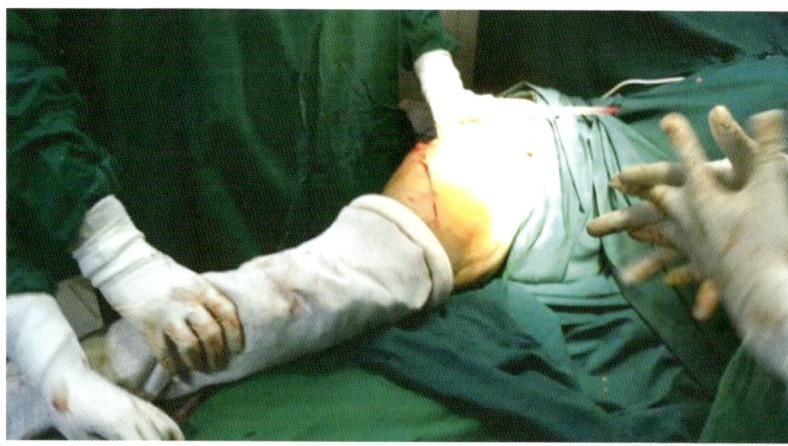

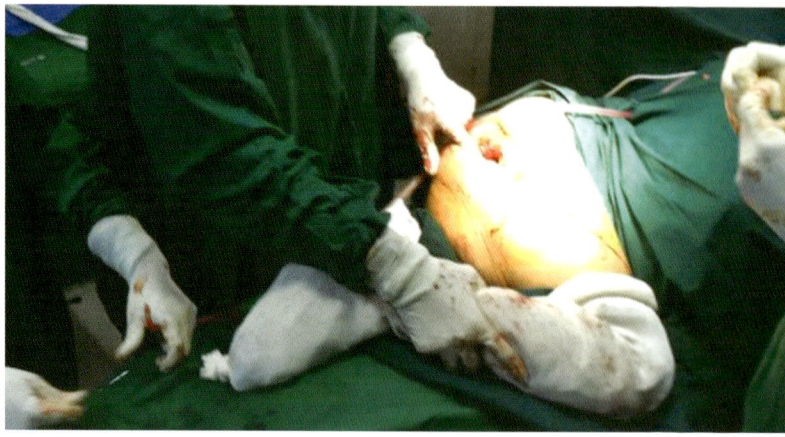

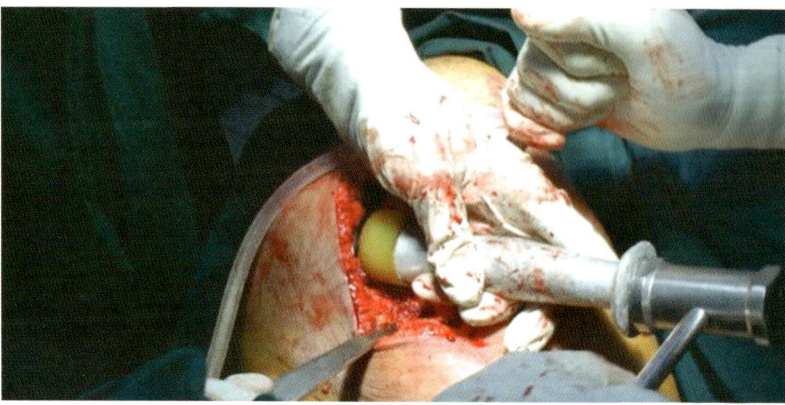

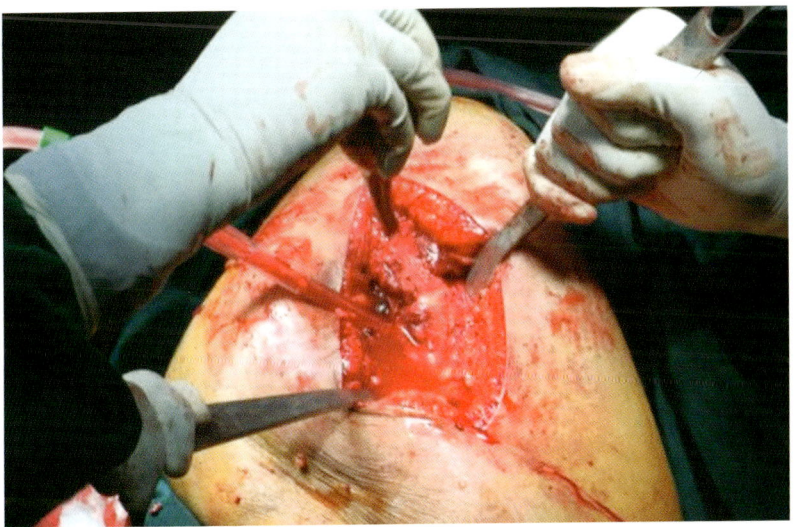

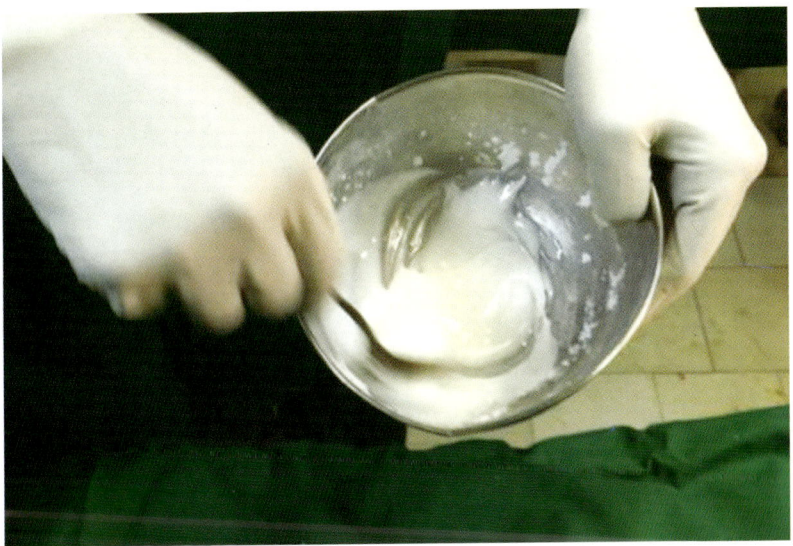

Cement is mixed and brought to a doughy stage after stirring and kneading.

The doughy cement is then finger packed into the medulla after the distal end is plugged with a cancellous bone block. This plug should be pushed to two cm below the proposed prosthesis tip.

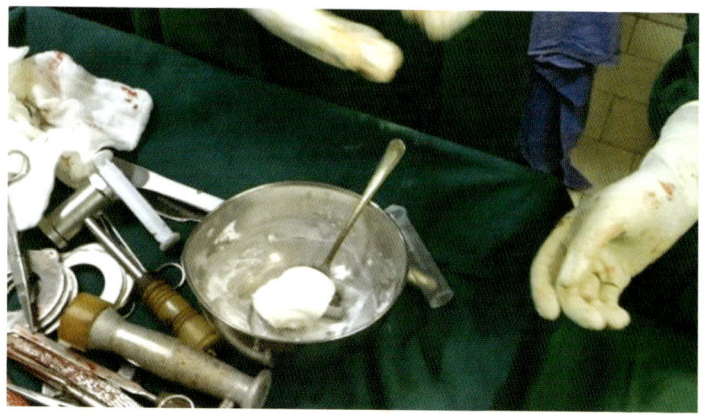

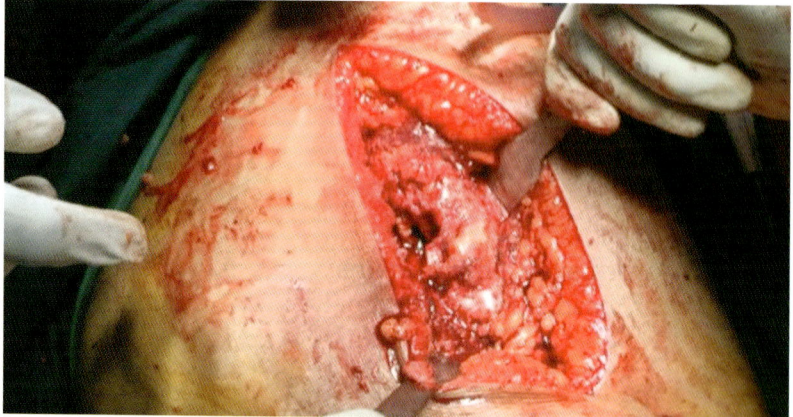

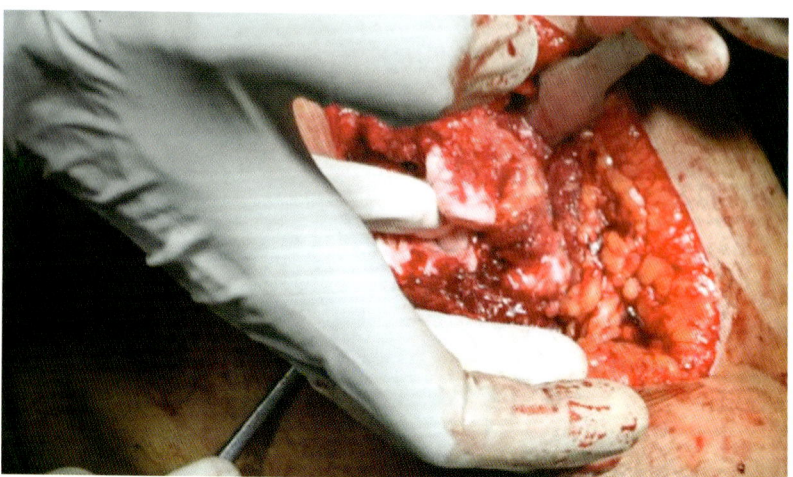

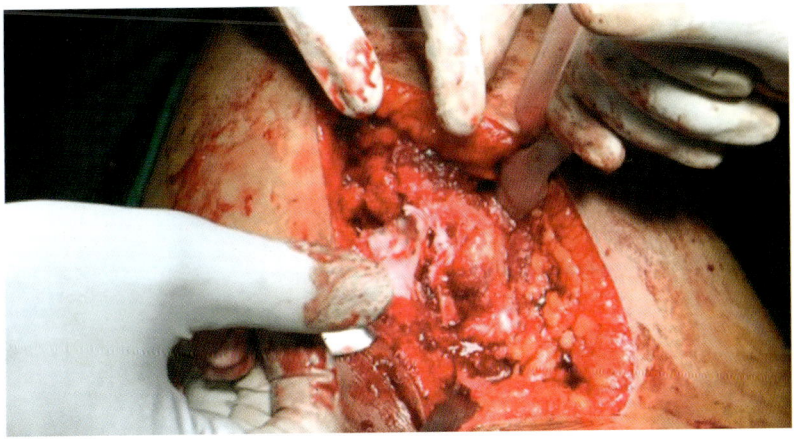

The prosthesis is inserted and a sustained pressure is applied until the cement sets. Special care should be taken to ensure that the implant is in the correct degree of version.

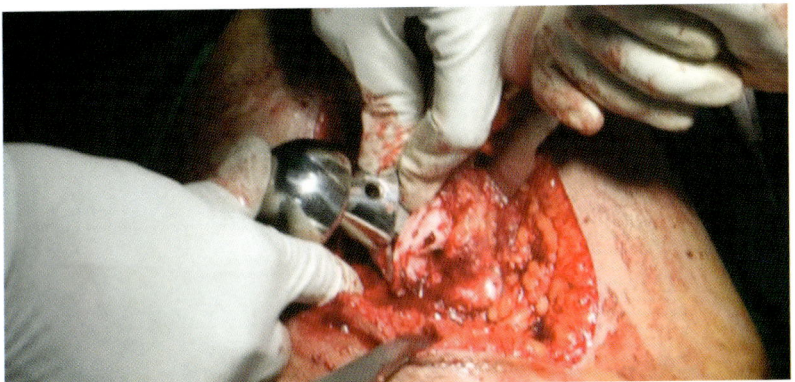

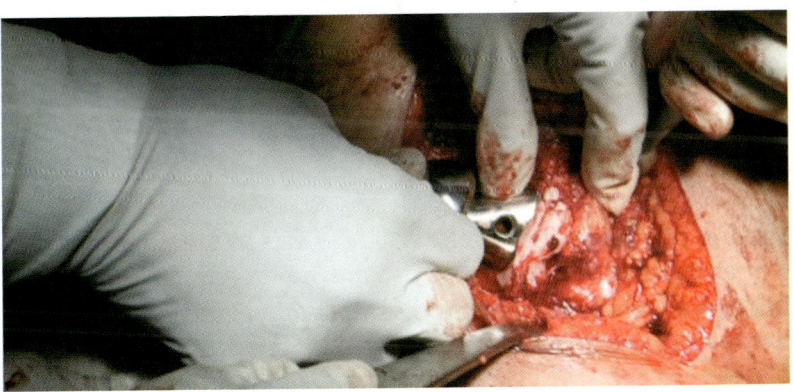

Either manually or with a head pusher, the sustained pressure is retained till the cement sets. Hammering of the cement is ill advised as it considerably weakens the cement mantle.

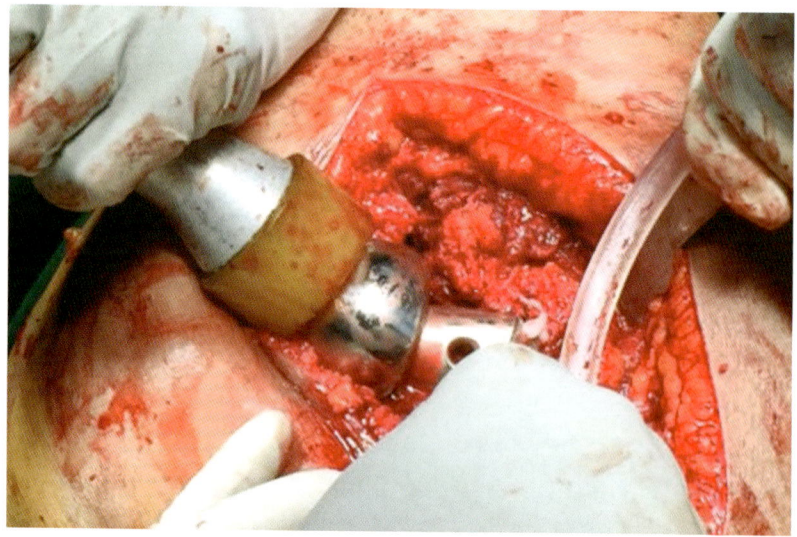

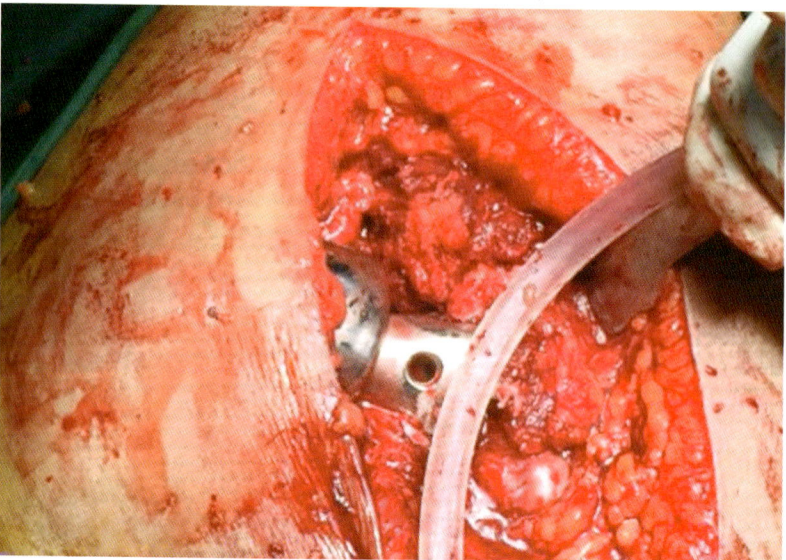

After the cement sets, the joint is reduced. It is put through full range of movements to evaluate its stability.

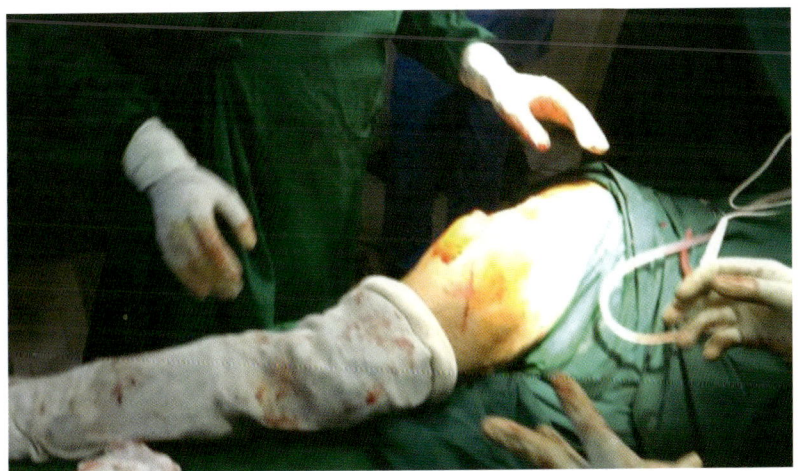

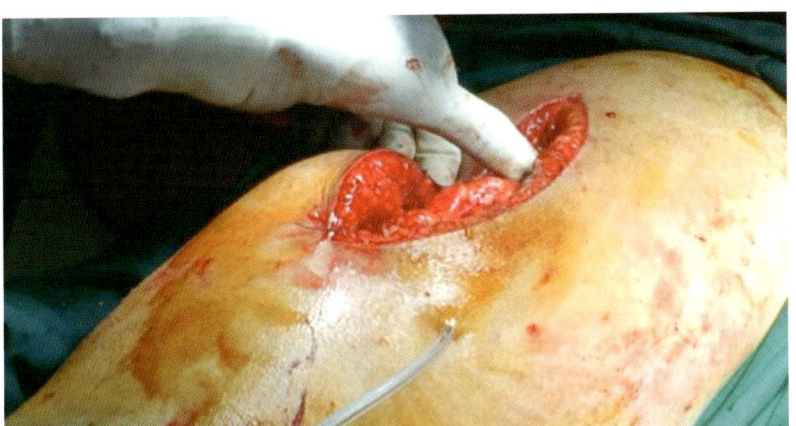

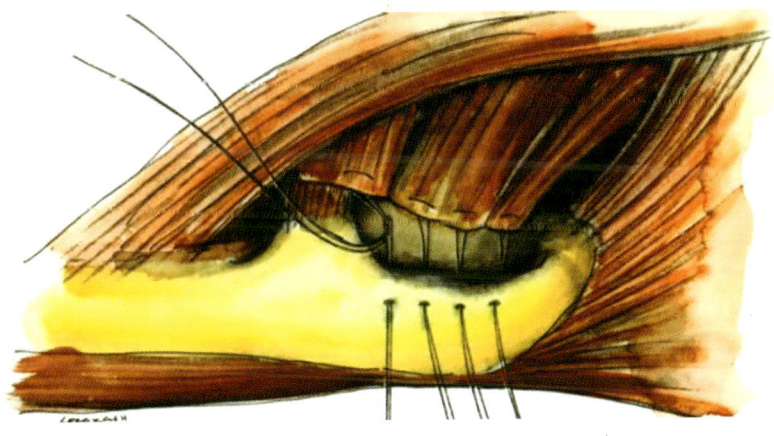

A suction drain is inserted, and the incision is closed in layers. The short rotators are reattached with hip in external rotation.

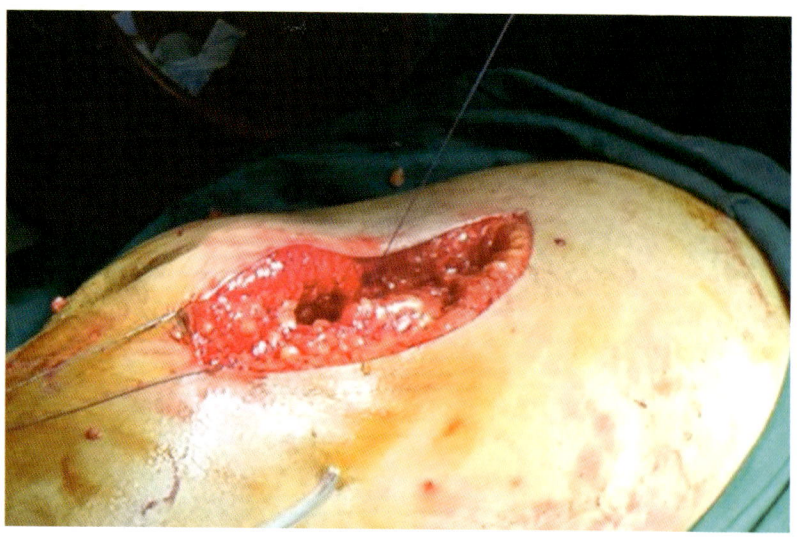

The suction drain is placed below the short rotators.

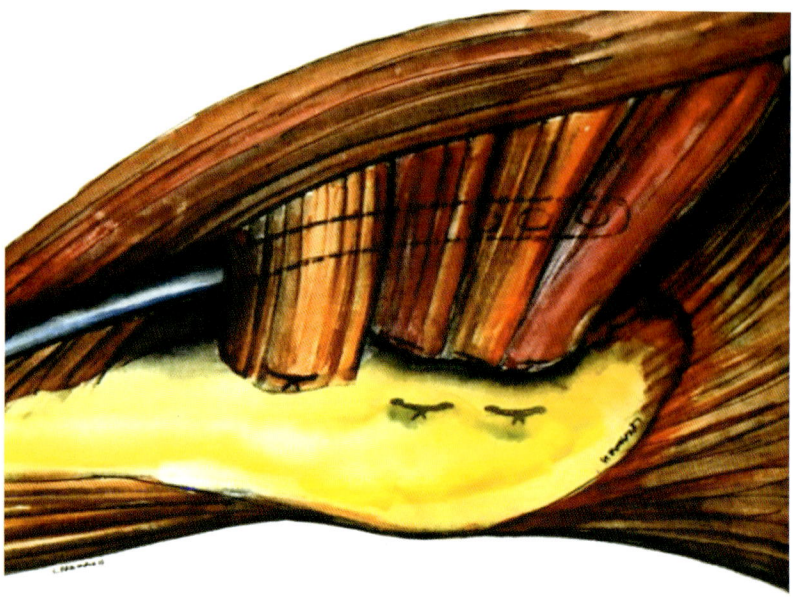

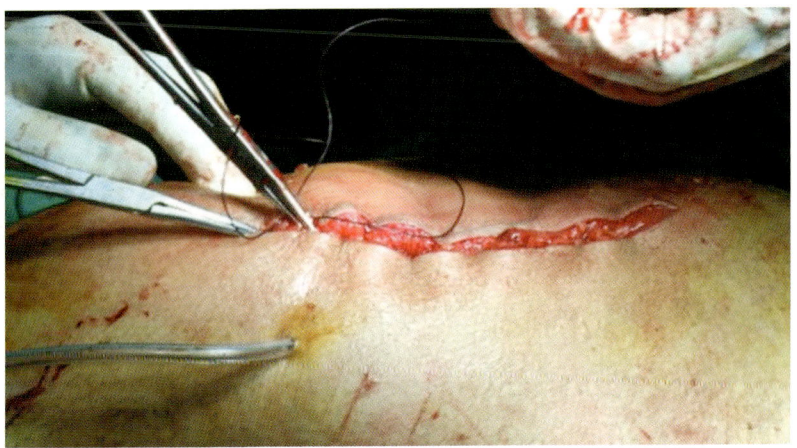

Use of staplers for skin closure speeds up the process, though simple nylon would suffice in most cases.

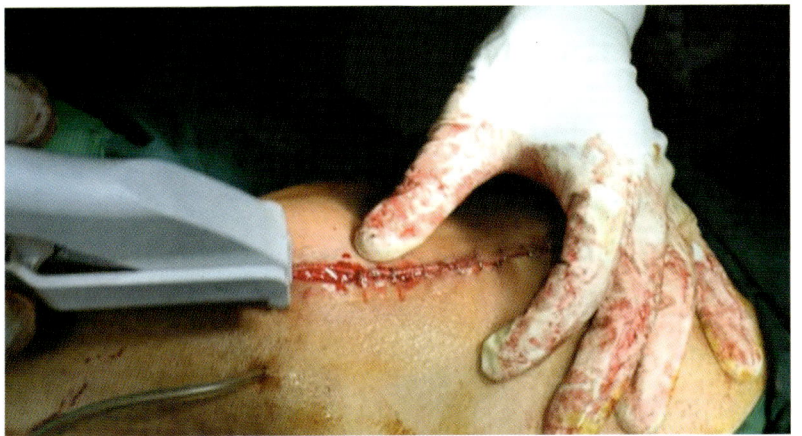

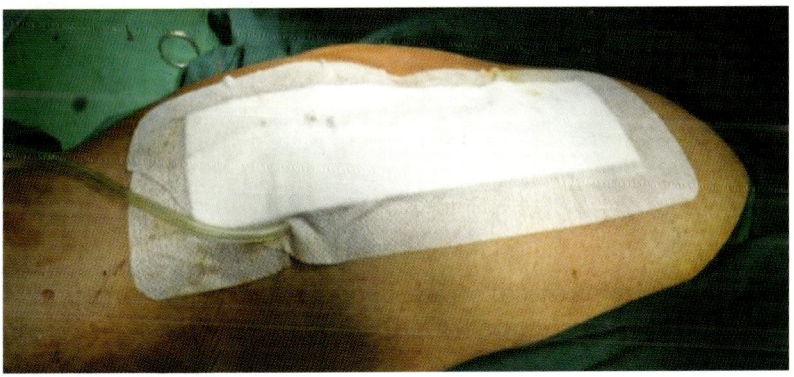

The incision is sealed with a porous sticky bandage and the suction drain is connected.

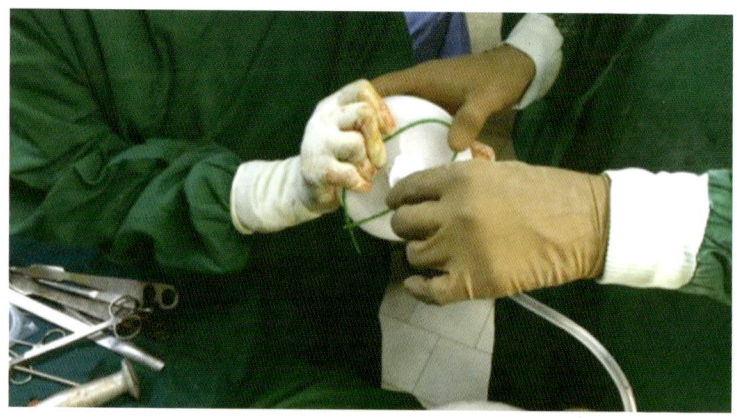

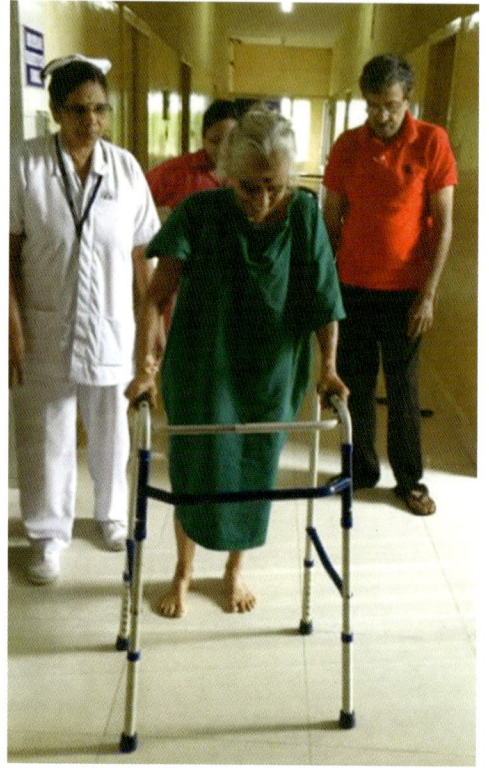

It is usual for the patient to walk the next day after drain removal.

7

Cemented Total Hip Replacement

Cement fixation of total hips has stood the test of time with long term follow ups or three decades or more showing excellent clinical and functional results. The literature is uniform in its comment thet long term failures are more due to plastic wear that cement failure.

Poly Methyl Methacralate has proved to be a satisfactory grout and space filler for hip replacements. Results of good cementation are good and vice versa. Liquid cement injected under pressure, a clean cement implant interface and sustained cement pressurization are the important tricks to be followed.

Complications from cement per se are relatively far and few. A catheter to remove pressure from medulla avoids thromboembolic complications. Monomer induced hypotension is easily managed by informing the anesthetist well in advance and administration of hypertensive drugs. Polymerization heat is not as big a problem as it is made out to be.

I have been using cemented hips for over three decades and find no reason to switch over to uncemented unless compelling reasons surface. The steps of a cemented hip are described below.

The surgery is performed under general or regional anesthesia.

As the average surgical time is a little under ninety minutes, even a spinal anesthetic can be used.

Epidural anesthesia is a safe option, allowing for post-operative analgesia.

First dose of prophylactic antibiotic is administered with the anesthesia.

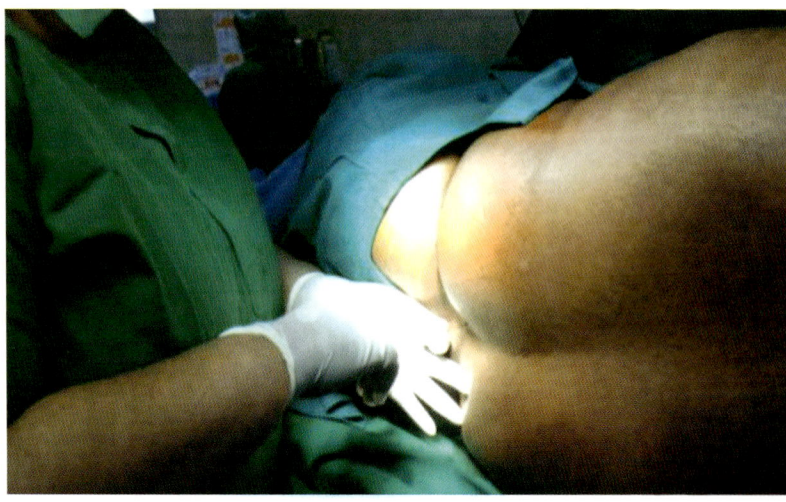

One unit of blood is usually reserved for use during surgery or during the post-operative period.

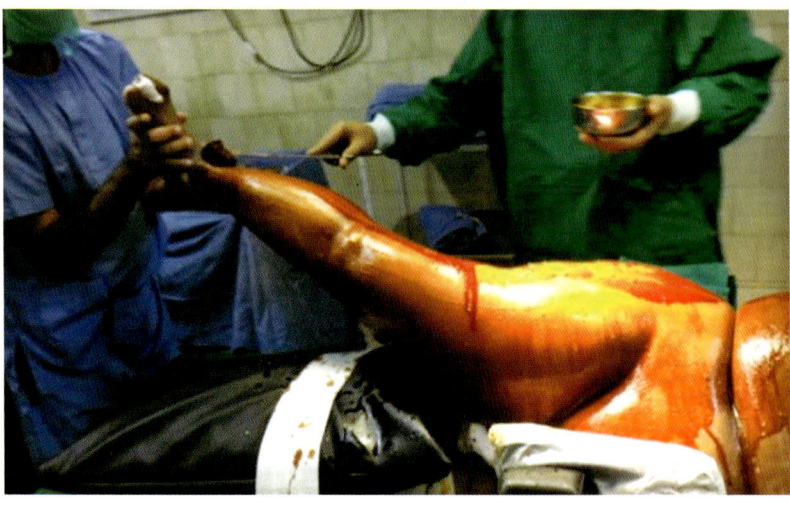

The patient is placed in lateral position with sand bags and table attachments to keep the patient stable. The leg is draped free for manipulations and dislocations.

The opposite limb is strapped to a pillow and the operating table.

The knee is flexed and kept flexed throughout the procedure to ensure that sciatic nerve is kept relaxed during the entire period.

The preparation extends from ankle to iliac crest.

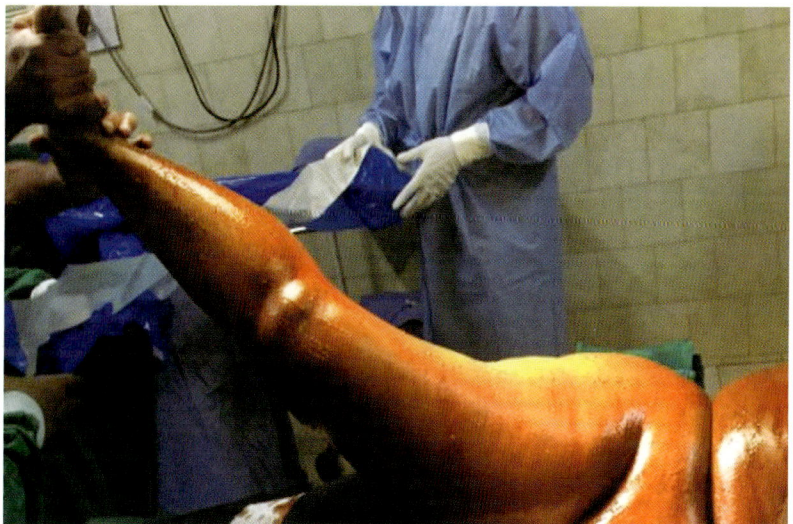

The area from ankle to groin below and iliac crest above are first cleaned with savlon and soap solution.

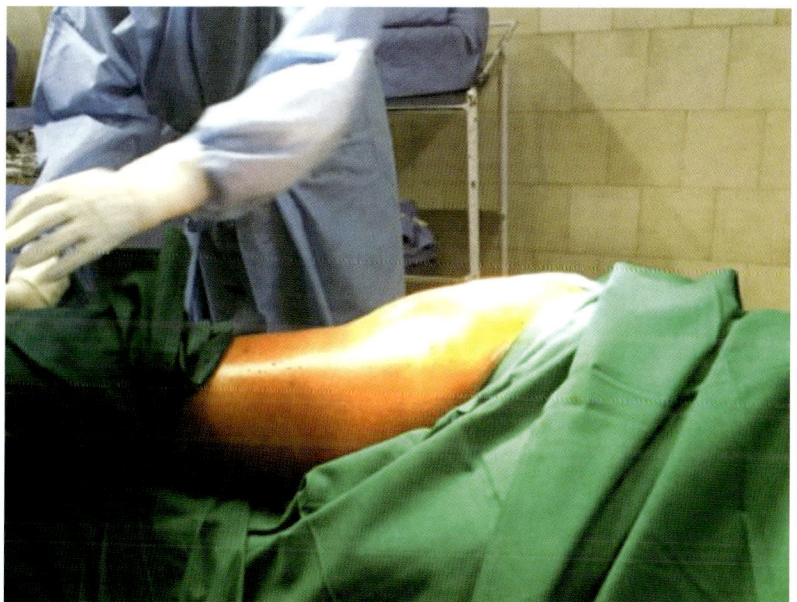

This is then swabbed with isopropyl alcohol solution.

A generous coat of povidine iodine paint is then applied to the above area.

As the patient has been fixed in lateral position with back supports, she stays in the same position throughout the surgery.

Large drapes are used. The drapes in the author's operating room are twelve feet square and cover the operating table floor to floor.

The area from iliac crest to a little above the knee are left exposed for the procedure.

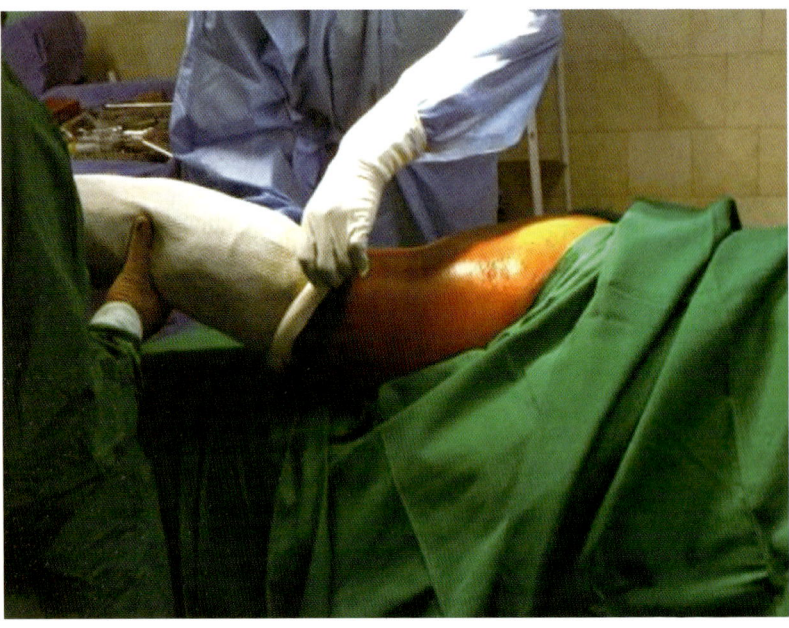

A stockinet is rolled over the draped leg to allow free knee movements during the entire procedure.

The knee is flexed at the beginning of the surgery and kept bent throughout the procedure to ensure that the sciatic nerve is relaxed and stays that way.

A flexed knee in addition provides a long lever arm to allow for easy internal and external rotations, so very essential for dislocation of the hip during the procedure.

At this stage the outer gloves are changed.

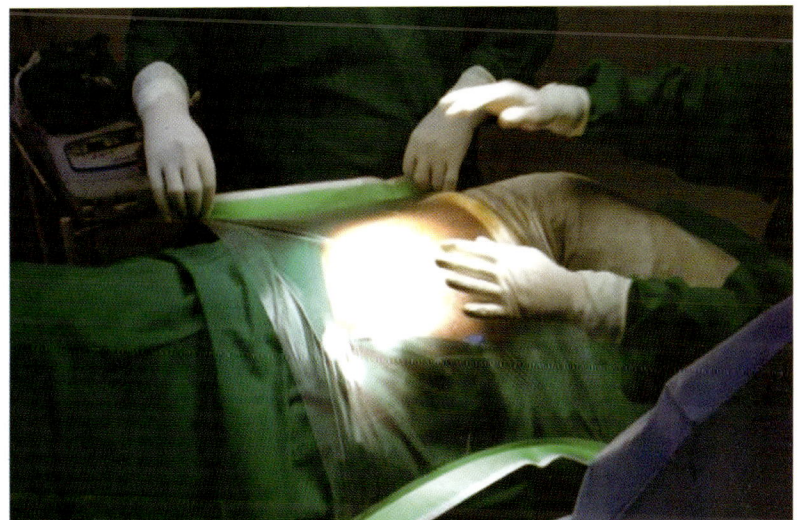

An adhesive opsite drape is now pasted over the operating area.

The surgeon feels the greater trochanter and the assistant rotates the hip internally and externally to assist the surgeon in identifying the landmarks.

In thin patients, both the greater and lesser trochanters can be easily palpated and identified. On the contrary, in obese patients. Only the outer edge of greater trochanter is palpably identifiable.

The surgeon plans for the skin incision.

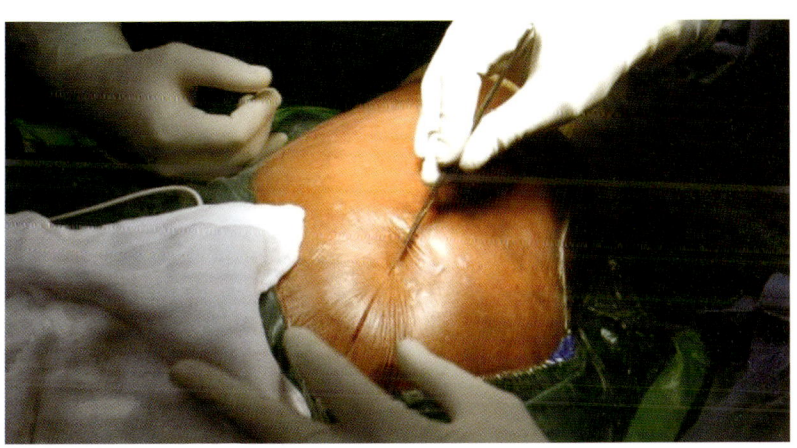

A straight lateral incision centred on the trochanter extends to equal distances proximally and distally.

The subcutaneous tissue and Fascia is cut in the line of skin incision.

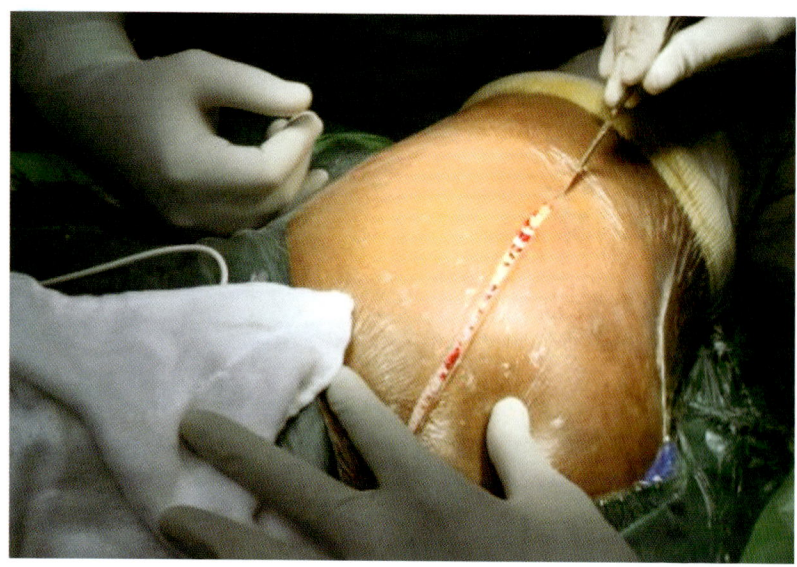

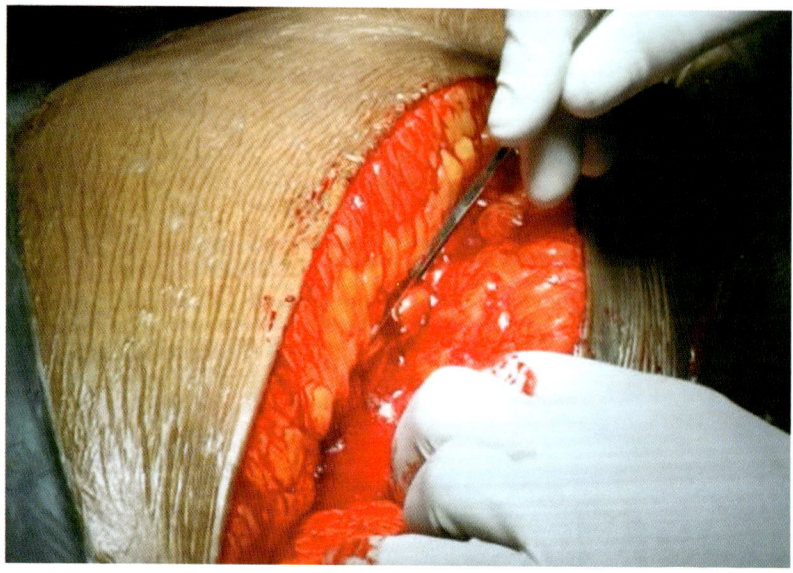

In this patient a large amount of sub cutaneous fat places the joint considerably deep down.

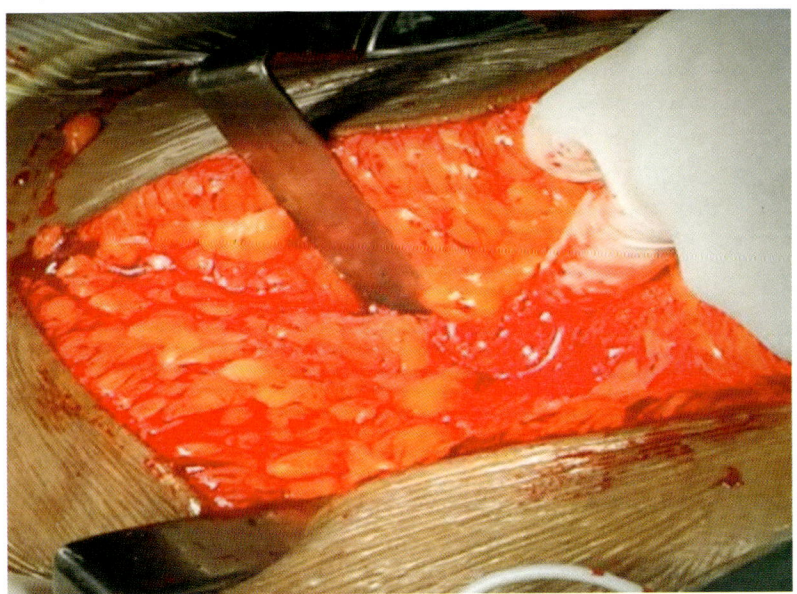

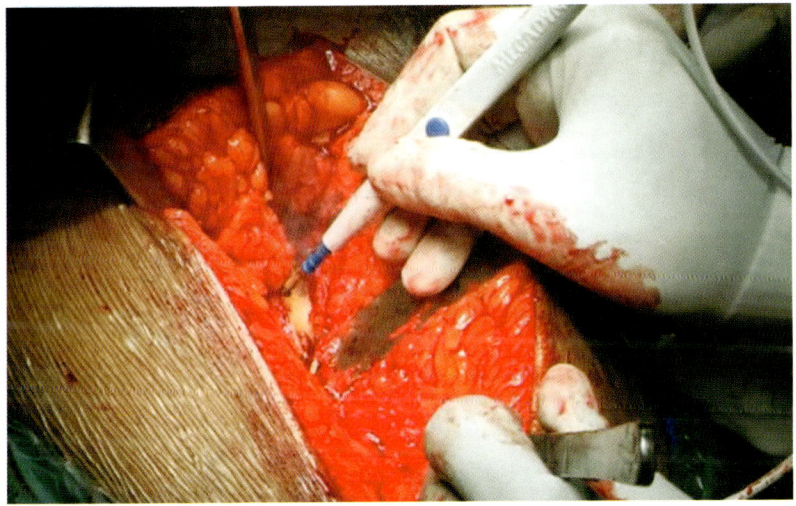

The fat is incised in the line of skin incision, and the fibres of glutei are split to expose the small lateral rotators of the hip.

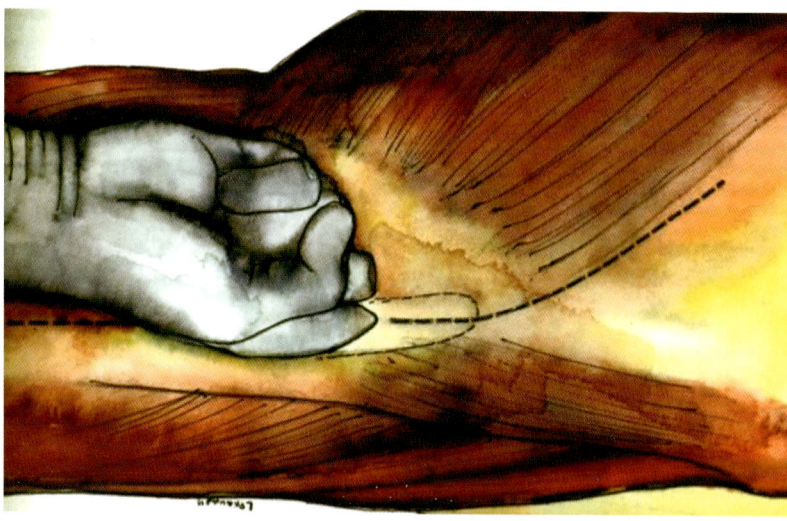

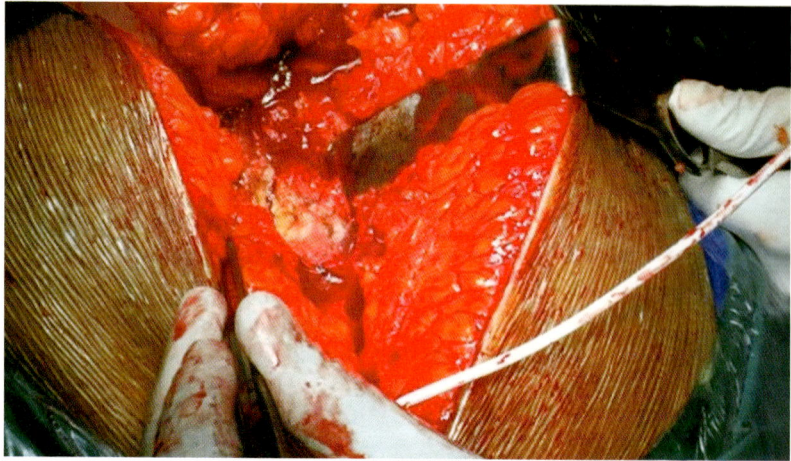

The assistant now internally rotates the hip and this tightens the short rotators.

The muscle belies of quadrates Femoris, superior and inferior gamelli, and piriformis are identified.

The lowermost part of the incision has the superior branch of lateral femoral circumflex artery and this has to be located, and coagulated. This vessel lies a little deep and will keep on oozing and irritating the surgeon is not dealt with early.

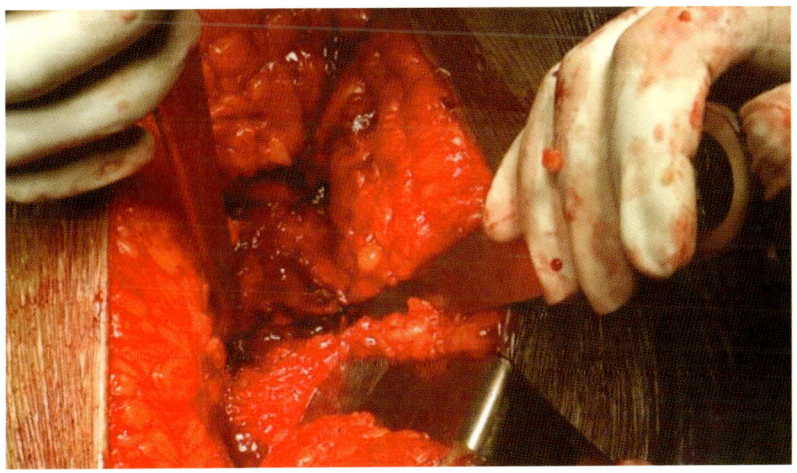

The short lateral rotators are now cut, leaving an attachment to the trochanteric flare for subsequent reattachment.

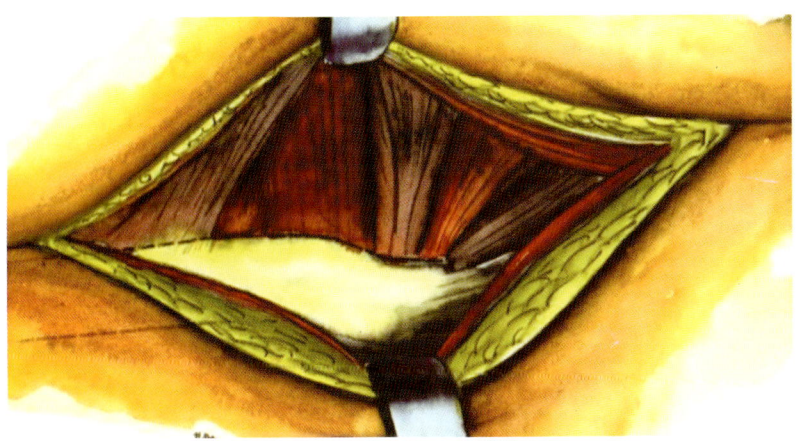

The inferior part if prifiormis is detached as well.

If the hip appears tight, additional soft tissue releases are performed.

The assistant internally rotates the hip, using the flexed knee as a lever, and this maneuver tightens the short rotators, making them prominent.

Some surgeons use stay sutures in the rotators to facilitate reattachment.

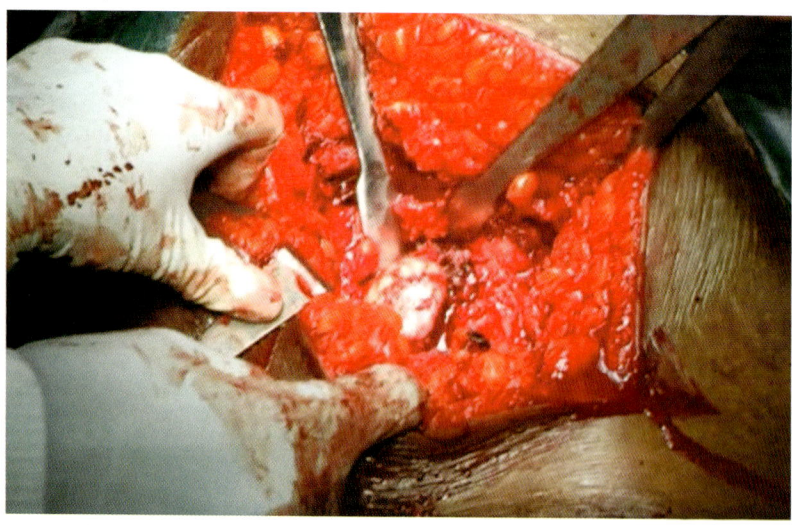

A gentle rocking movement of the flexed knee towards internal rotation exposes larger areas of the head.

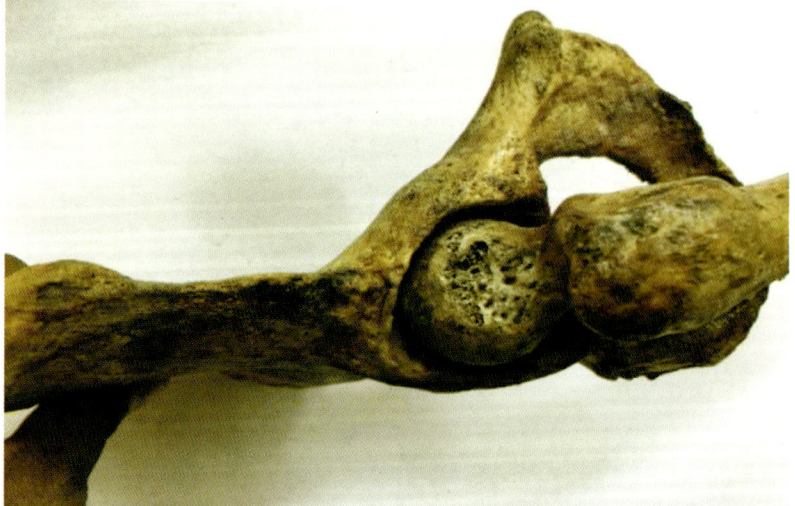

The surgeon levers out the head, as the assistant continues to slowly externally rotate the hip.

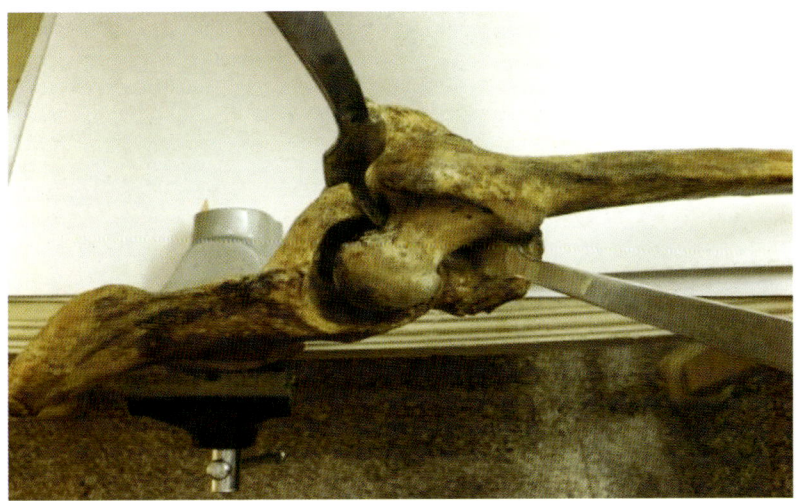

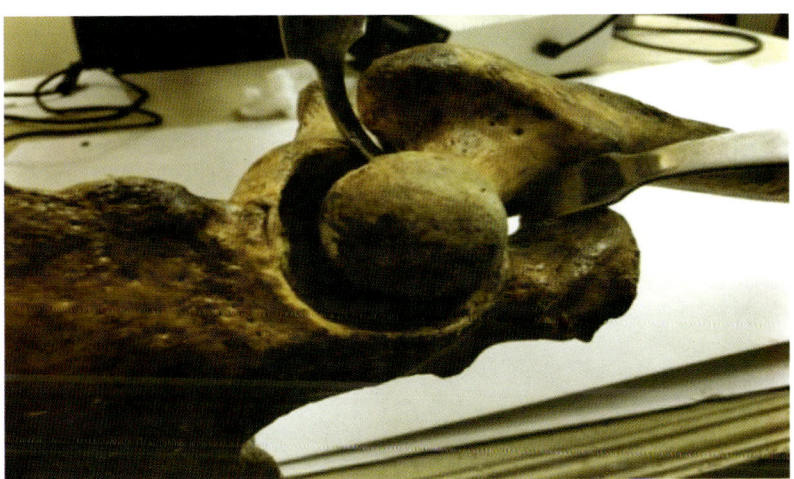

Additional soft tissue releases are done to facilitate an easy dislocation of the head. Homman retractors placed above and below the neck help this maneuver.

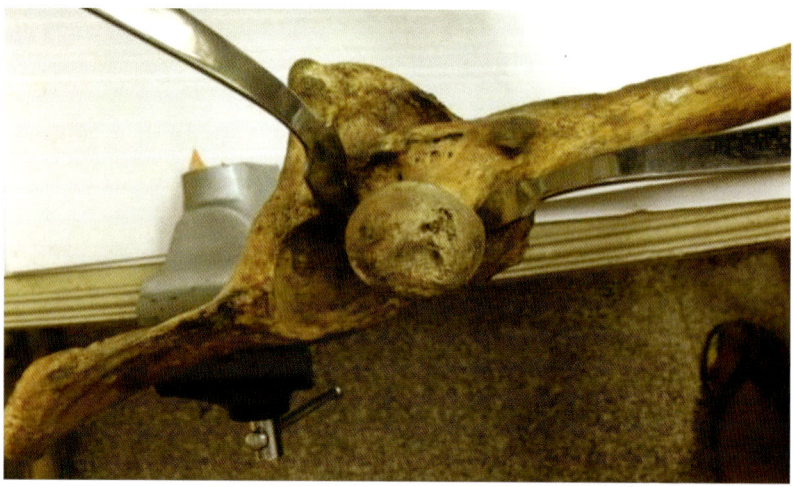

The assistant should not use excessive force during internal rotation, especially in patients with osteoporosis and rheumatoid arthritis, because there is a risk of spiral fracture of the shaft of femur.

As the limb is internally rotated, greater areas of the head become exposed.

Adduction and further internal rotation dislocates the hip joint.

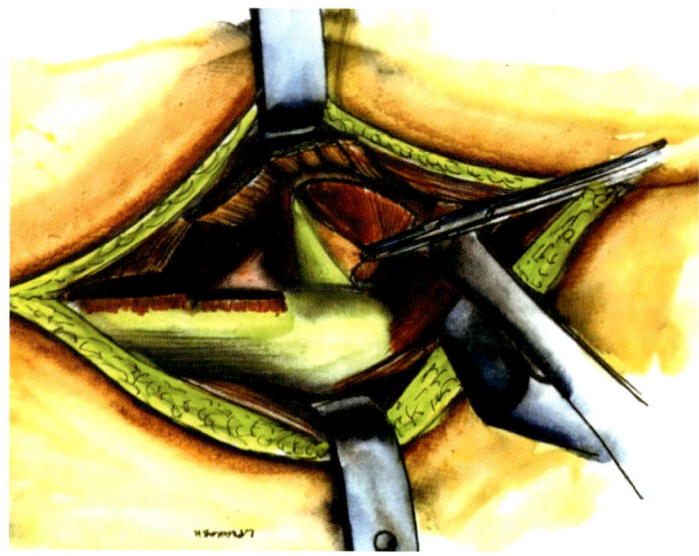

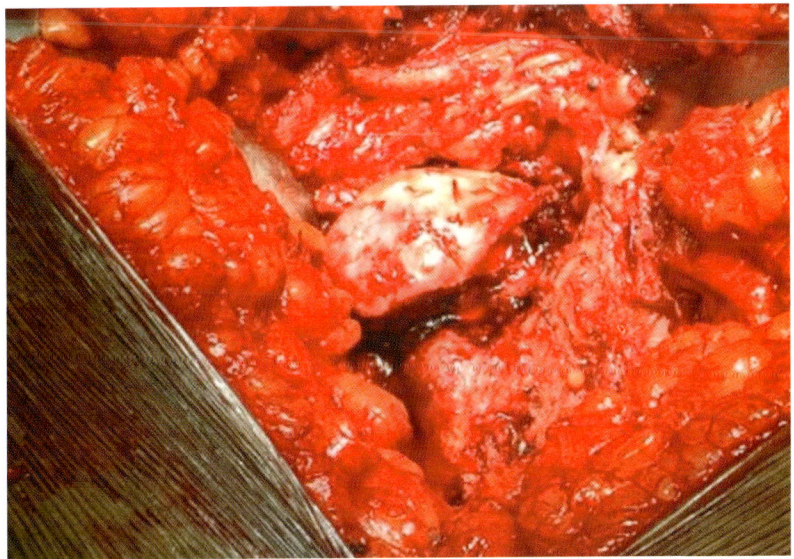

The dislocated head is now visualized completely.

In this case, the head is completely deformed, and overhanging Osteophytes are hiding the neck.

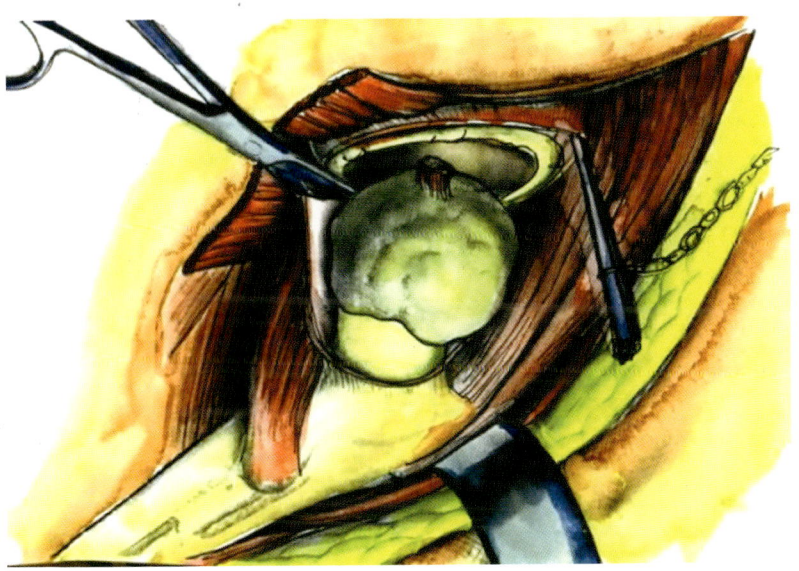

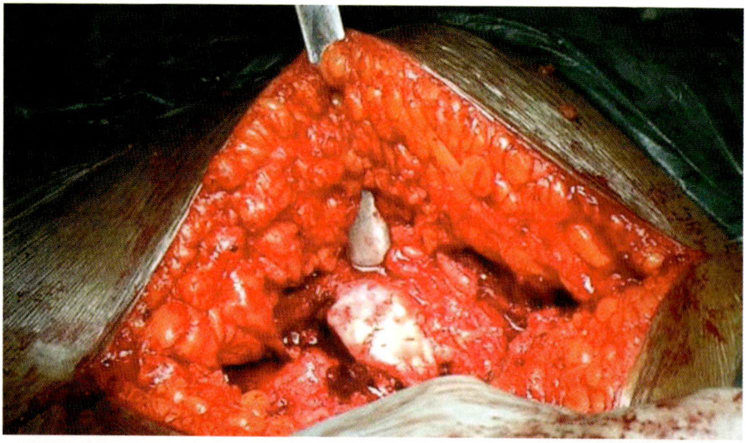

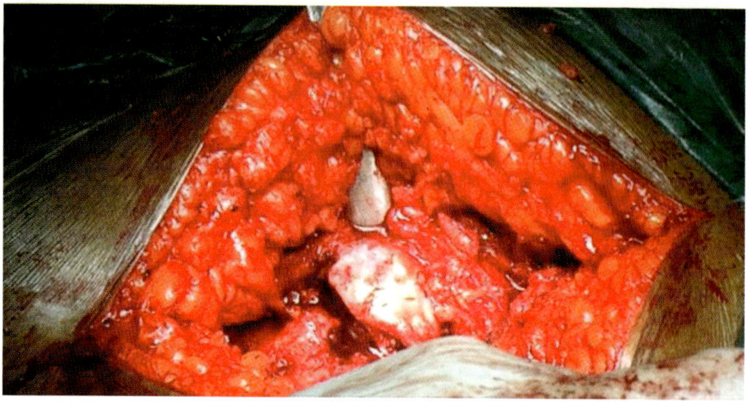

Appropriately placed homman retractors will allow the head to be visualized in its entire extent.

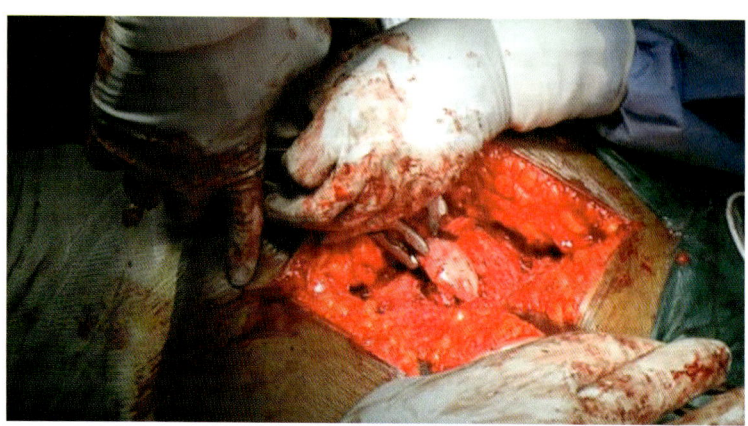

The overhanging Osteophytes are nibbled to allow a proper visualization of the neck.

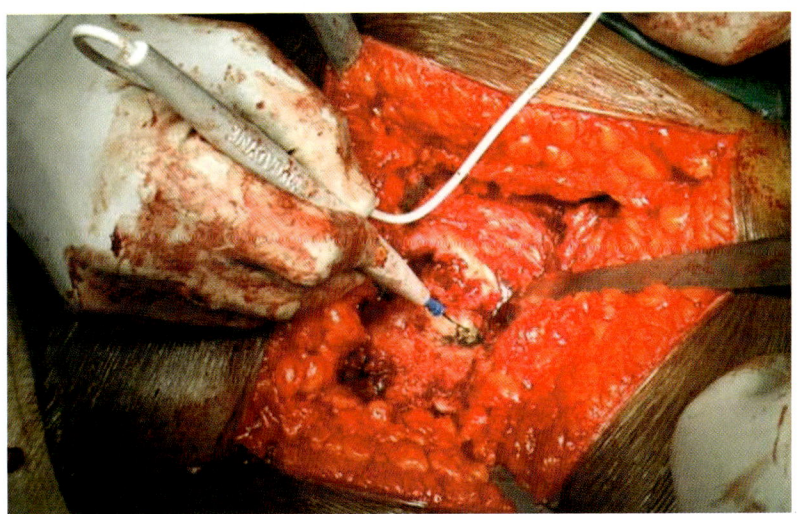

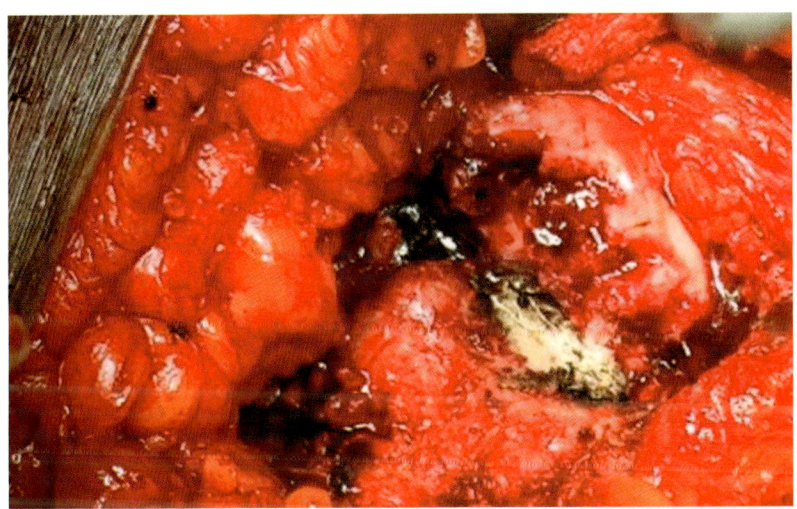

Using a cutting diathermy, the line of correct neck osteotomy is marked. Many companies provide templates for marking the correct cut angle.

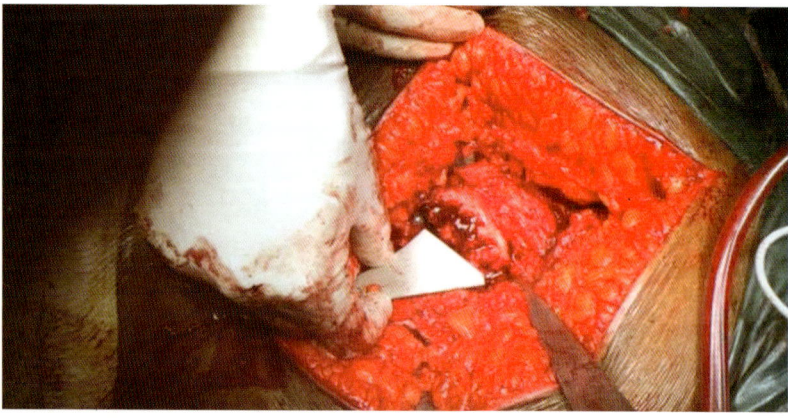

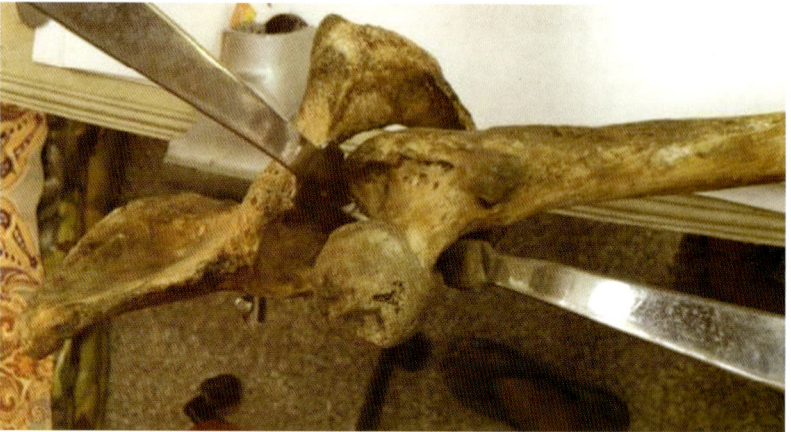

Some surgeons use a trial prosthesis aligned with the femoral shaft for marking the cut, instead of using a template.

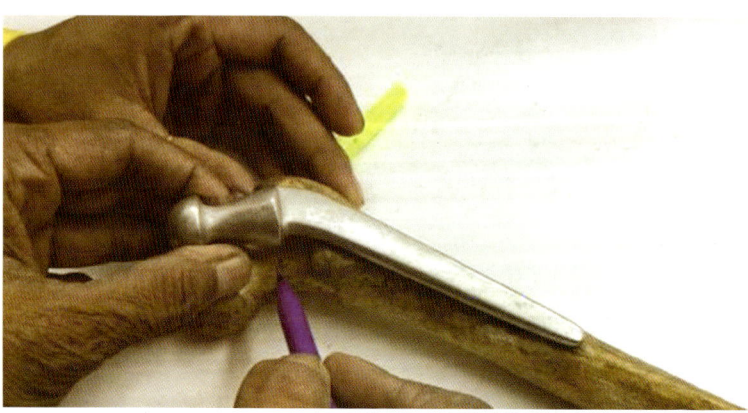

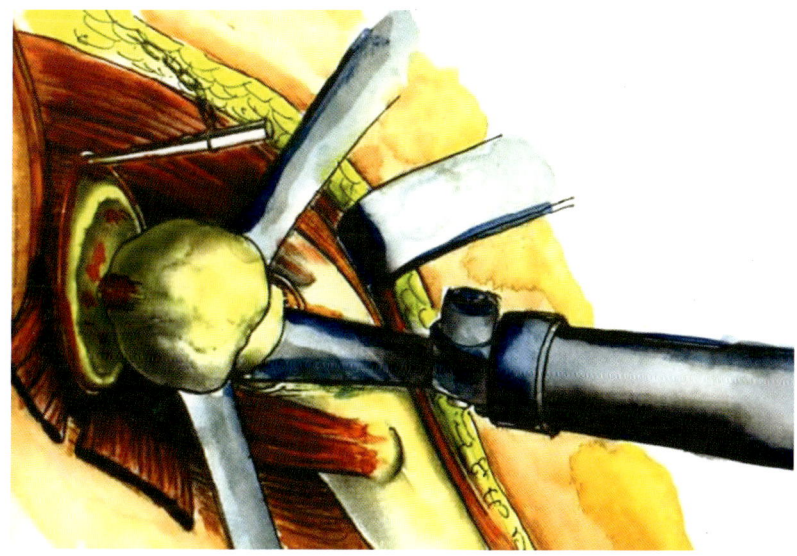

The inferior point of the cut should be one cm above the lesser trochanter, and go upwards at an angle of about forty degrees towards the greater trochanter.

As the version angle differs in different hips, it is best to follow the version angle of each hip during the procedure.

Homman retractors on either side of the neck will allow for support as the oscillating saw is used to cut the neck.

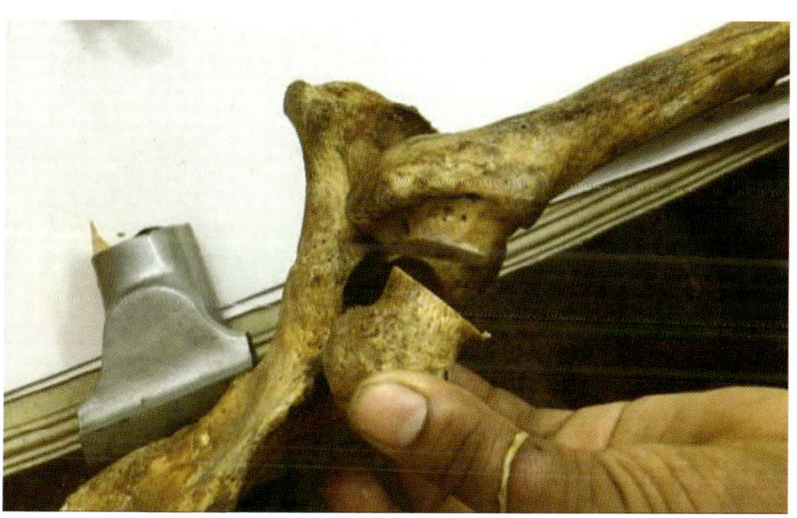

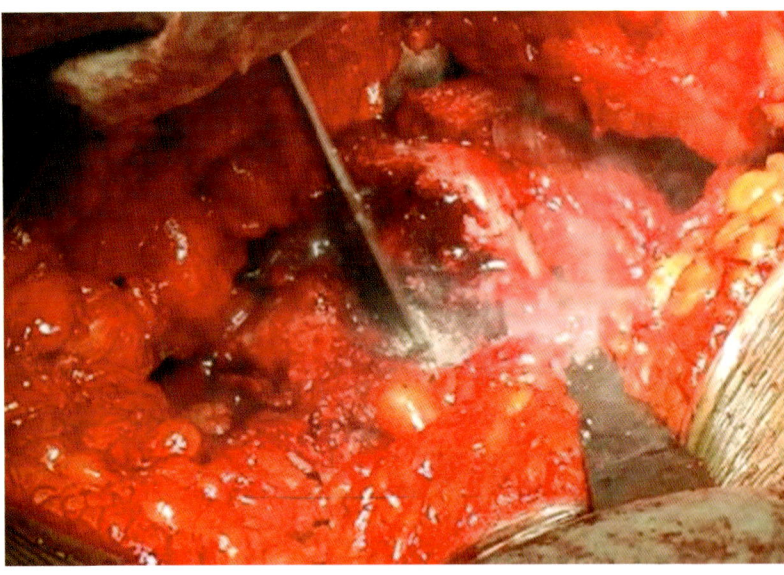

With a power saw the neck is osteotomized at the correct angle.

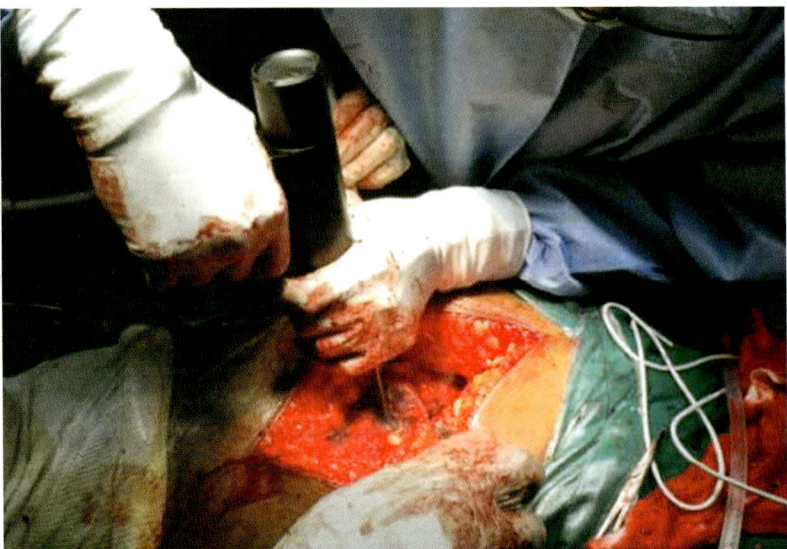

The head is now removed and measured. However in such deformed heads, it is better to measure the acetabulum.

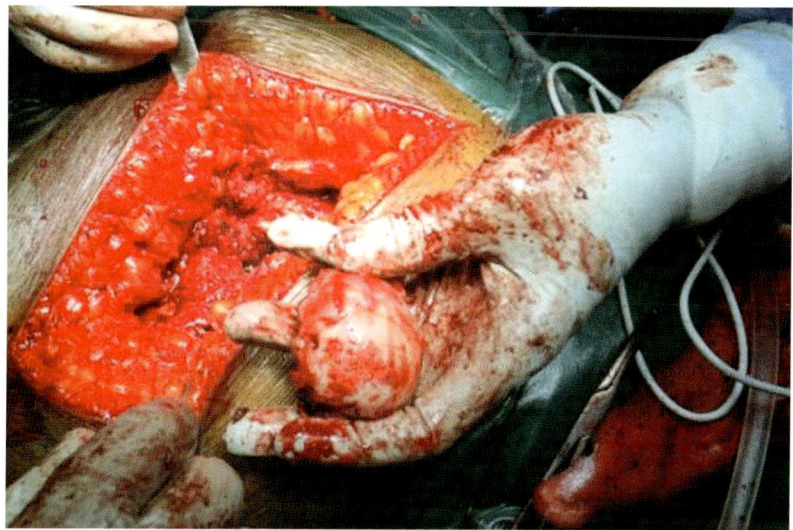

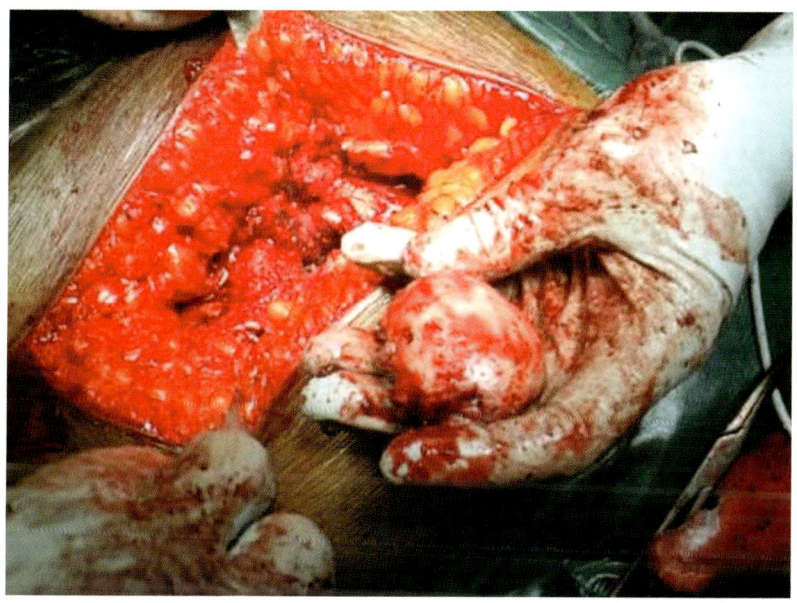

Examination of the deformities of the head, tell us about the shape of the acetabulum and would guide the surgeon towards the correct areas to be reamed.

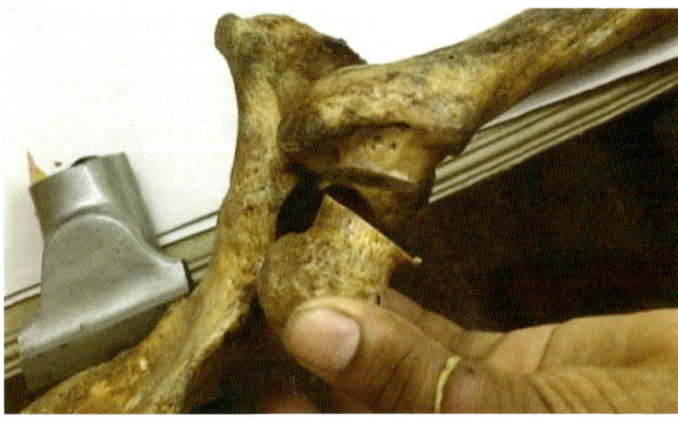

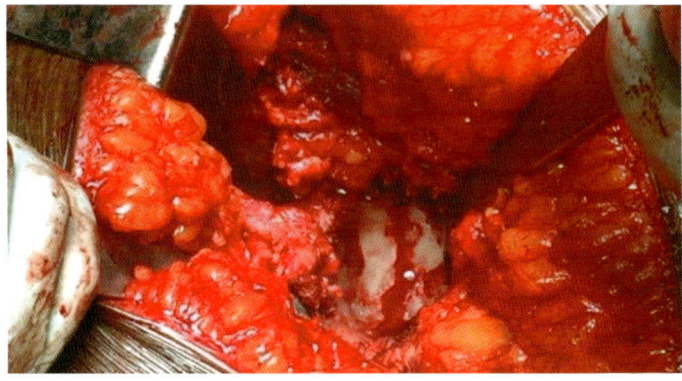

Judicious placement of Homman retractors, will ensure that the femur is pushed out of the way and the acetabulum is visualized 360 degrees.

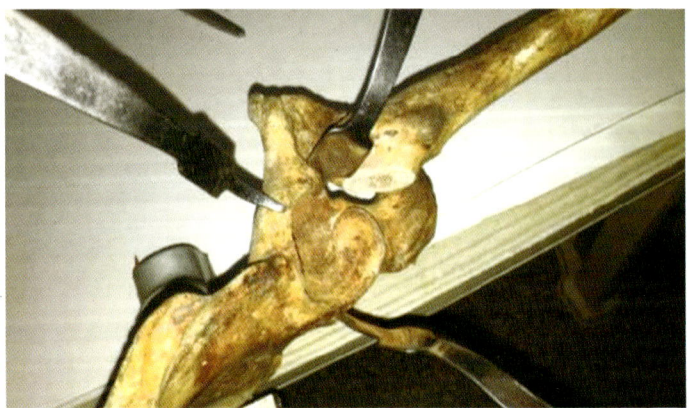

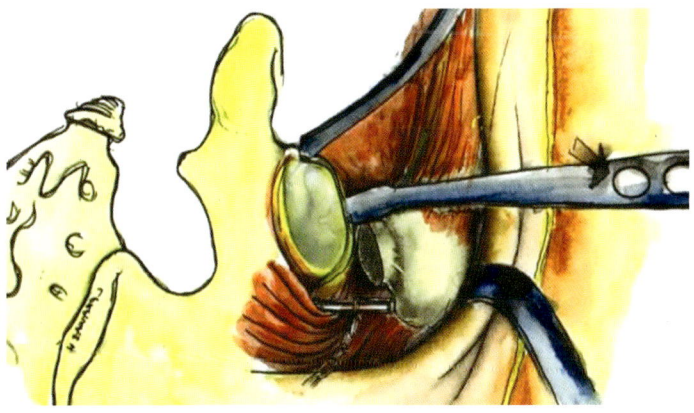

The acetabulum is inspected to evaluate its true extent and to distinguish between the true acetabulum and the false, with which subluxed heads usually articulate.

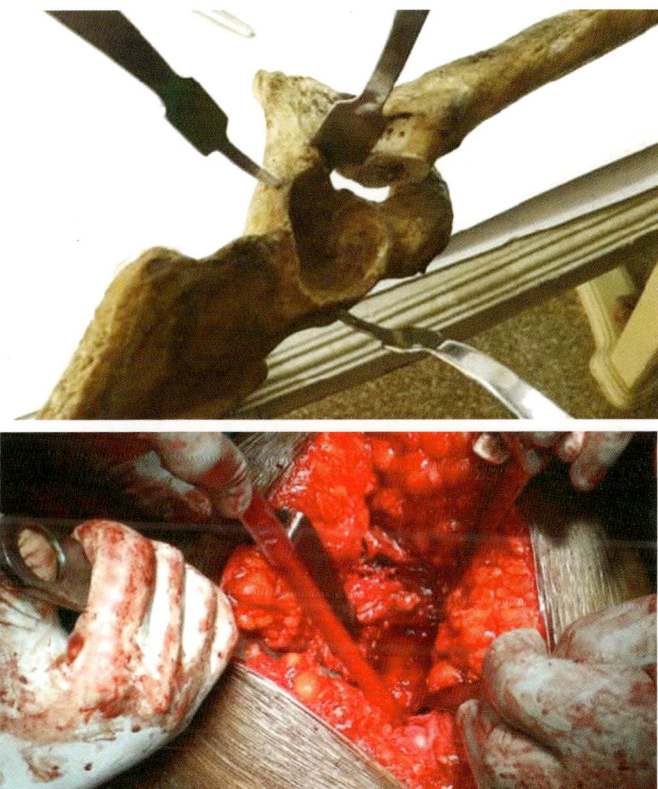

The hip capsule and surrounding soft tissue is now excised to allow the use of acetabular scraper spoons to scoop and clean the interior of the socket.

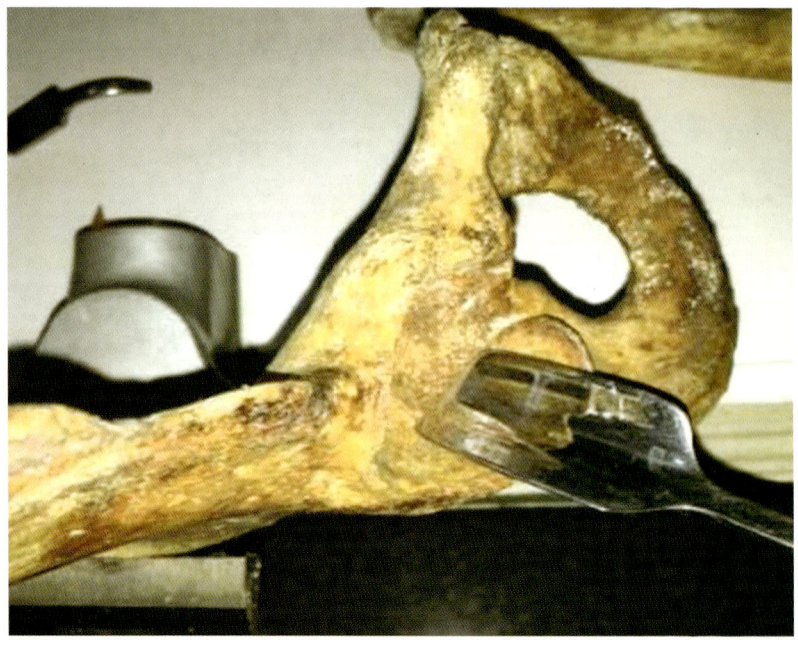

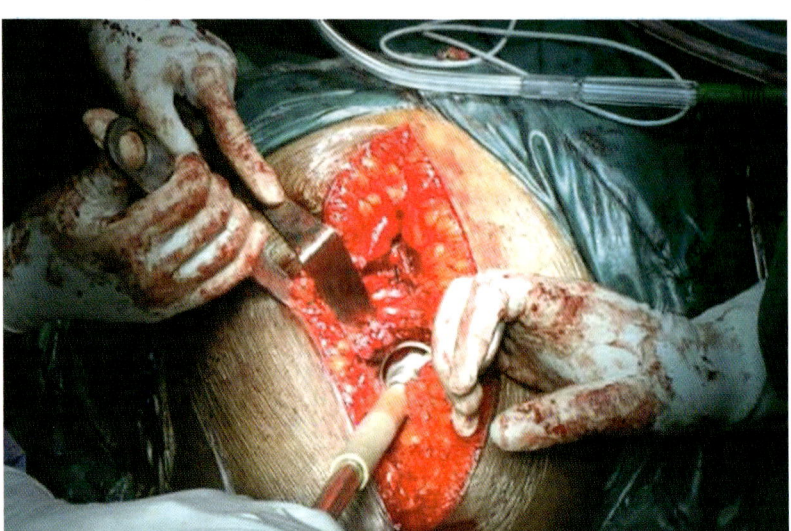

Power reamers are available in various sizes and designs. Increasing sizes are used to ream the acetabulum in the correct direction.

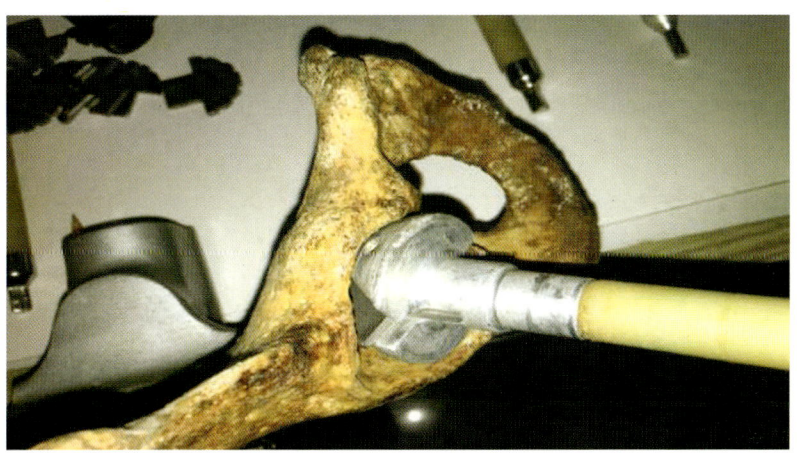

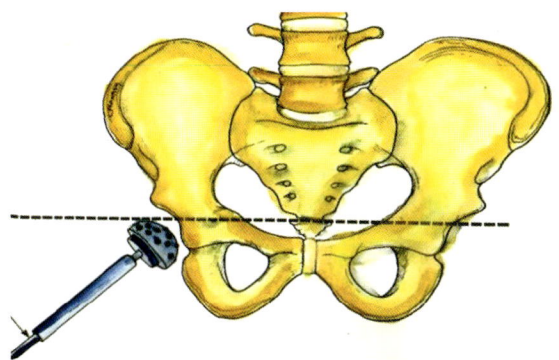

The version of an acetabulum is between 43 to 48 degrees in saggital and fifteen to twenty degrees in coronal plane.

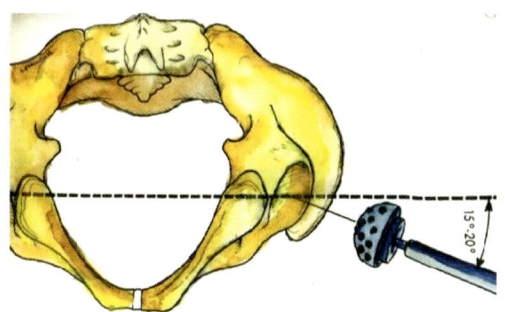

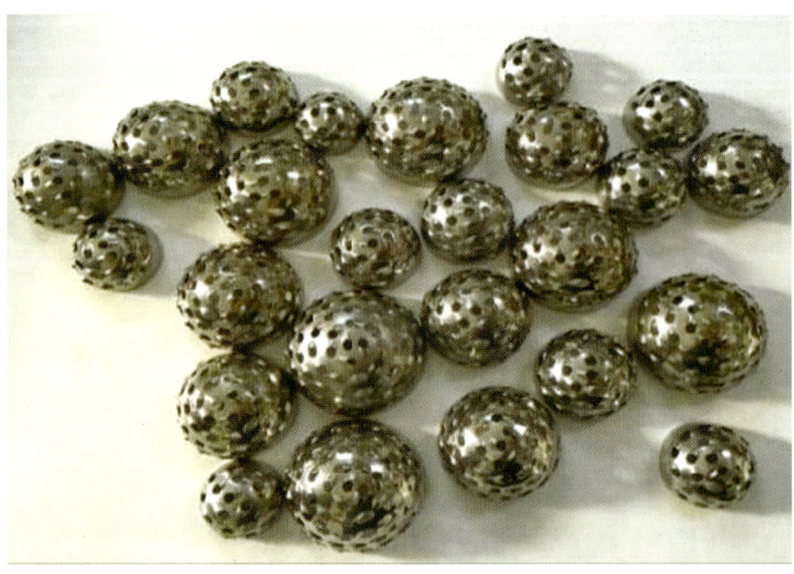

Acetabular reamers are available in various designs and in increasing sizes from the smallest to the largest to ream any acetabulum.

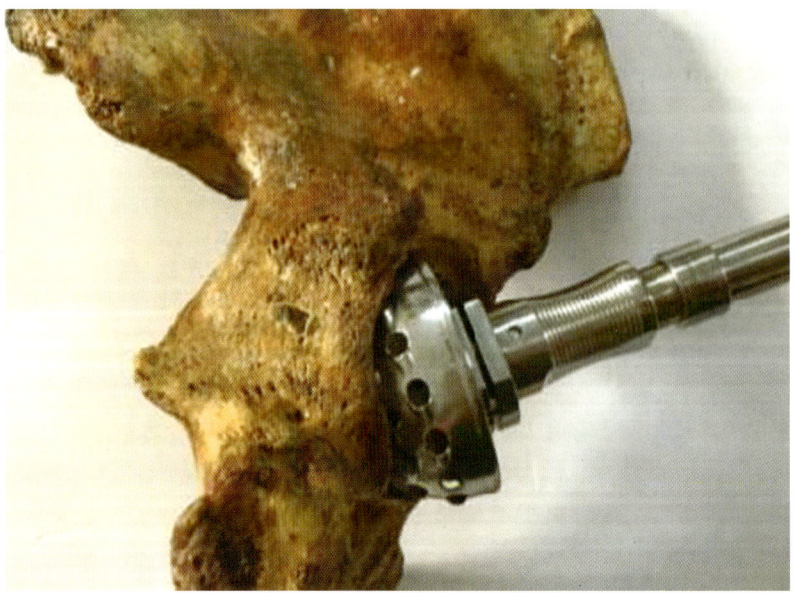

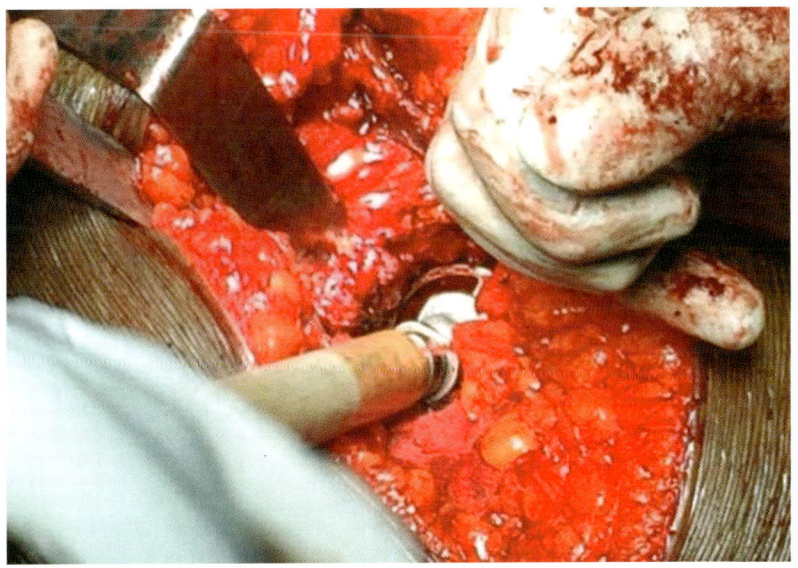

Progressively large reamers are now used to enlarge the acetabulum. It is essential to ream up to the sub chondral bone

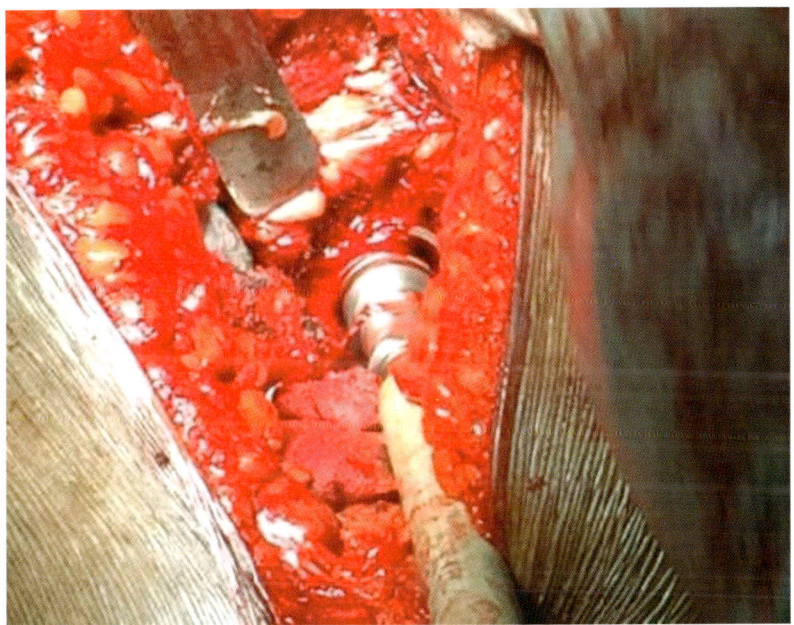

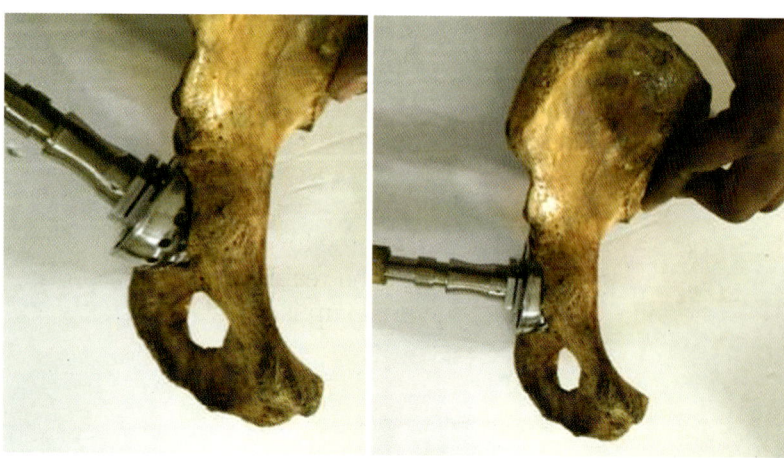

The sequence of reaming is inferior, middle and then superior, with an attempt to get the position as close as the normal acetabulum as possible.

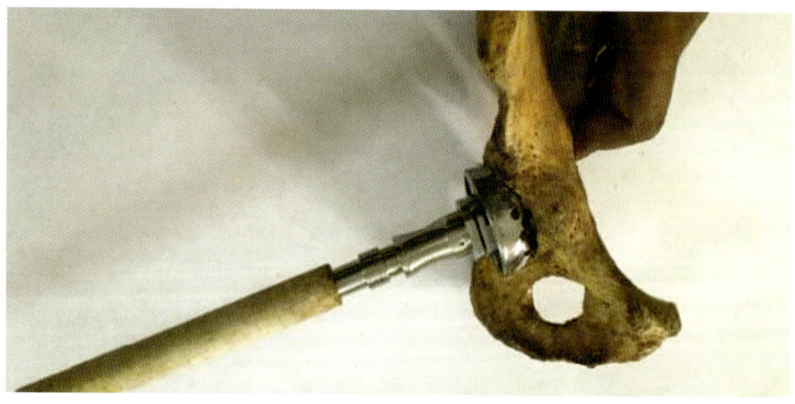

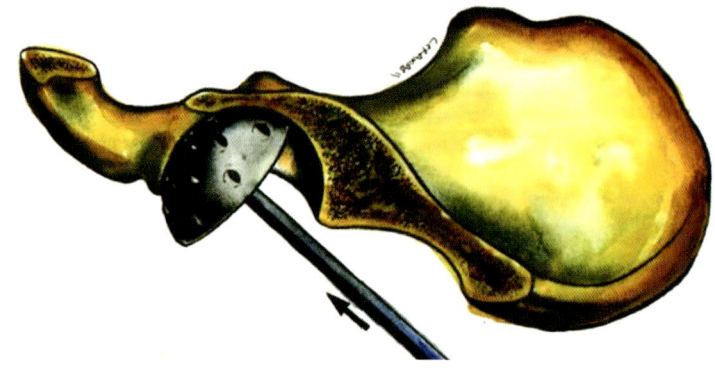

It is necessary to ream the true acetabulum and get the margins correctly.

In many cases, including the one demonstrated here, the subluxed hip deforms the acetabulum over the years and a false acetabulum is created posterior-superiorly in which the flat deformed femoral head is articulating.

The true acetabulum begins from the fovea acetabulis, where the ligamentum teres is attached. The reaming should begin in this direction to ensure that the final cup is placed in the correct level.

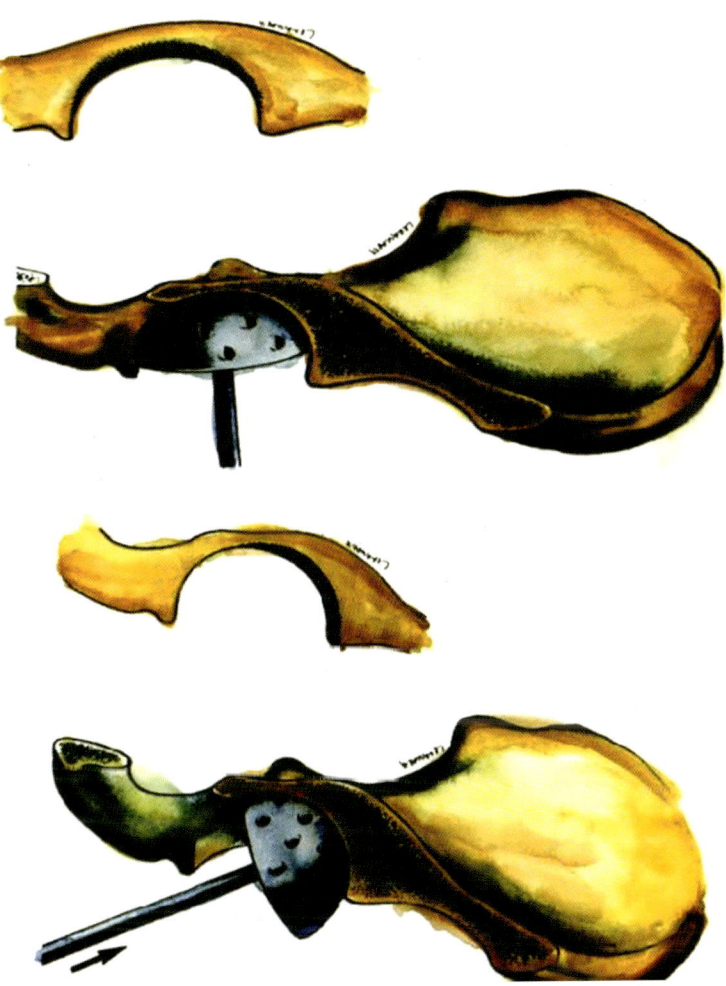

The order of reaming is inferior, central and then superior, all the time ensuring that the final cups position would be accurate anatomically.

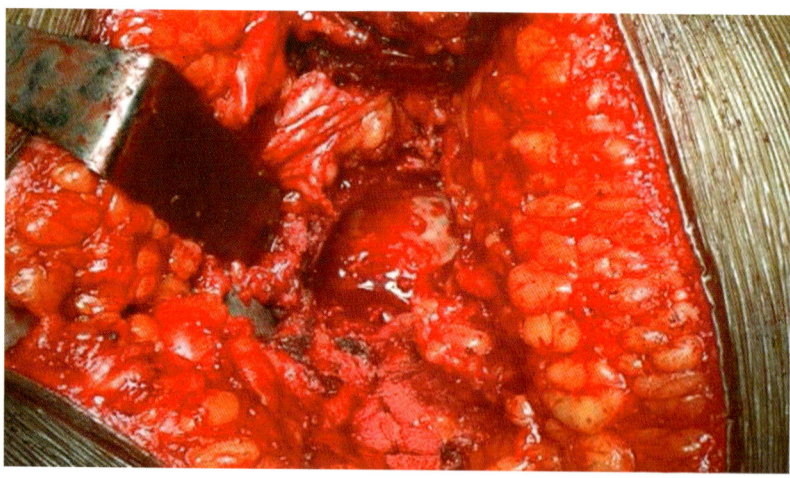

Once the true acetabulum is identified it is reamed till all cartilaginous tissue is removed and bleeding cancellous bone is visualized.

The interior of the acetabulum is now inspected to ensure uniform bleeding cancellous bone all around.

Judicious placement of Homman retractors, allows a three sixty degree visualization of the acetabulum.

Using a large mop, the interior of the acetabulum is packed dry and re-inspected to ensure uniformity and adequacy of reaming.

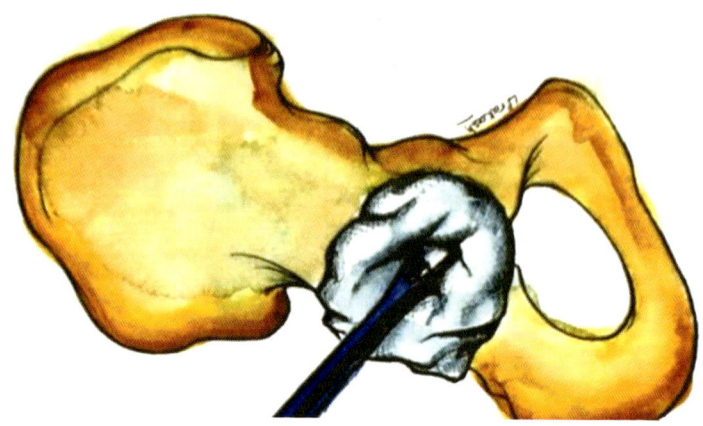

Using measurement gauges, the acetabular dimensions are measured. The outer diameter of the cup to be used would be 3 to 4 mm smaller than the reamed interior of acetabulum to give a two to three millimeter of uniform cement mantle.

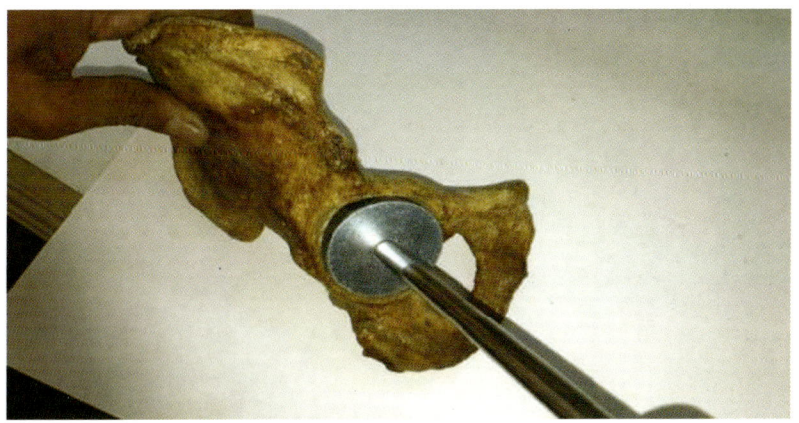

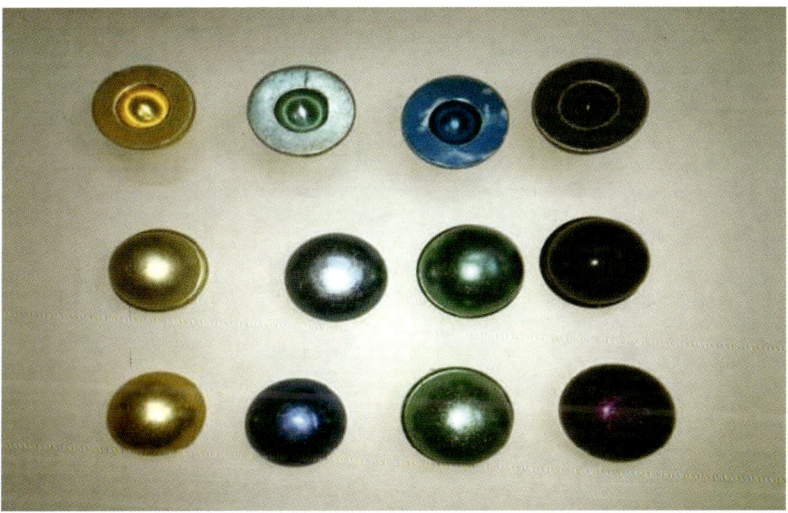

Trial cups are available in various sizes and at this stage the surgeon decides on the appropriate cup size that is eventually going to be cemented.

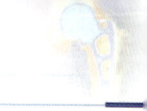

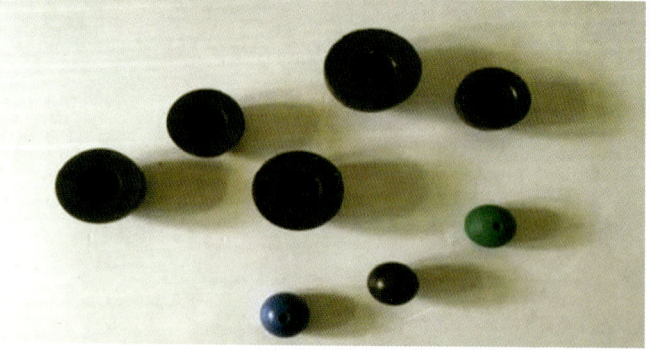

Using a 6.5 mm drill bit with a stopper, 12 to 16 holes are made in the acetabulum in all directions.

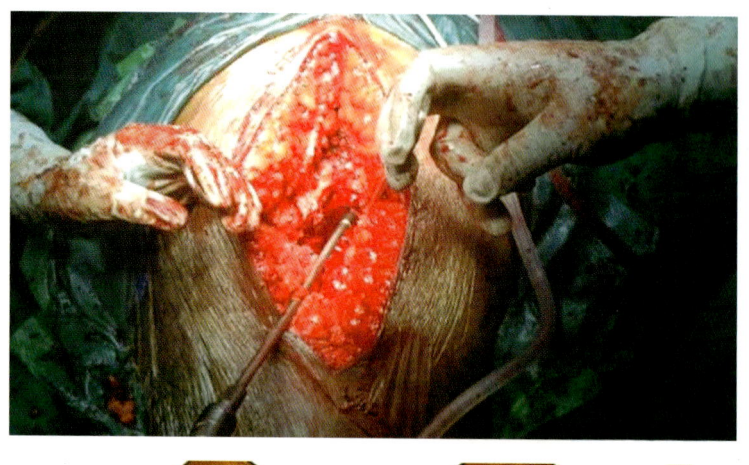

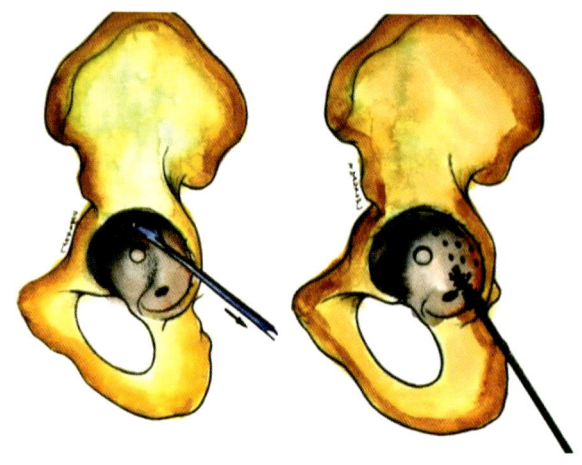

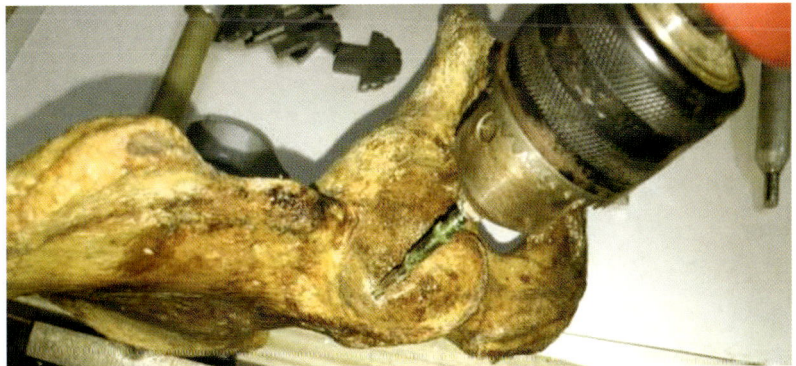

Some surgeons defer this step to just before cementation because they feel that the cancellous holes will bleed. The author drills them at this stage itself and packs the cavity.

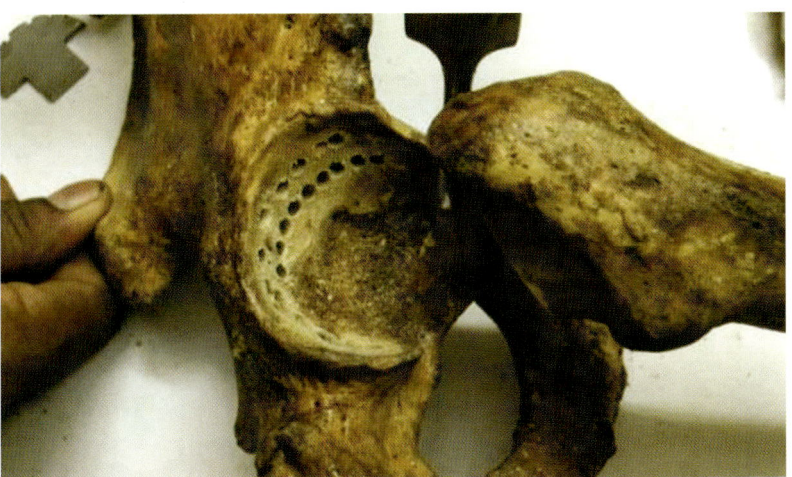

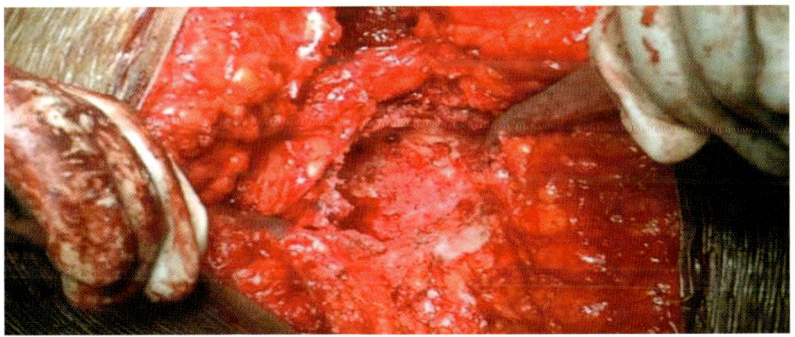

If cement anchorage holes have been drilled into the acetabulum, a large mop soaked in adrenaline saline is packed into the cavity to reduce bleeding from the reamed and drilled cancellous areas.

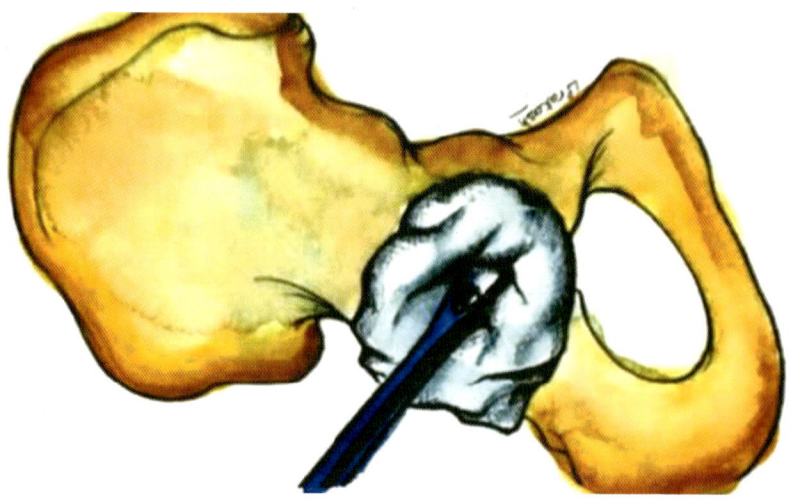

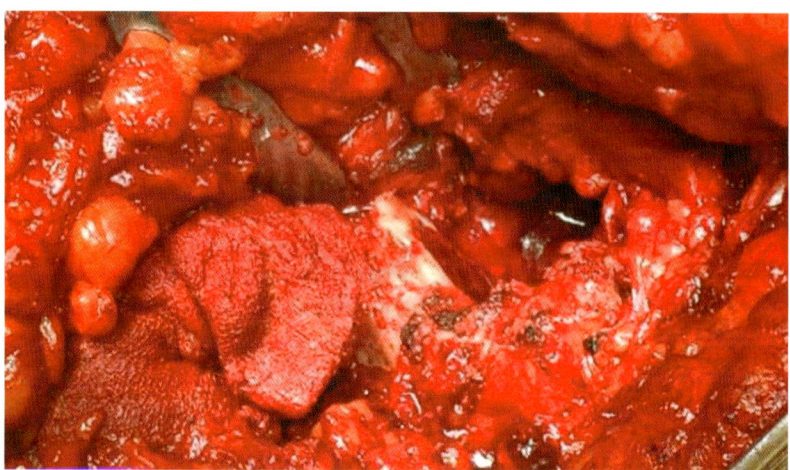

Correct placement of Homman retractors, and full internal rotation, brings forth the neck in the correct position for reaming.

The point of femoral entry in the posterior aspect of neck is identified.

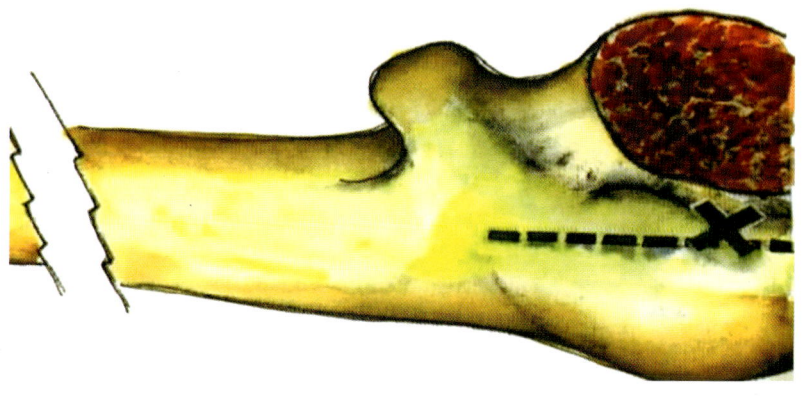

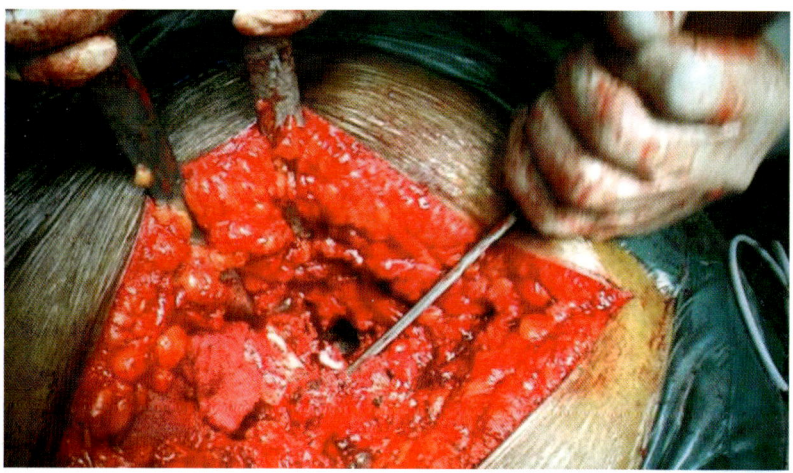

Using a long chisel, the posterior aspect of the neck is gouged, producing an entry point for the box chisel to be used in the next step.

During femoral reaming, the assistant keeps the knee flexed, controls the rotation and pushes it upwards to produce counter traction during reaming and broaching.

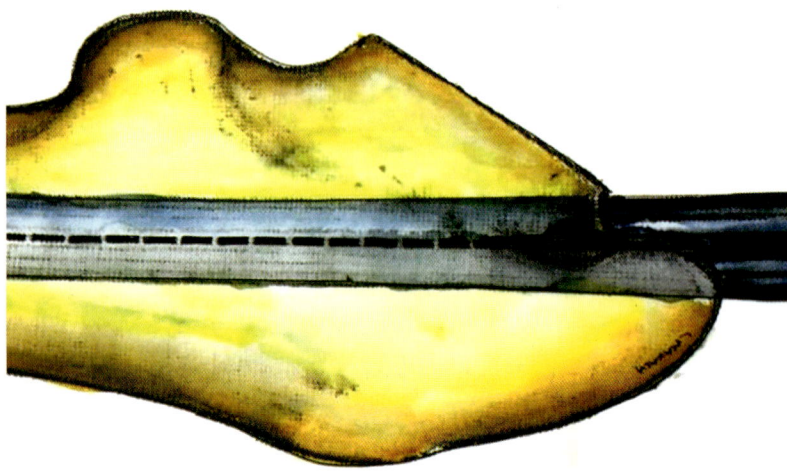

The femur is reamed and broached to allow a smooth entry of the prosthesis and permit an uniform 2 mm cement mantle all around the femoral component.

This is an important step, and any mistakes here would result in a varus prosthesis which is unacceptable.

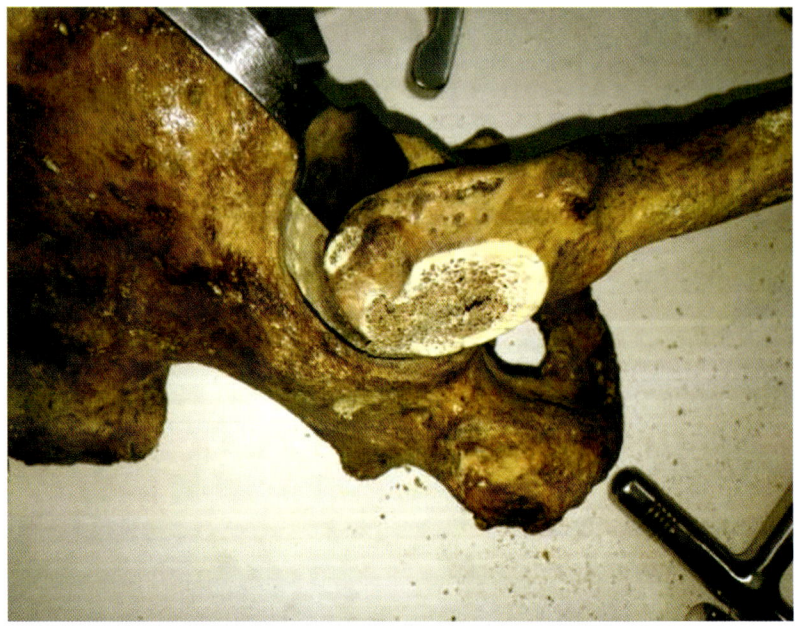

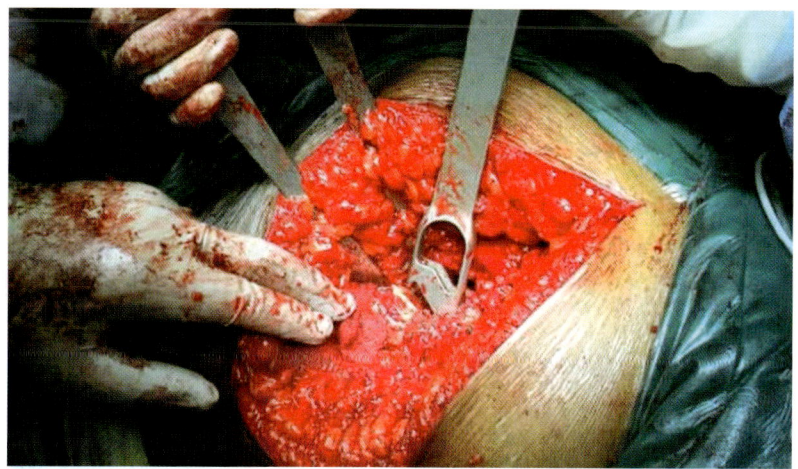

A box chisel is now introduced. The first push is posteriorly towards the trochanteric fossa. It is then brought down in line of the femur.

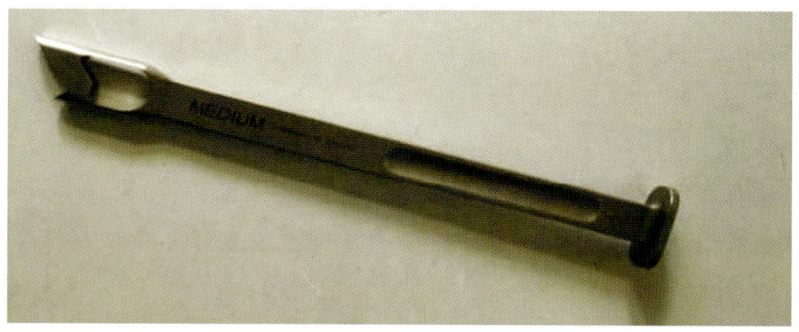

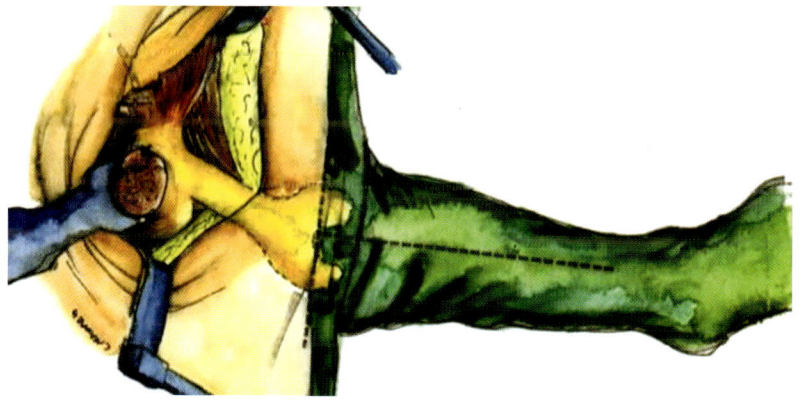

It is essential to go far back into the trochanteric fossa and remain ten to fifteen degrees deviant from the lesser trochanter to get the position and version correct.

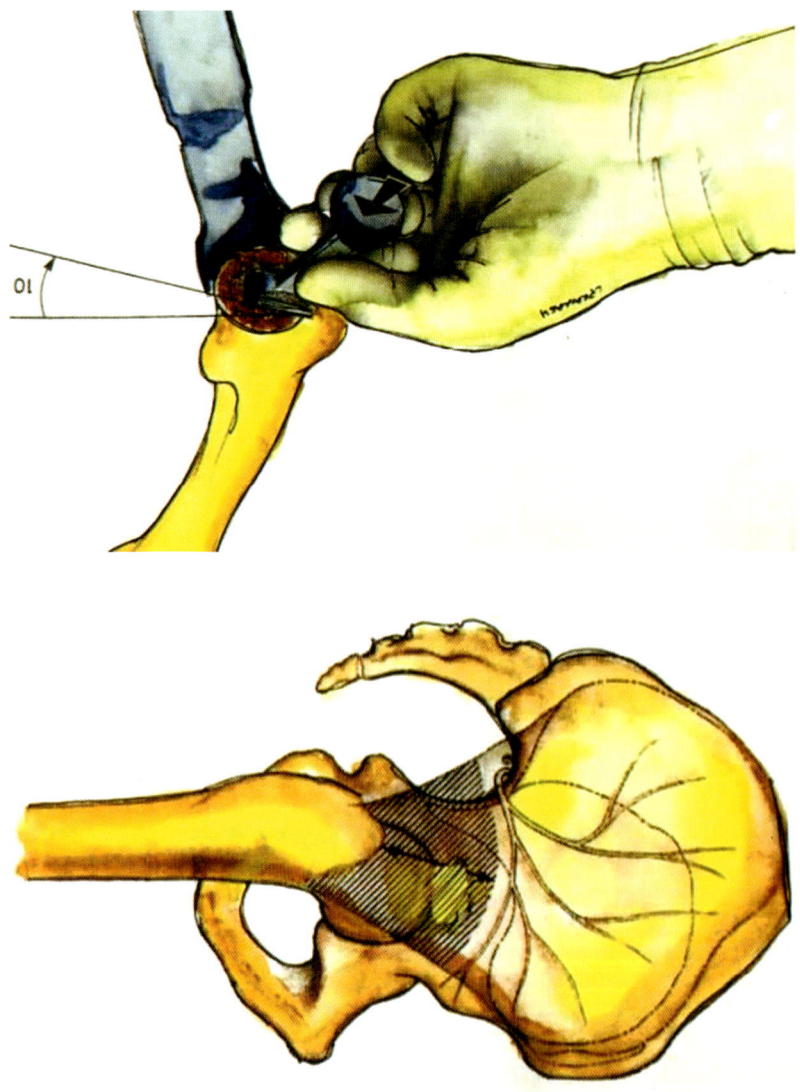

This is a fairly important step because the box chisel introduction inclination defines the femoral version.

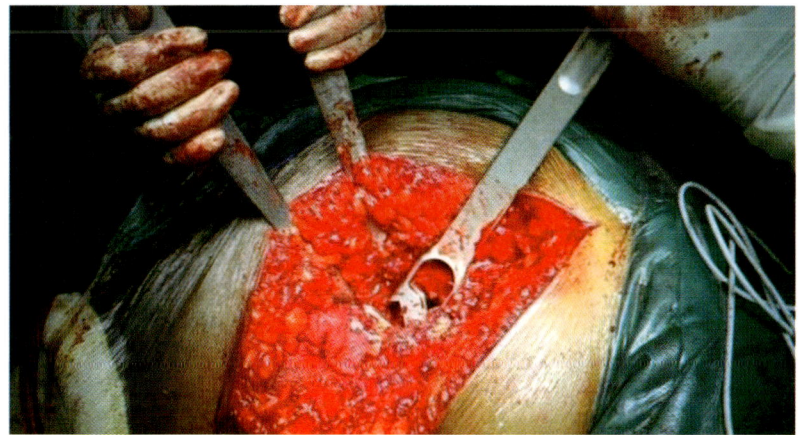

A rule of thumb is to stay fifteen degrees deviated from the direction in which the lesser trochanter points. This would provide a fairly satisfactory version.

It is important to remember that femoral anteversion differs from person to person and varies between males and females. Rather than use precise guides to give the perfect degree of version, a more scientific methiod is to follow the version trhat the patient already posseses.

The femoral neck is a fairly accurate indicator of the femoral version.

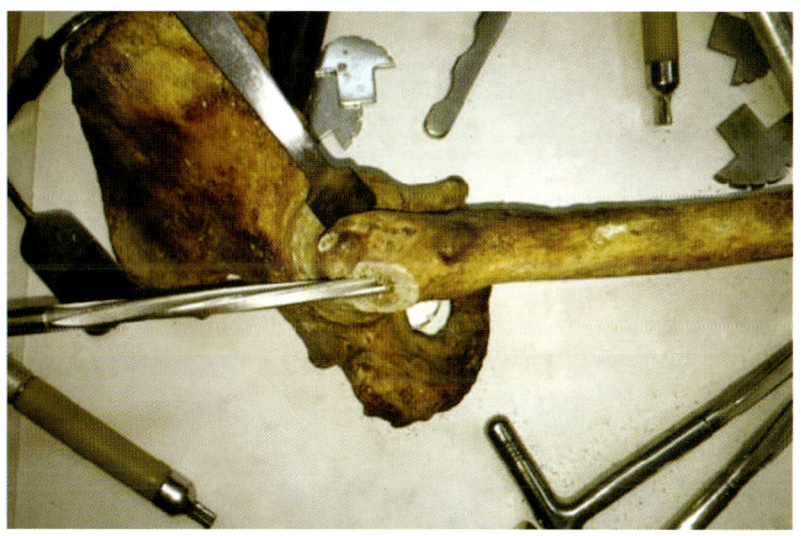

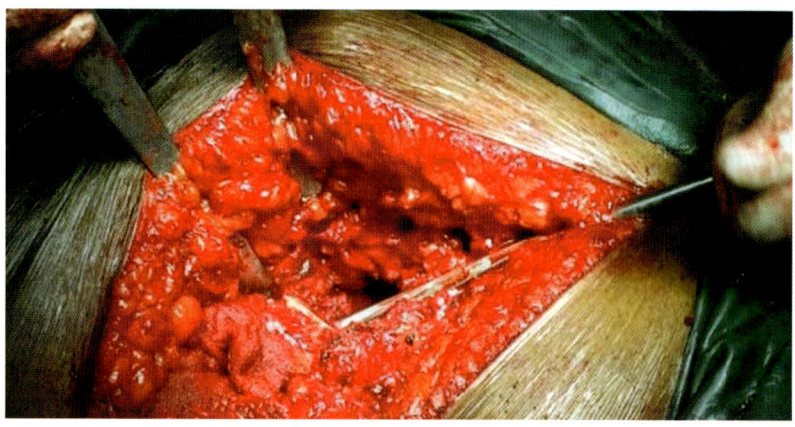

Using progressively large broaches, the femoral medulla is expanded to accommodate the prosthesis of choice.

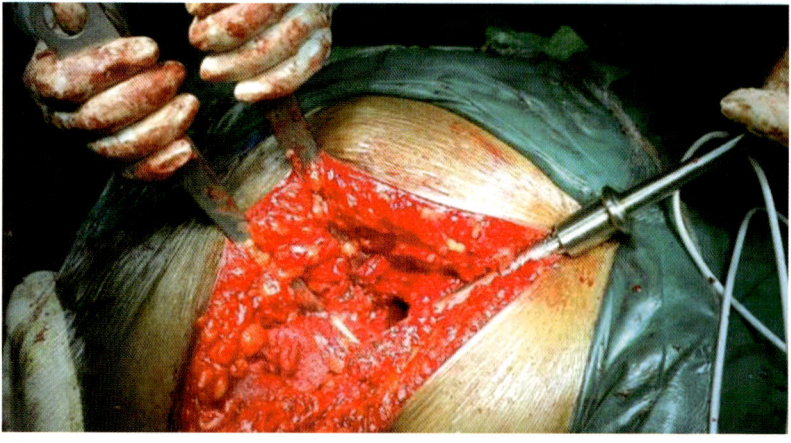

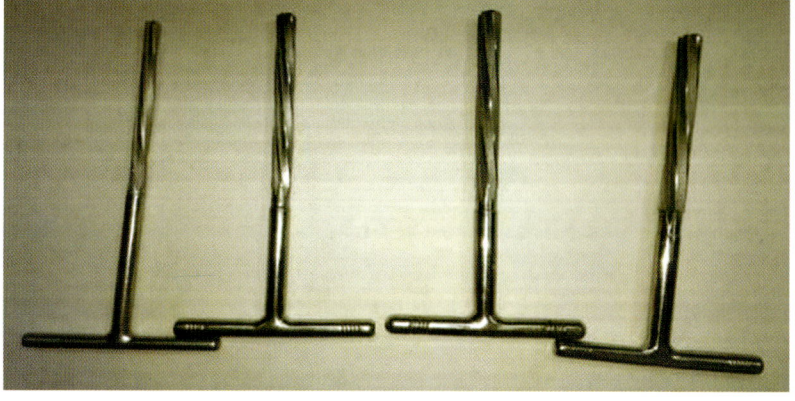

Femoral broaches are available both manual and power driven. The authors person preference is manual unless the bone is very sclerotic.

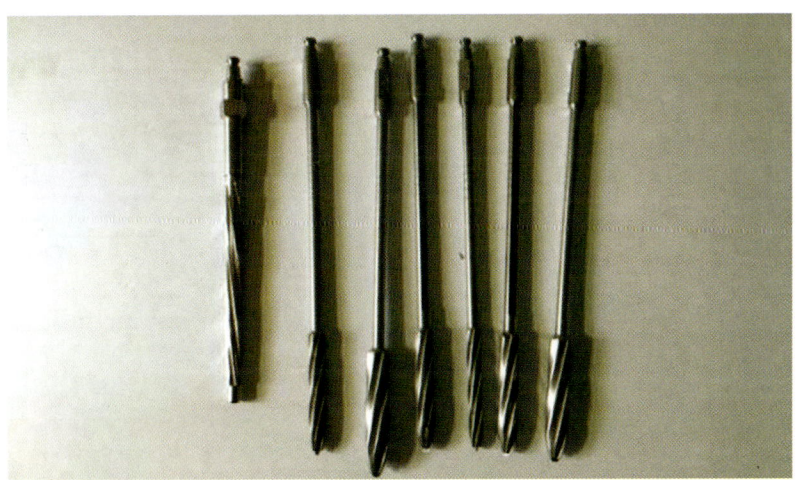

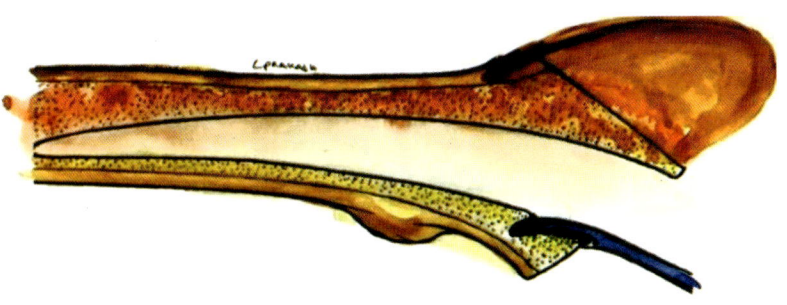

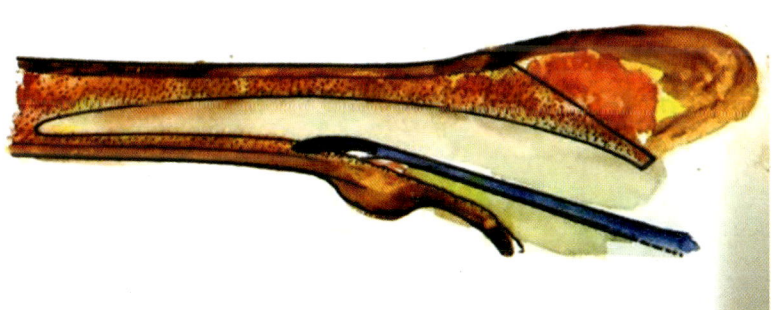

Using a sharp curette, the cancellous bone in the calcar area is expanded on all sides. This will ensure that the subsequent step if insertion of the femoral rasp becomes pain-free and easy.

The cancellous bone, spongy in nature has a tendency to grab the teeth of the femoral rasps necessitating hammering it out. A judicious use of curette before beginning rasping will ease the procedure.

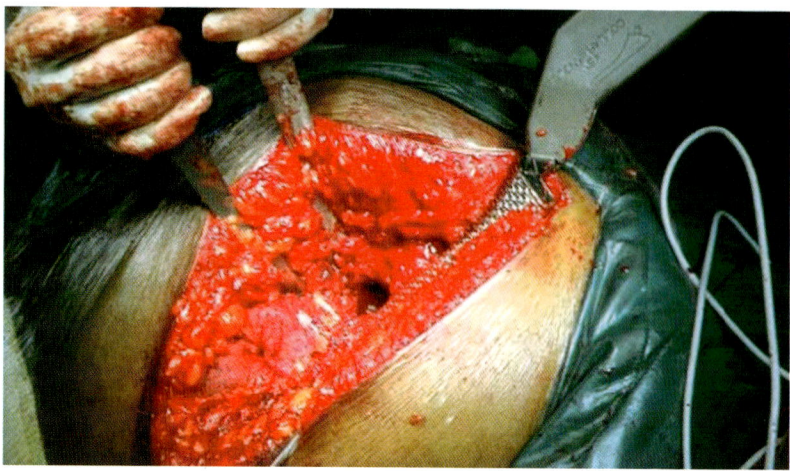

Appropriate sized rasps are used to decide the best fit and best size of the prosthesis.

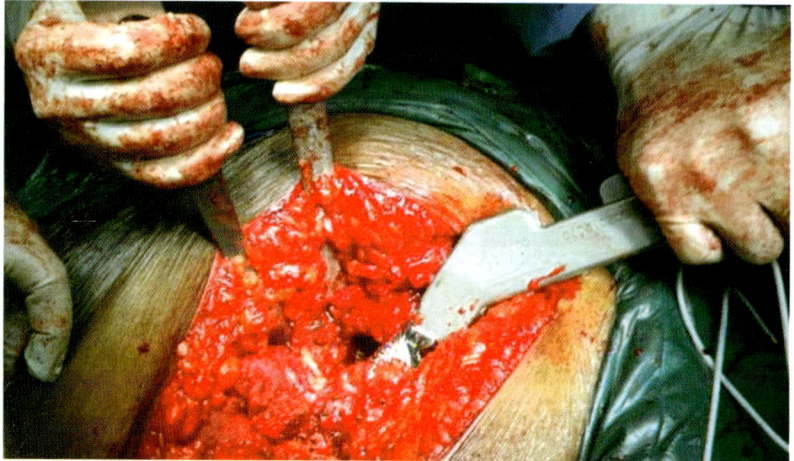

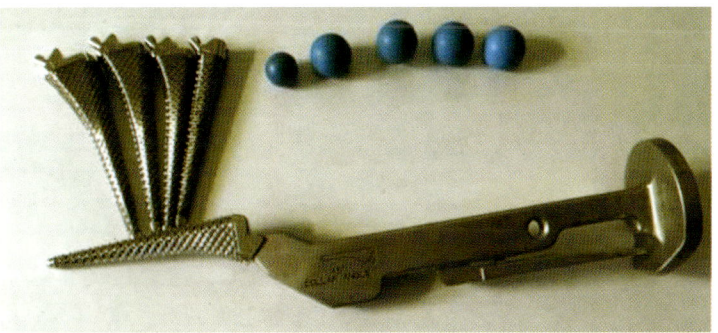

Different companies provide different designs of rasps to suit the prosthesis. They all have sharp spikes to open up the femur.

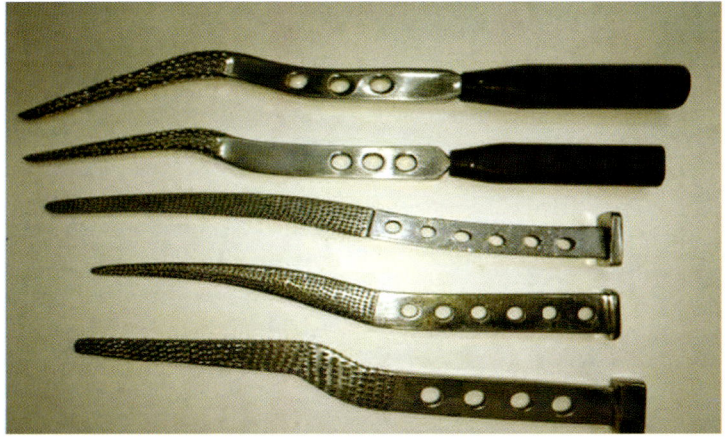

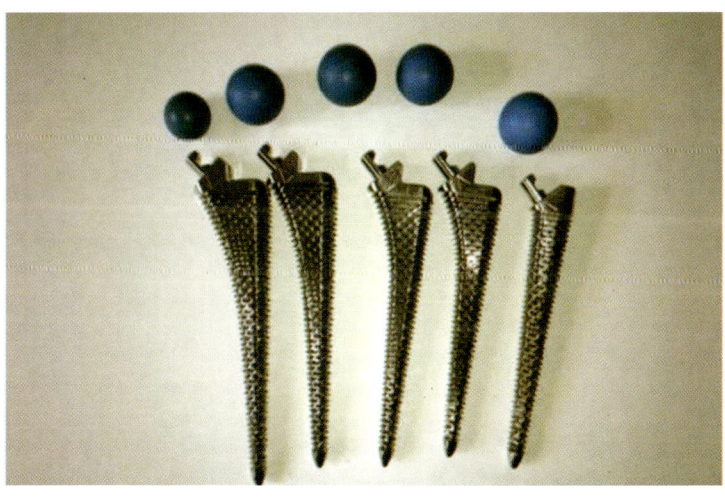

In most cases the rasps themselves can be used as femoral trials, by attaching the head balls.

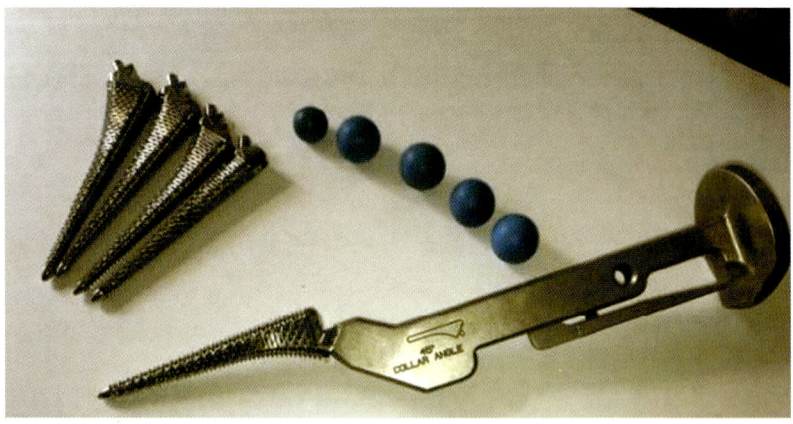

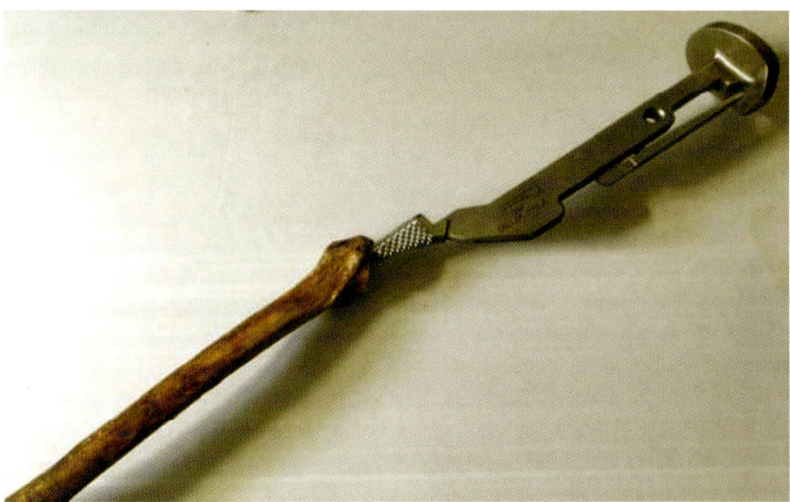

The rasp should seat well into the femoral stem with a good calcar fit, valgus orientation, in a correct degree of valgus, with a uniform space all around; for a decent cement mantle.

The rasp follows the pathway cut by the box chisel earlier.

It should enter as far back posteriorly as possible in the trochanteric fossa to enable a valgus placement of prosthesis.

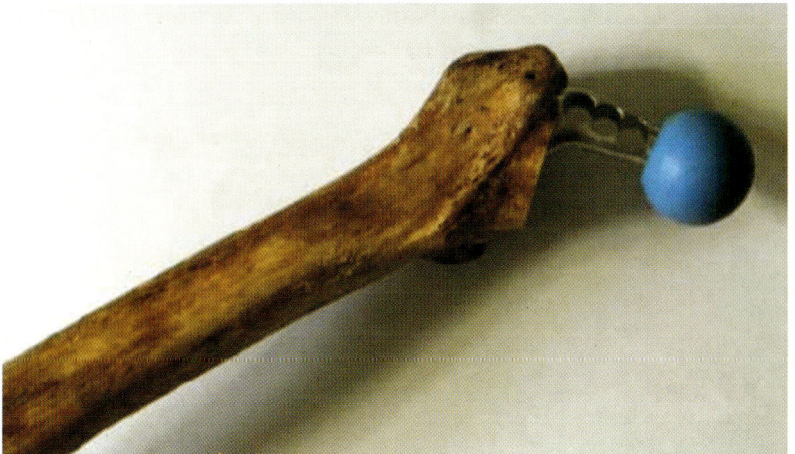

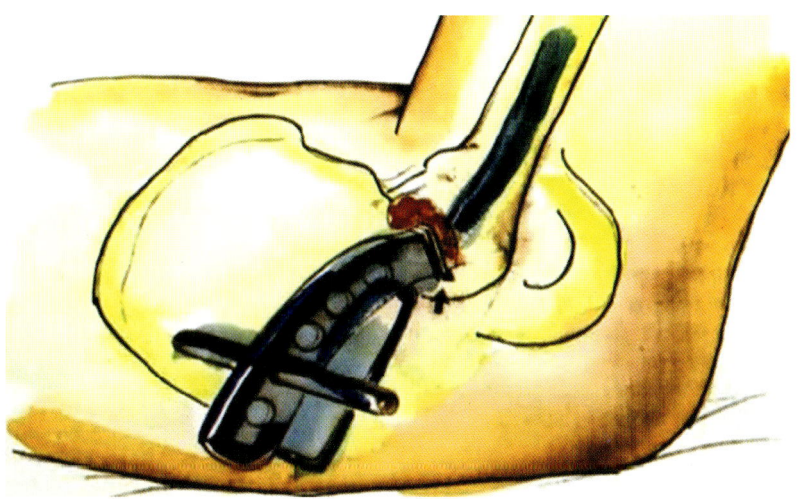

The assistant flexes the knee and applies counter traction against it as the rasp is pushed it.

It is preferable to use repeated filing movements to enlarge the femoral cavity, rather than use hammer and extractors.

In some instrumentation designs, the rasp doubles as a femoral trial, where after the handle is removed, a trial head is snapped on.

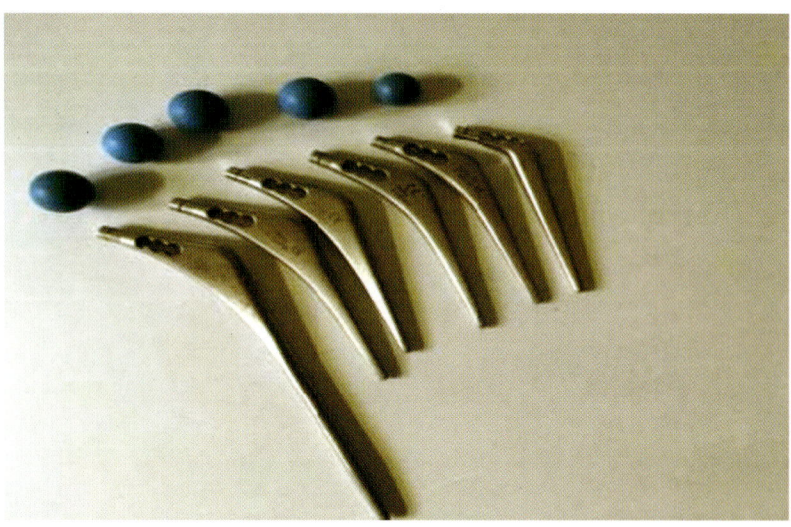

Depending on the prosthetic design, appropriate trials are available in the instrumentation set. An appropriate trial is now selected.

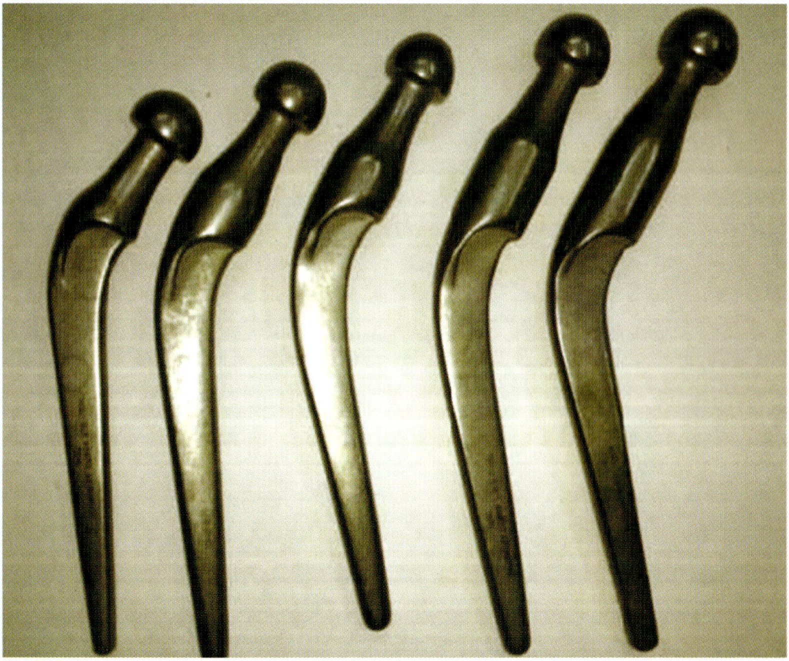

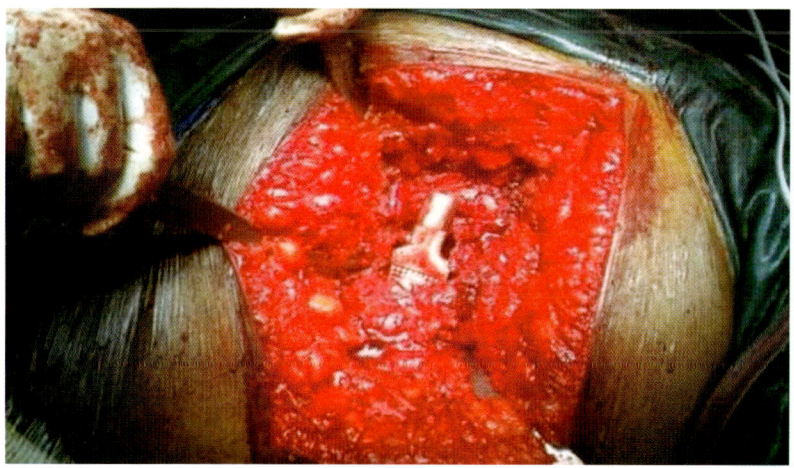

Acorrect trial prosthesis is now inserted and it is ensured that the stem gets deep down and allows a snug fit at the calcar. Also the proximal stem has to be positioned posteriorly to ensure a valgus orientation of the prosthesis.

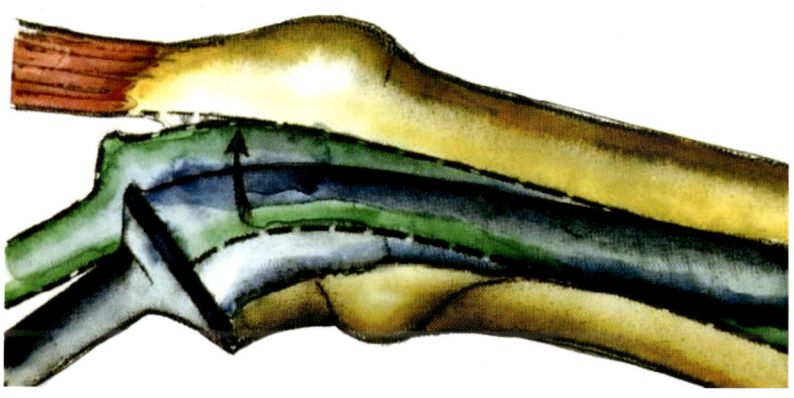

Here it has to be ensured that the anteversion of about fifteen degrees is maintained. Anteversion in hips varies between 12 and 16 degrees, and it is best to position the prosthesis in the same degree of version as the patient's earlier hip.

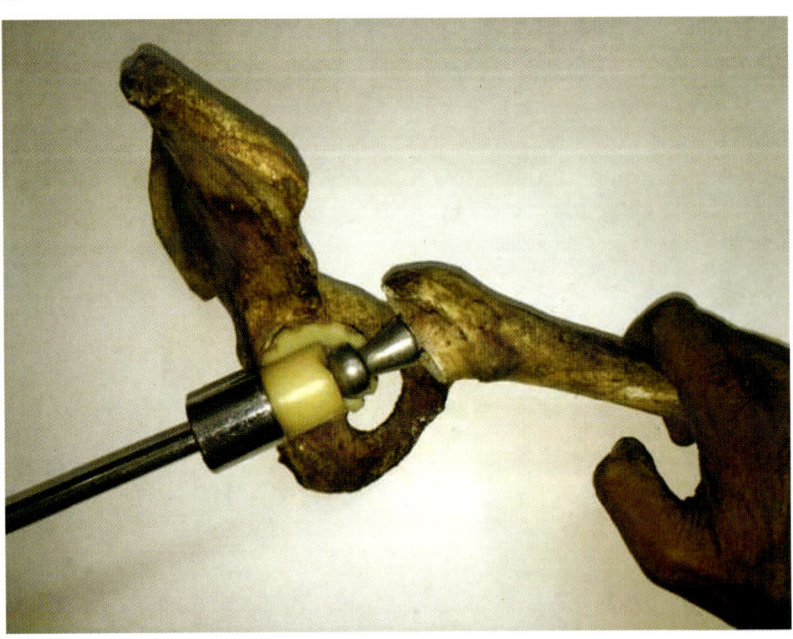

Error in prosthesis version is a sure recipe for disaster, and will certainly lead to an unstable hip and recurrent dislocations.

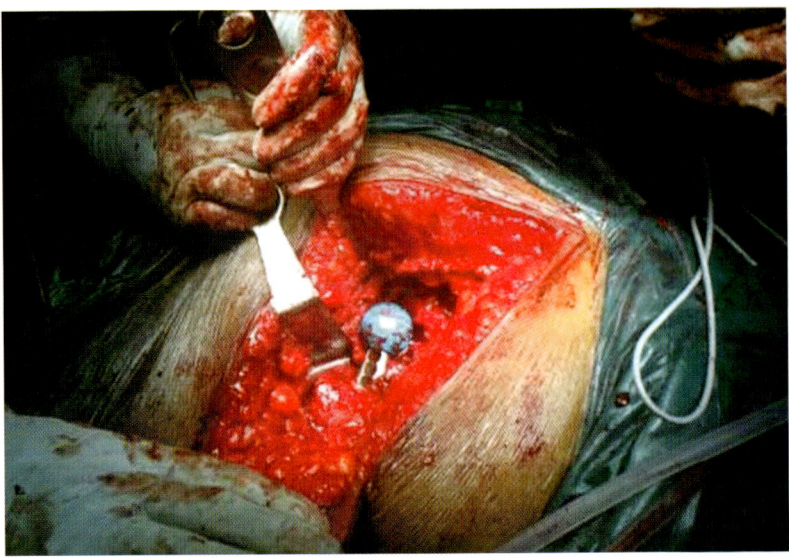

The trial femoral and acetabular components are inserted and a trial reduction is performed checking stability in motion in all directions.

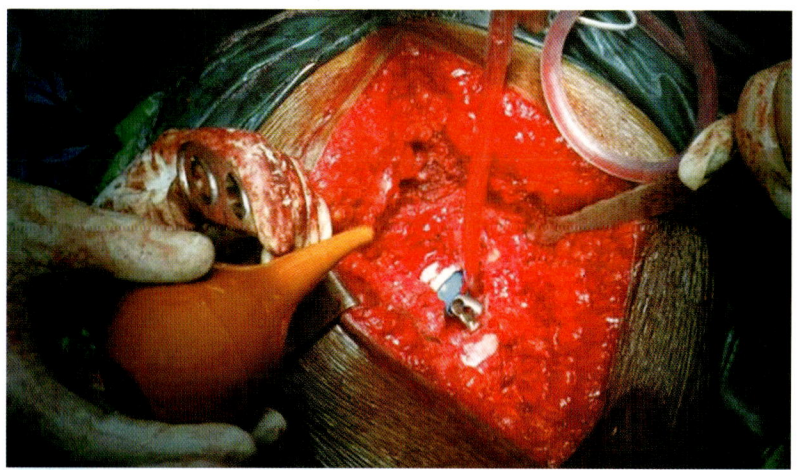

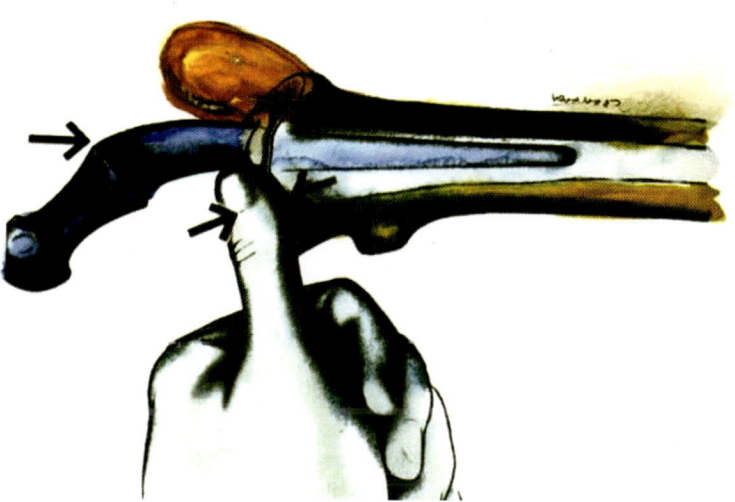

In cemented hips, it is necessary to make sure that the prosthesis is a loose fit, allowing a decent cement mantle all around the stem.

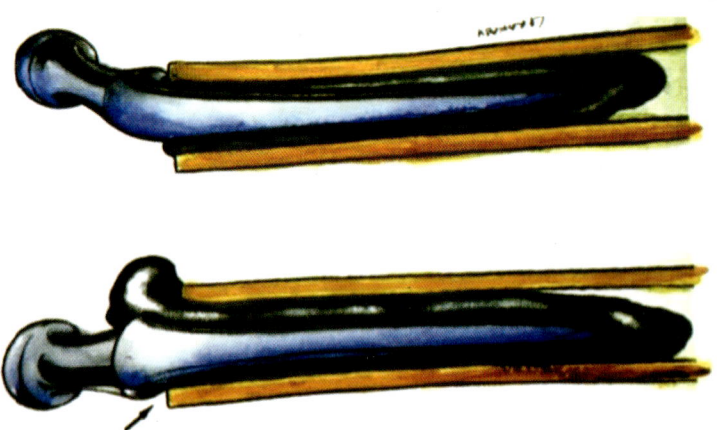

The acetabulum is now cleaned and swabbed. The cavity should be clean and dry during cementation.

A guaze soaked in adrenaline is packed tightly into the acetabular cavity and kept in place to produce a bone dry area prior to cementation.

The actual stem and cup are now unpacked from the boxes.

In the present case an Ogee cup is being used, and this requires templating. The cup template is placed on the rim of the acetabulum and the surgeon decides on the amount to be trimmed from the periphery.

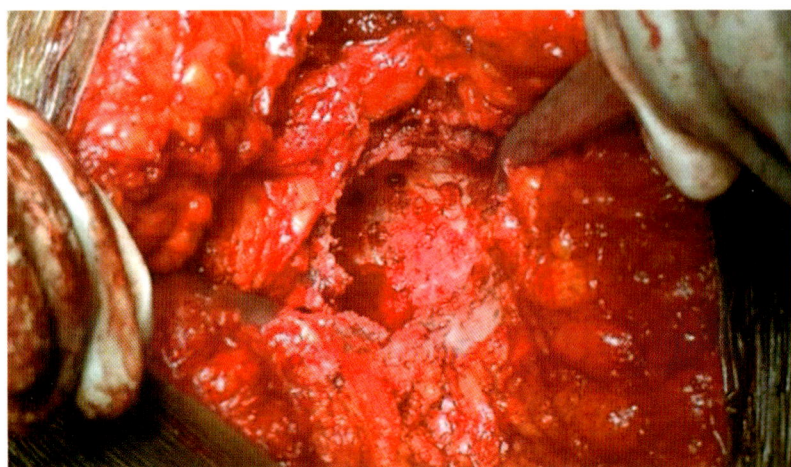

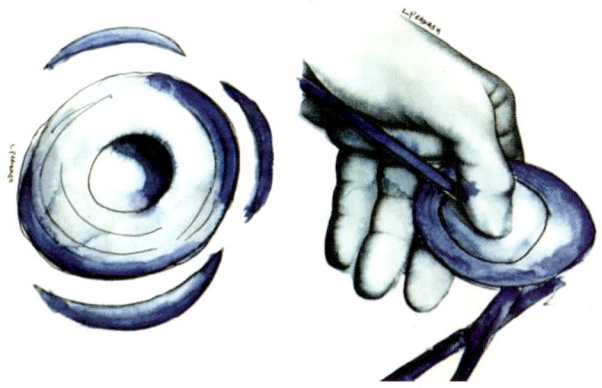

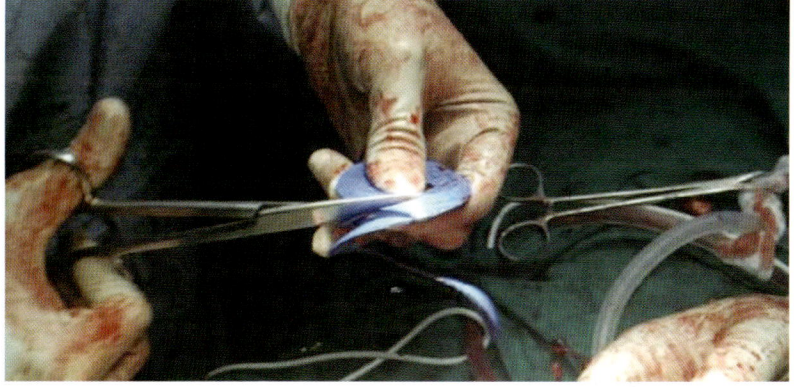

The markings on the blue plastic template allow for a precise cut and placing it on the acetabular margin allows the surgeon to fine tune the edges ensuring that there is no overhang.

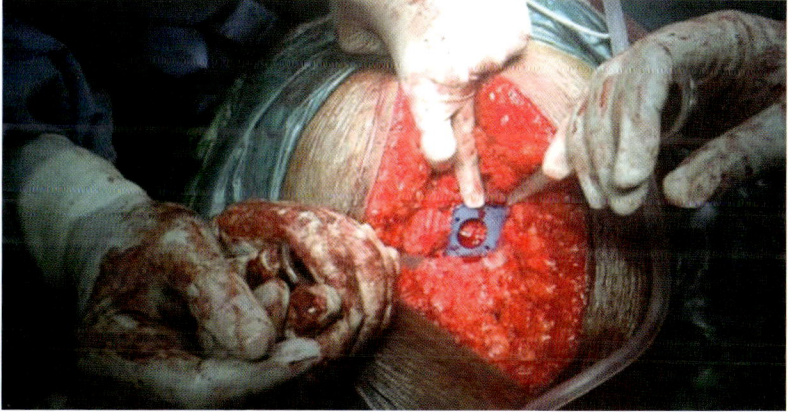

Placing the template on the cup, the flange is precisely trimmed. The cup is placed in the socket and the flange coverage is inspected.

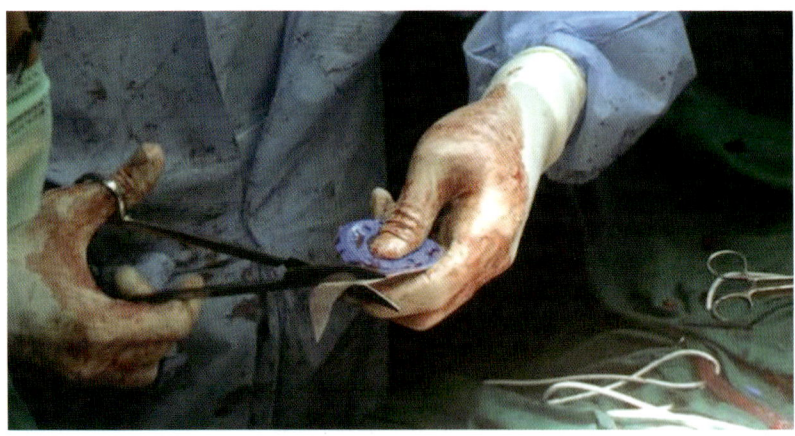

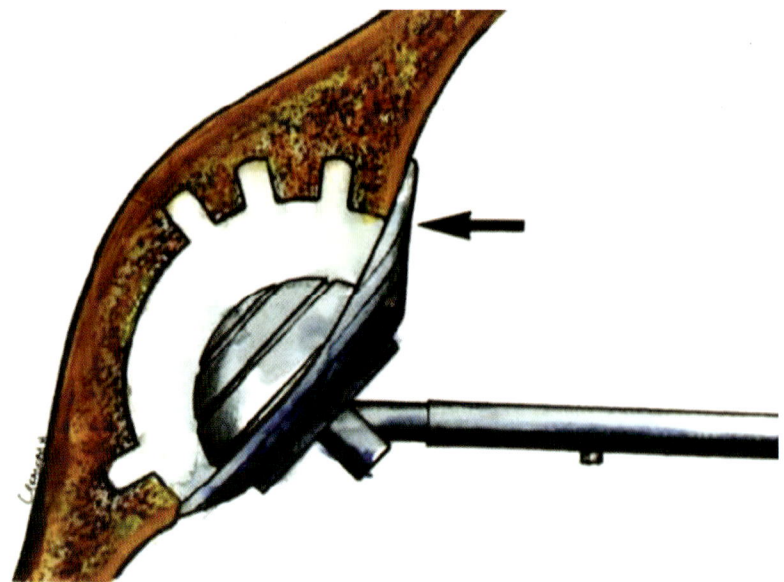

The flange should seat well along the entire perimeter of the well reamed acetabulum.

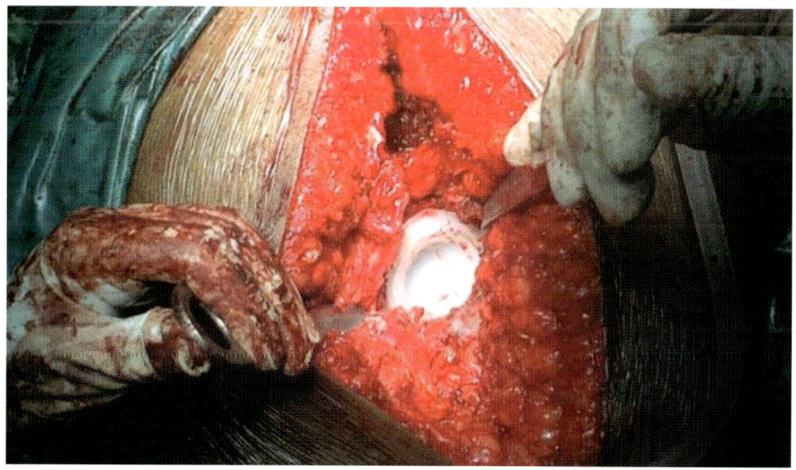

A flanged cup has an advantage that it pressurizes the cement circumferentially and allows for excellent cement bondage.

Another advantage which flanged cups possess for cementation is that; by looking at the resting of the flange over the rim of the acetabulum, we can ensure that the socket version is matched by the cup position. This acts as an additional aid to the acetabular positioning guides available in the instrumentation set.

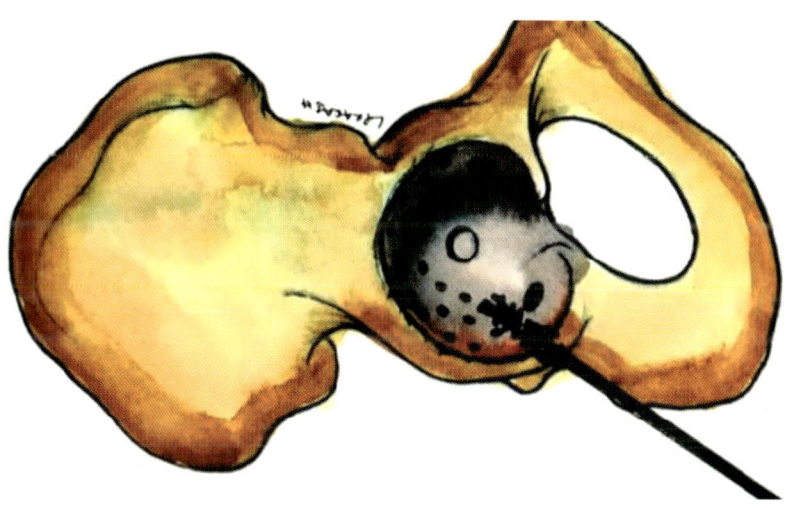

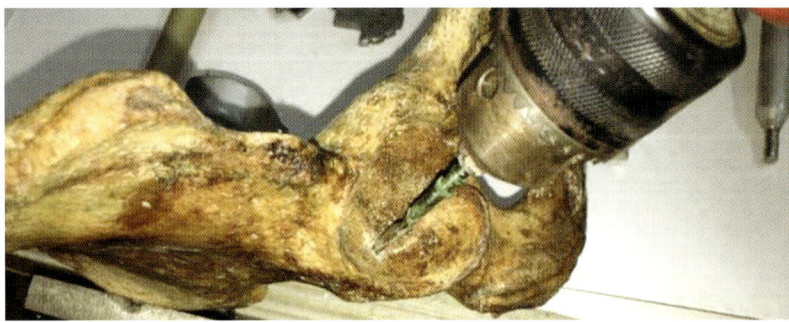

If the cement anchorage holes had not been drilled earlier, they are done at this stage.

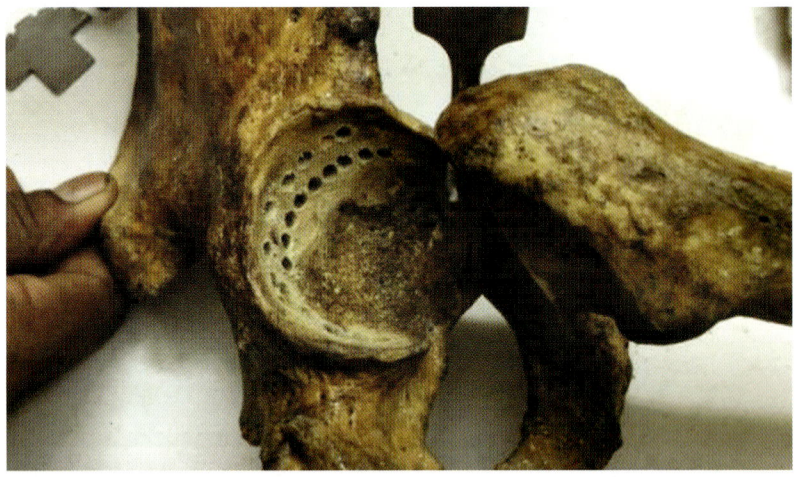

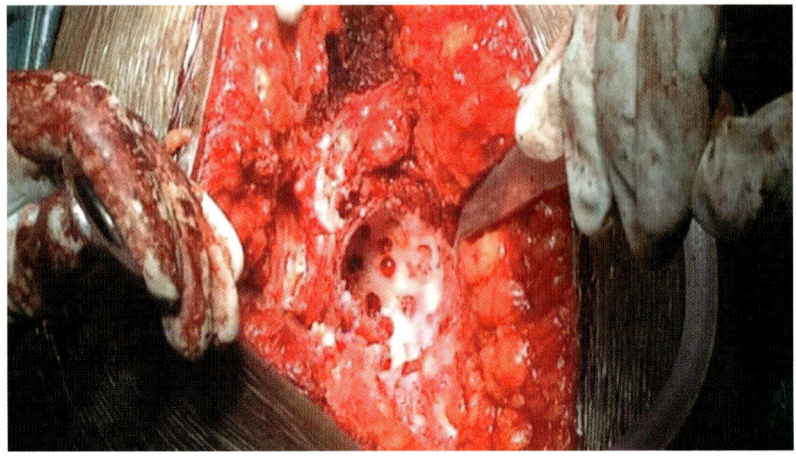

The acetabular cavity is tightly packed with adrenaline soaked pad to make it blood free and dry.

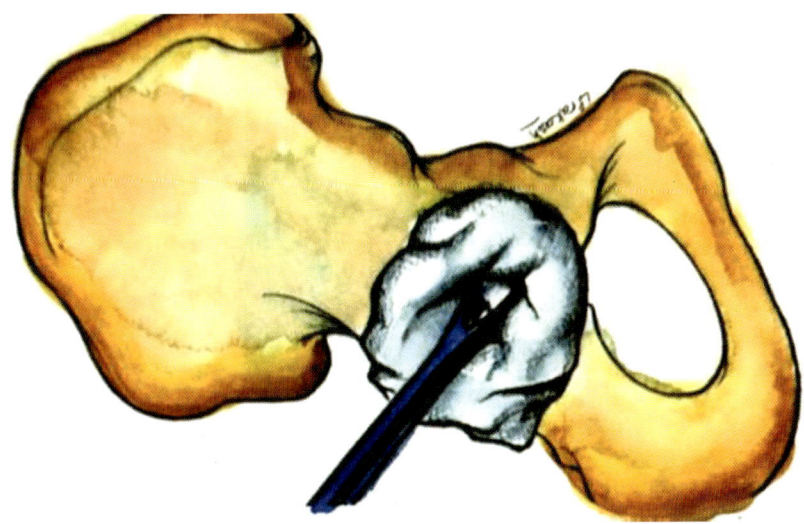

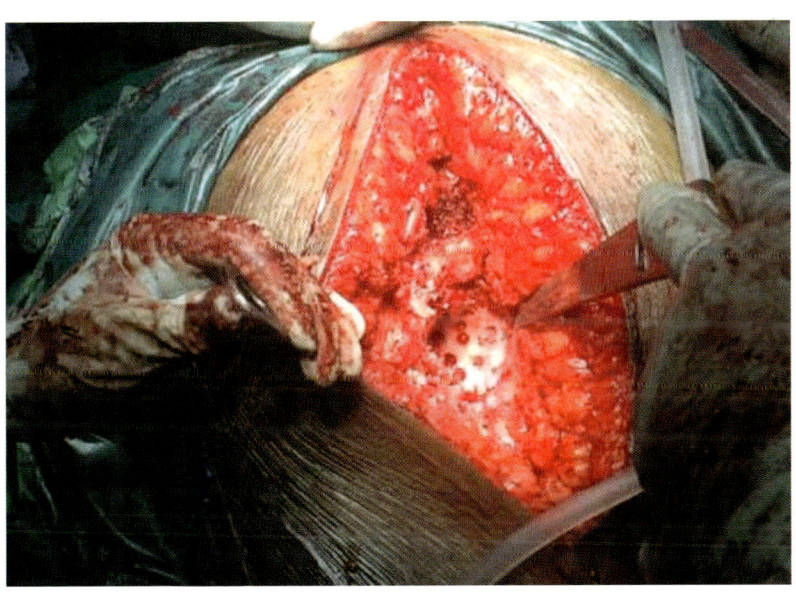

On removal of the swabs the acetabular cavity should be clean and dry. No blood or oozing should be present.

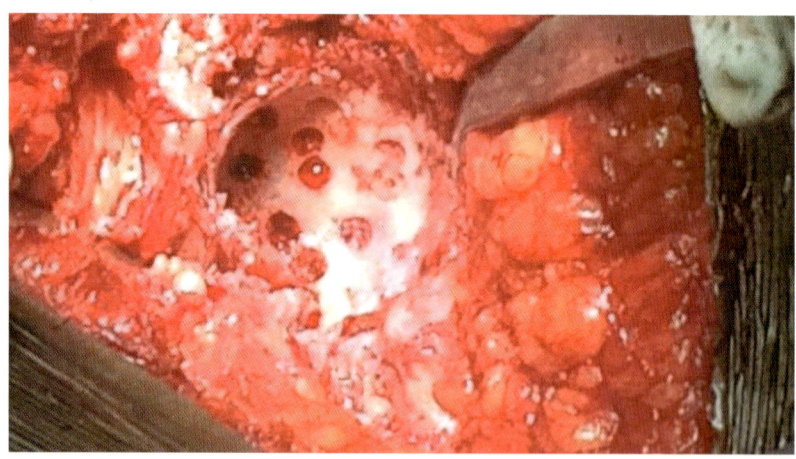

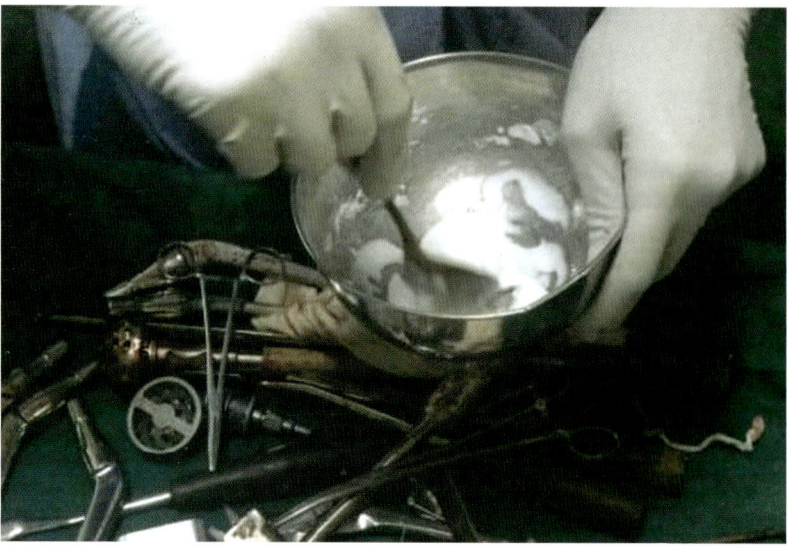

Cement is mixed and when it is in a fairly doughy stage, poured into a twenty cc syringe. A makeshift nozzle may be attached to the syringe.

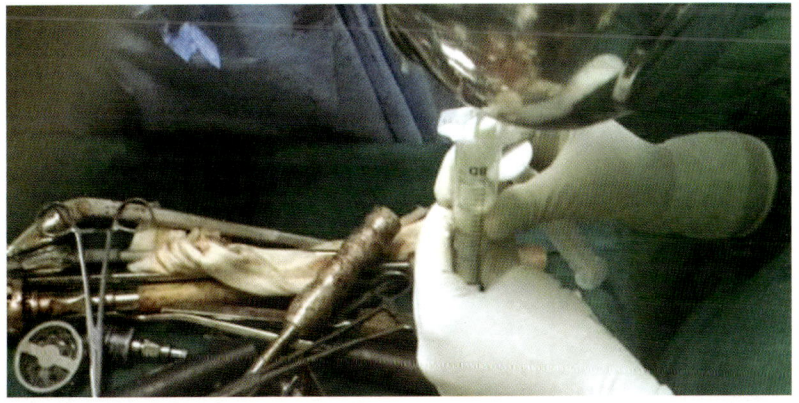

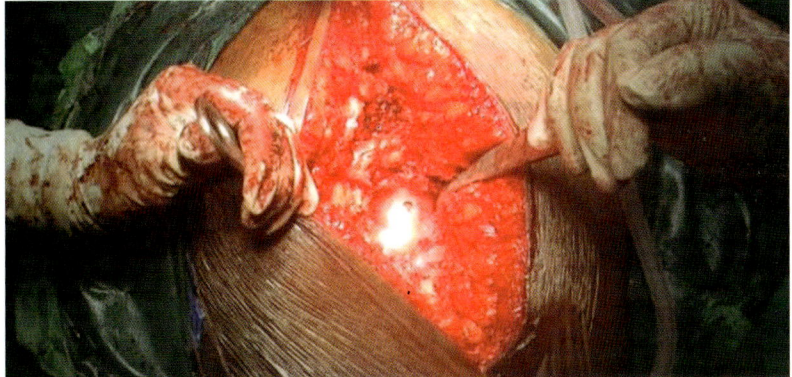

The acetabular pad is removed and cement is injected into the socket. Liquid cement flows into the anchor holes drilled earlier.

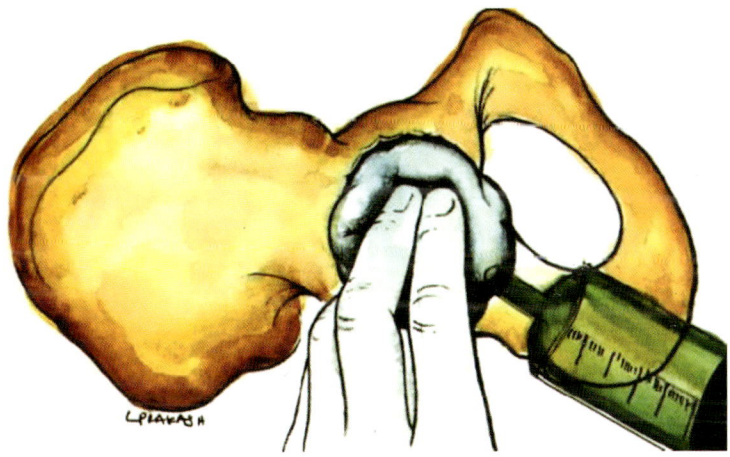

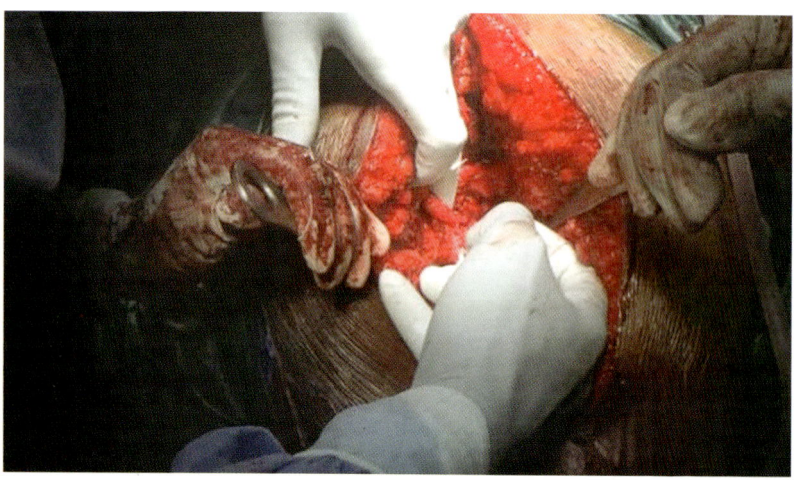

Using a syringe ensures that the cement surface is blood free and the HDPE – PMMA bondage will be firm.

Using liquid cement ensures that the acrylate flows well into the numerous cement holes for a better cup anchorage.

Using a flanged or Ogee cup ensures that the cement is presurrised without leaks as it sets to allow for a firm anchorage.

A dry acetabular cavity before cement introduction is essential for a deceent cement cancellous bone bondage.

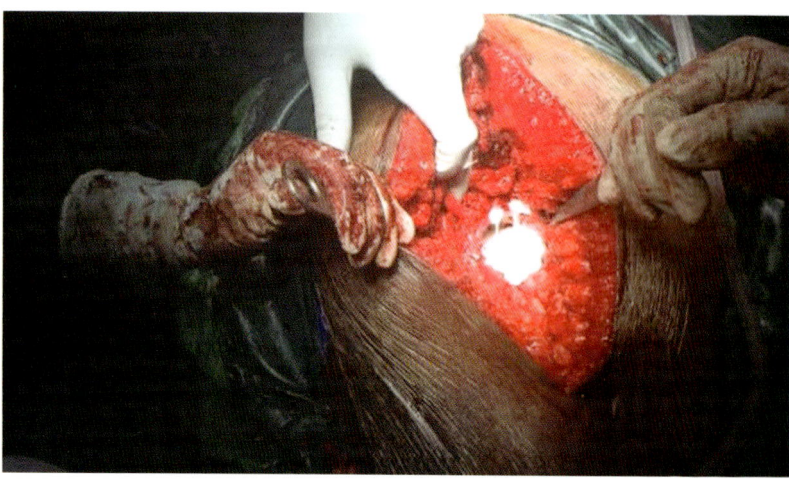

After ensuring that the cement surface is totally blood free, the cup is inserted in the correct orientation. A sustained pressure is maintained as the cement sets.

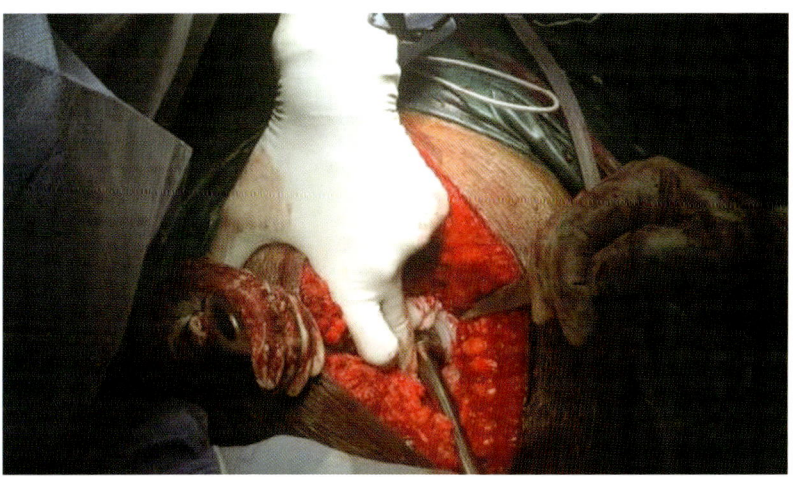

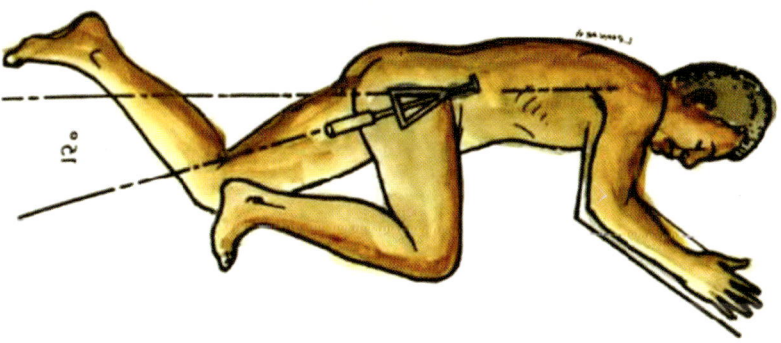

Precise and proper orientation of the cup is probably one of the most important aspects of this procedure.

The trick is the cup orientation in 45 degrees tilt and fifteen degrees version. An acetabular guide locates this position.

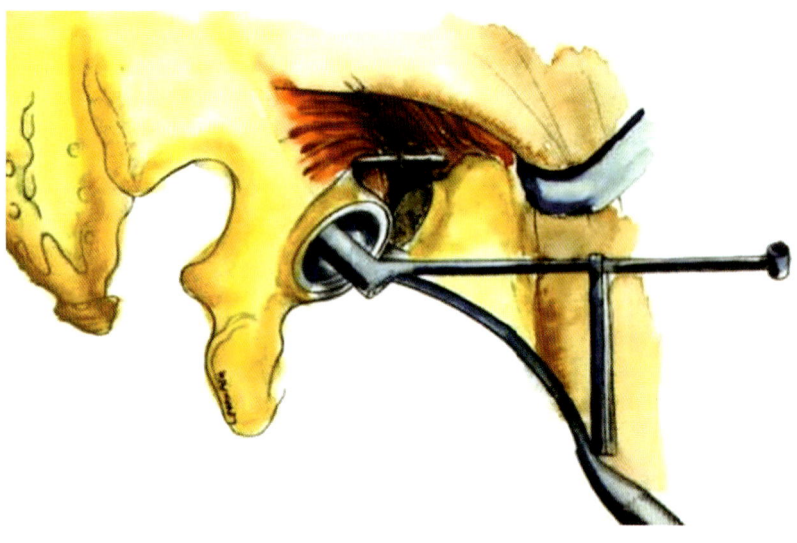

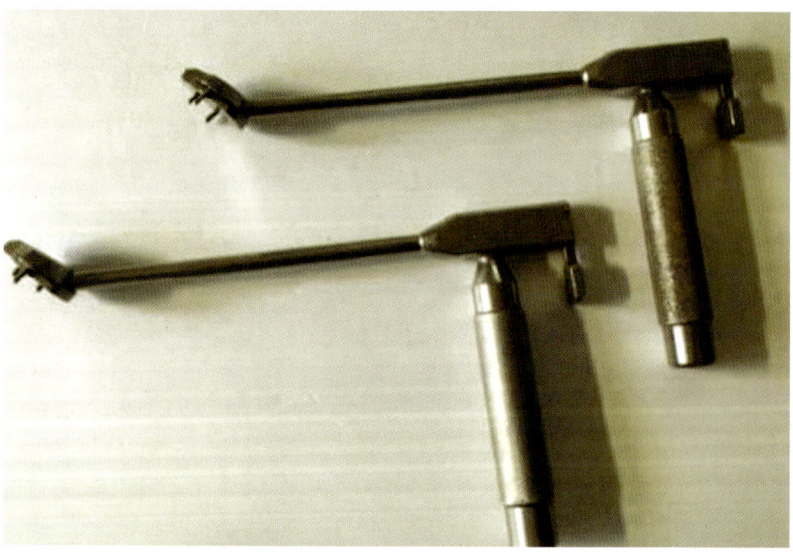

Most instrument sets have acetabular guides, which will seat the cup in this position.

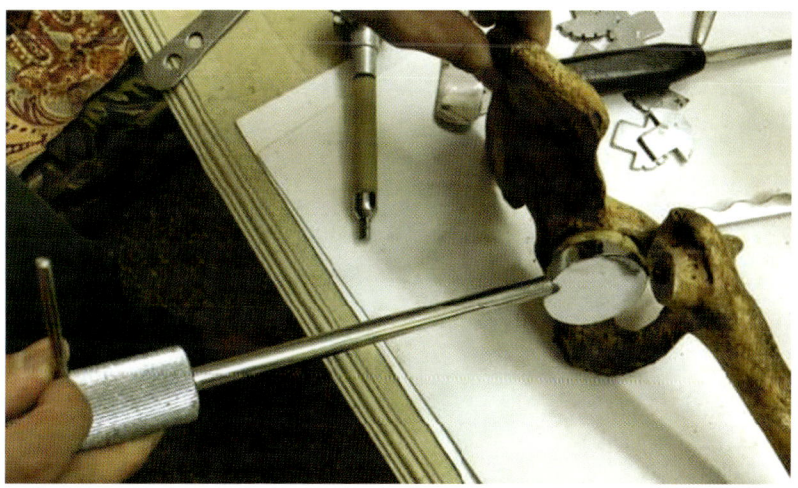

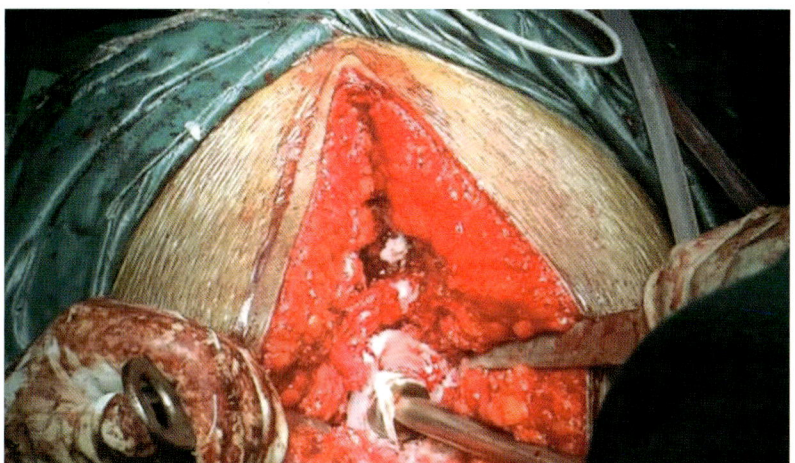

Many instrument sets have guides to align and position the cup precisely; however the rule of thumb is to keep the cup at forty five degrees to the pelvic axis and with a fifteen degree posterior overhang.

Long posterior wall cups, as in this case provide additional stability.

It should be ensured that the cup seats well in the acetabulum and the cup is well contained and has a uniform acetabular rim around it. Use of a flanged cup facilitates this.

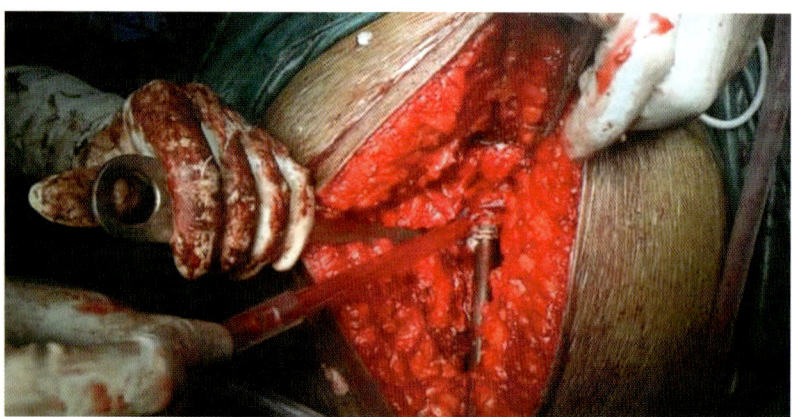

Sustained pressure is applied over the cup as the cement sets. Hammering of the cement weakens the mantle and should be avoided at all costs.

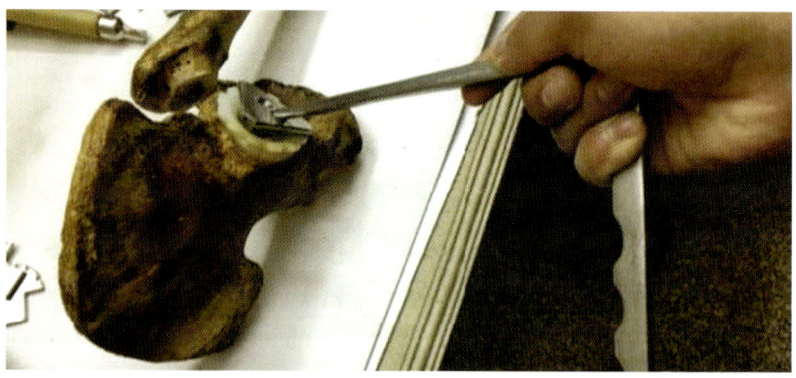

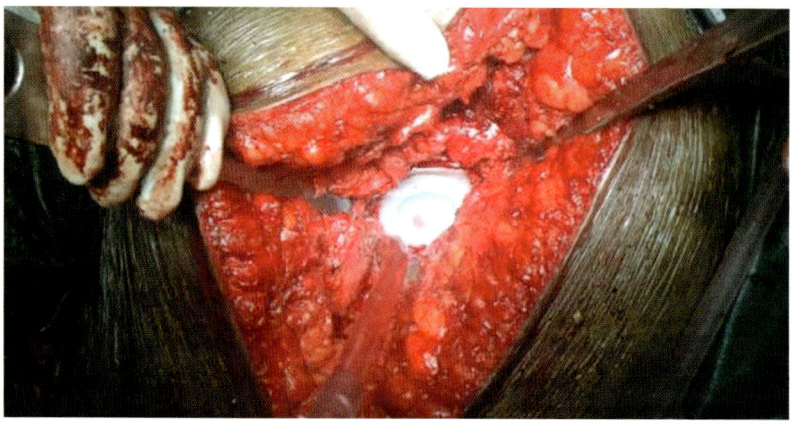

The cup is washed and loose cement bits are removed. It is inspected once again to ensure that the cementation has been done in the correct alignment and version.

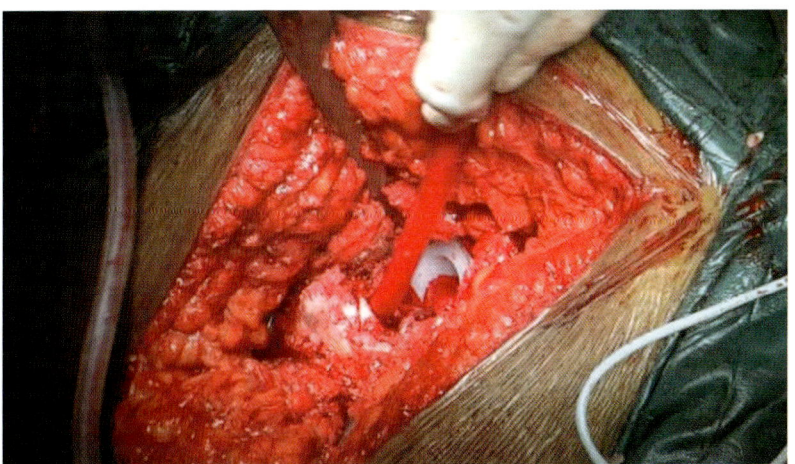

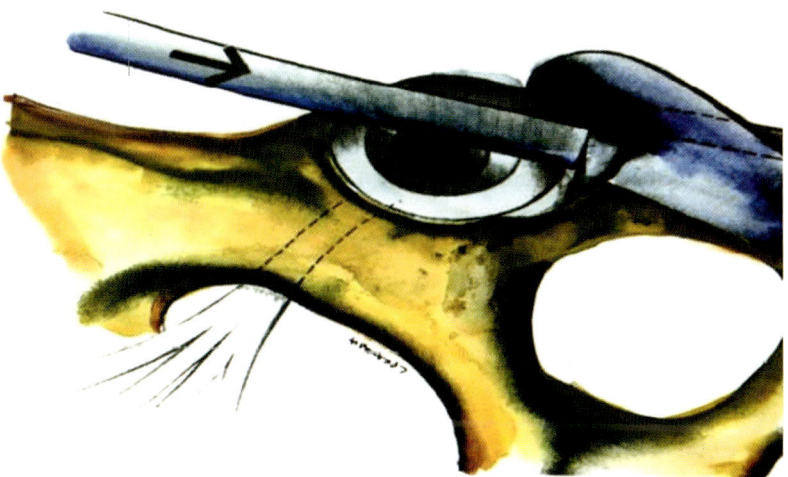

Excess cement which has set is now removed with a fine chisel. All overhanging, and loose cement should be meticulously removed.

This is one of the most important steps for the long term survival of the hip joint. Though metal on HDPE is an excellent bearing surface with less than half a millimeter wear in a year, an addition of the hard and rough methyl methacralate debris, floating bits or pieces, acts like a sand paper or file augmenting the wear tremendously and scratching the polyethylene cup interior.

A few minutes spent at this stage will give the patient a few years of extra life for the implasnt.

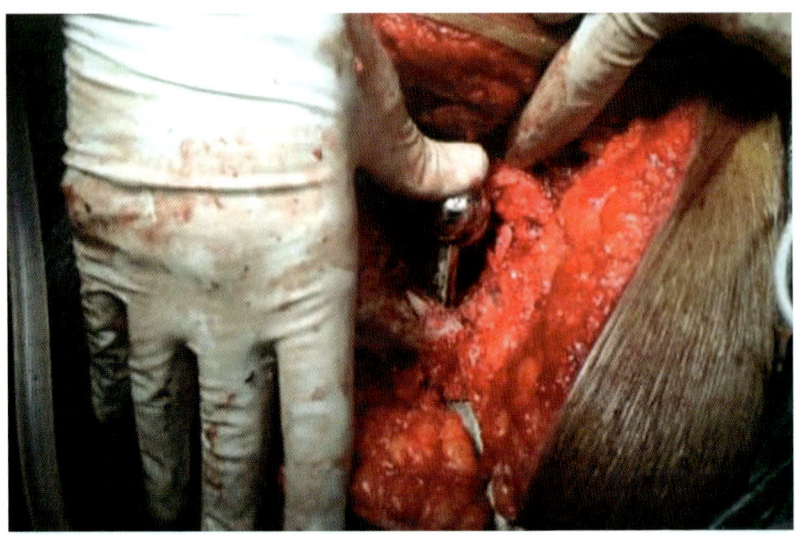

The femoral medulla is now sucked dry and cleaned.

The actual femoral component is inserted without cement, its position checked, and a trial reduction performed.

The hip should be stable in all ranges of movement and should allow twenty degrees of internal rotation in ninety degrees flexion, without uncovering more than 20% of the head.

As the neck sizes can be adjusted due to neck modularity, the right tightness of the hip is checked. If it is too tight, a shorter neck is used and vice versa.

Small defects in acetabular orientation can now be corrected by corresponding adjustments of femoral anteversion.

Using the lesser trochanter as a landmark, the femoral version is checked once again after reduction.

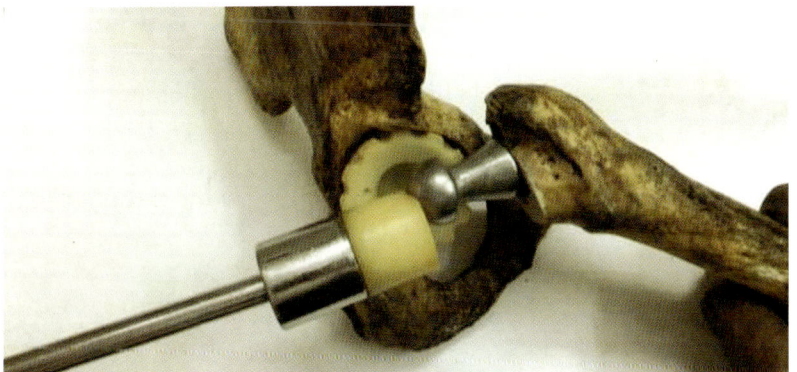

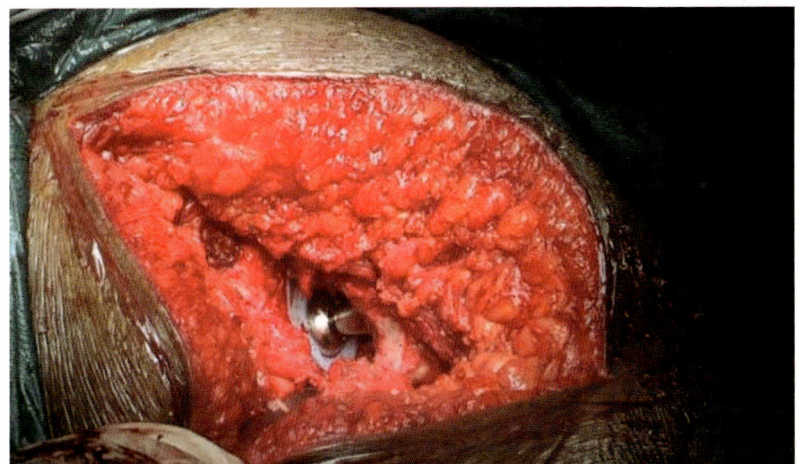

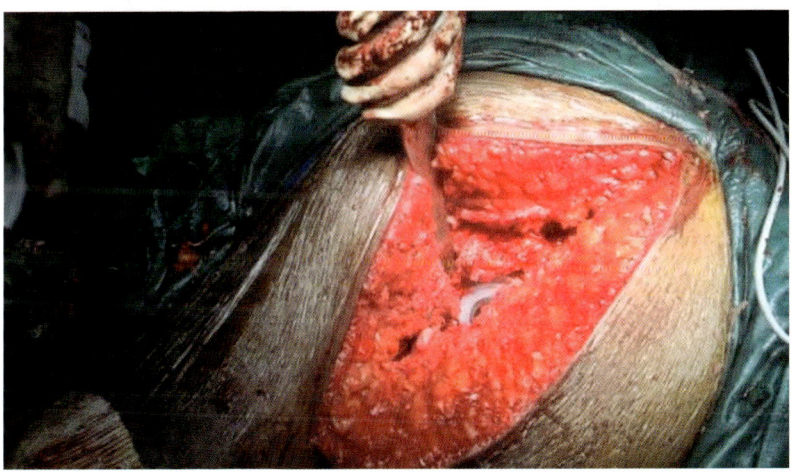

The hiup is put through full range of motion to ensure its stability.

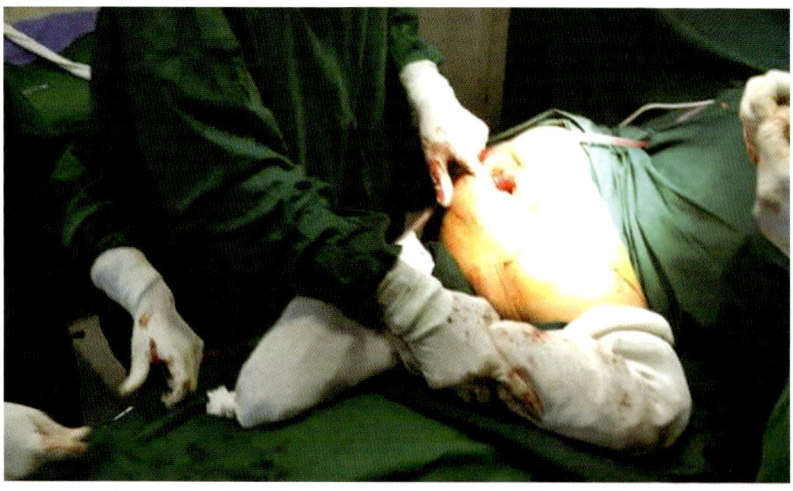

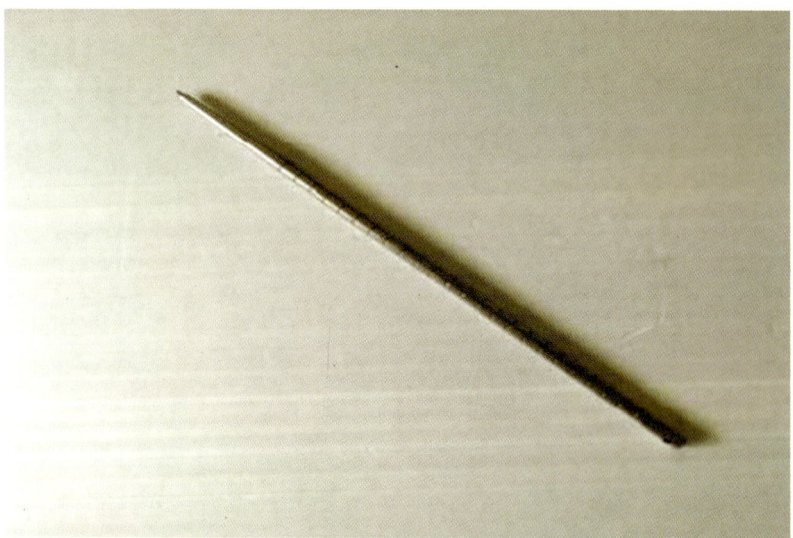

One can use either a conventional cement restrictor with a plastic plug, else a piece of cancellous bone removed from the head and cut into the appropriate shape.

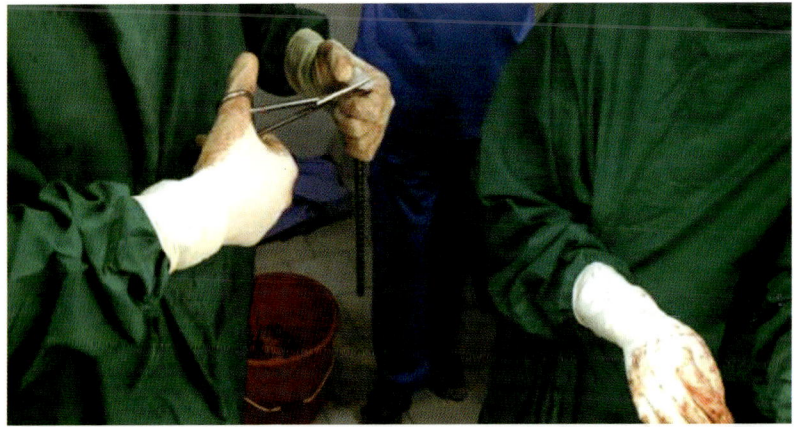

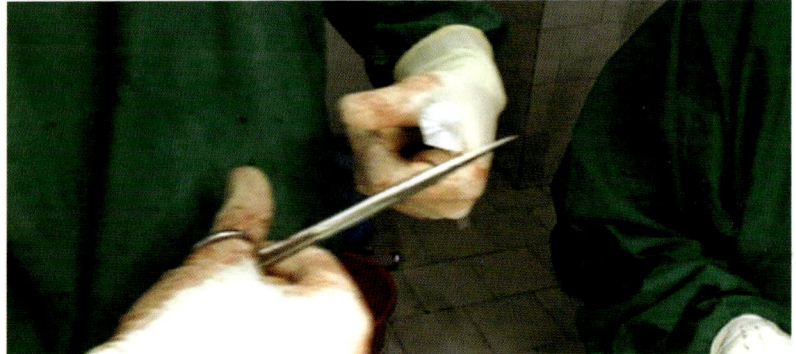

The restricter is inserted dep into the medulla, and the instrument markings read out the depth.

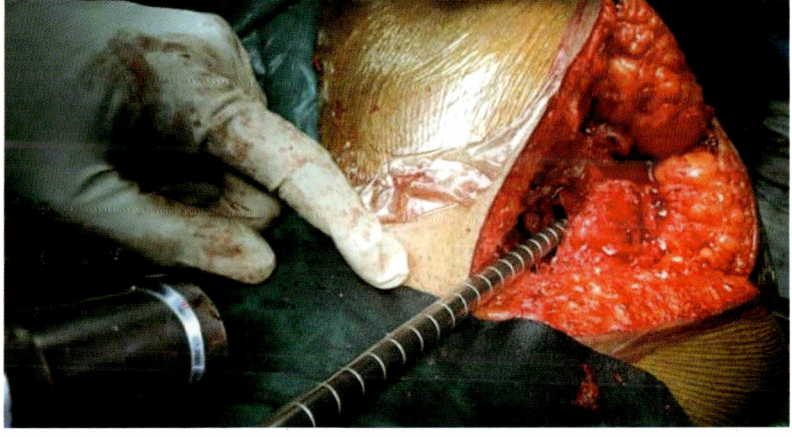

The purpose of the restrictor is to ensure that the cement mantle does not remain beyond an inch on the distal tip of the prosthesis.

A plug primarily helps in keeping a closed compartment where a gun injection of cement will allow for acrylate pressurization, and allow its permeation into the interstitial cancellous areas.

A good well distributed and integrated cement mantle is the secret of long term success of a total hip arthroplasty.

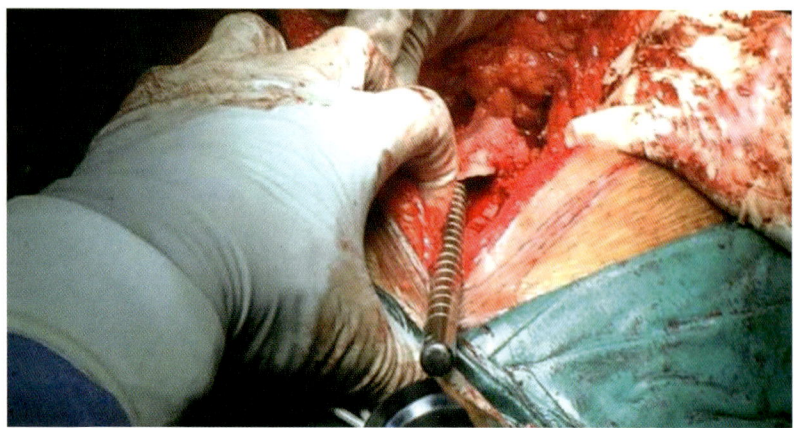

A cement restrictor is now screwed on to the introducer and pushed into the medullary canal.

This instrument has markings and can be pushed to the desired length.

The restrictor is pushed so that it lies about one centimeter below the tip of the prosthesis.

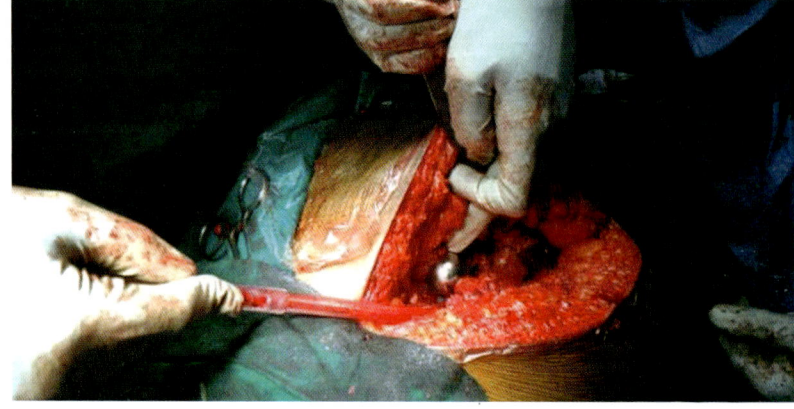

The femoral component is reintroduced once again to ensure that it sets well and there are no obstructions to the stem passage.

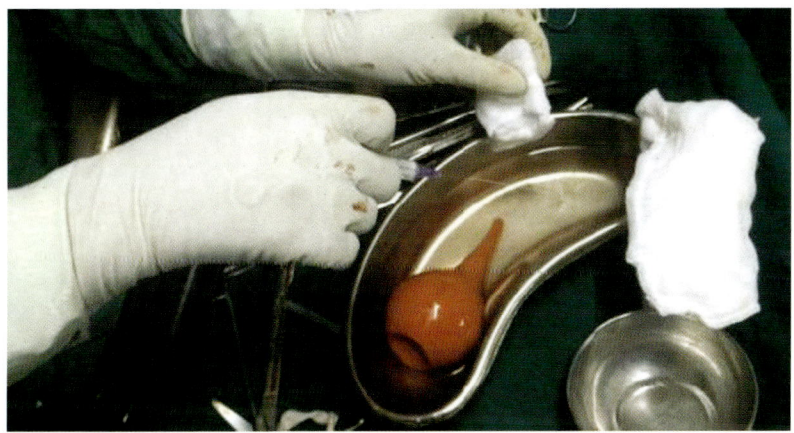

Preparation for cementation is begun.

The femoral medulla is packed with adrenaline soaked tape gauze.

Two or three ml of adrenaline are mixed with a hundred ml of saline and ribbon gauzes are soaked in them.

These are counted and introduced one by one into the medullary canal packing it tightly.

It is essential to keep the cavity clean, dry and blood free to allow for the best integration between the bone cement and the femur.

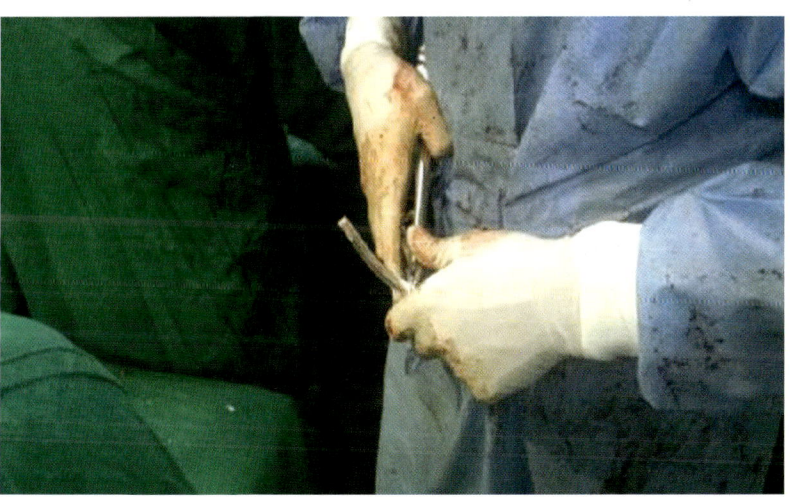

Either a cement gun is used or the same is fabricated intra operatively by attaching a drain tube trip to a 20 ml syringe.

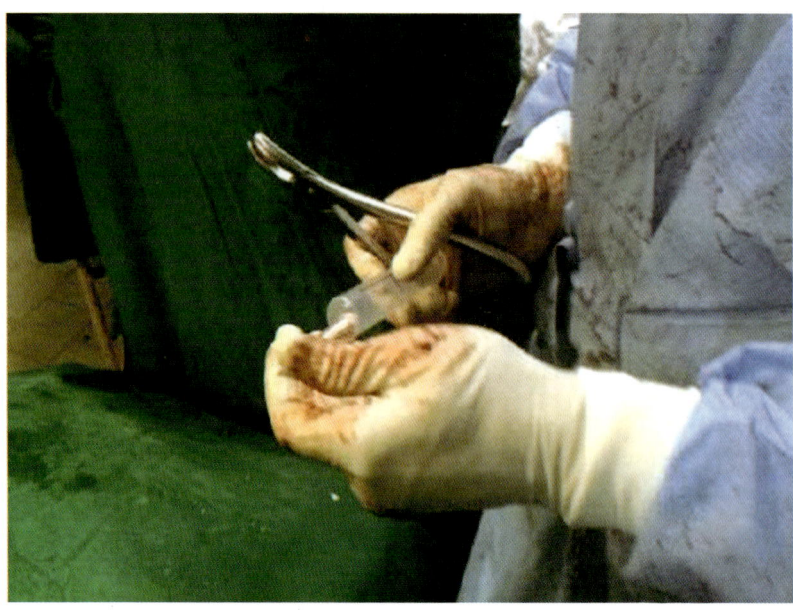

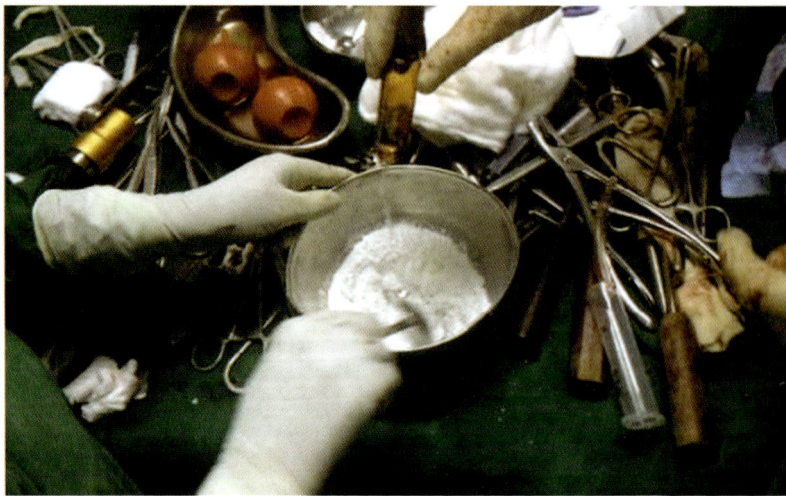

Low viscosity cement is mixed and when still liquid is poured into the syringe.

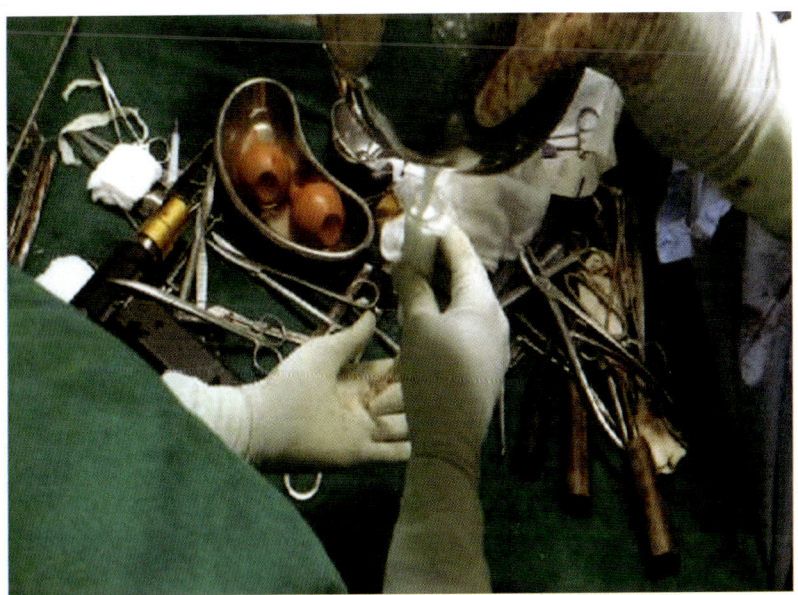

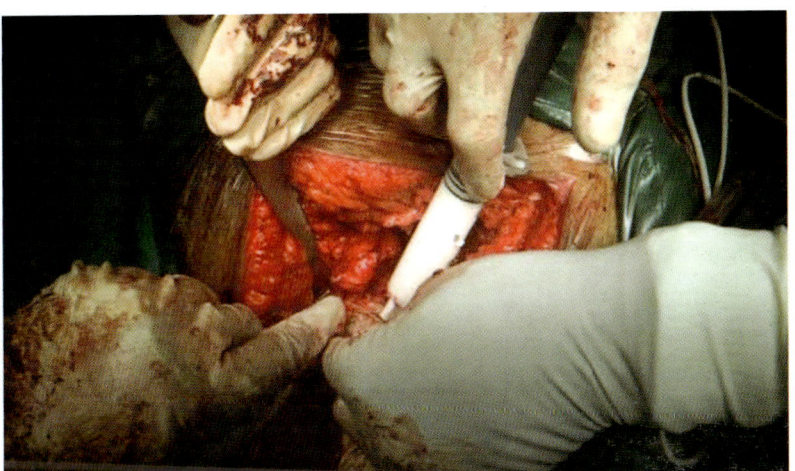

A catheter is inserted into the medulla after removal of the tape gauzes which are re-counted to ensure that none has been left behind in the medullary cavity.

The nozzle is pushed deep into the medullary canal and cement is injected under pressure.

As the cement is pressurized, the catheter is removed.

The exposed surface of cement is swabbed to ensure that it is totally dry and blood free.

The femur is now ready to accept the prosthesis.

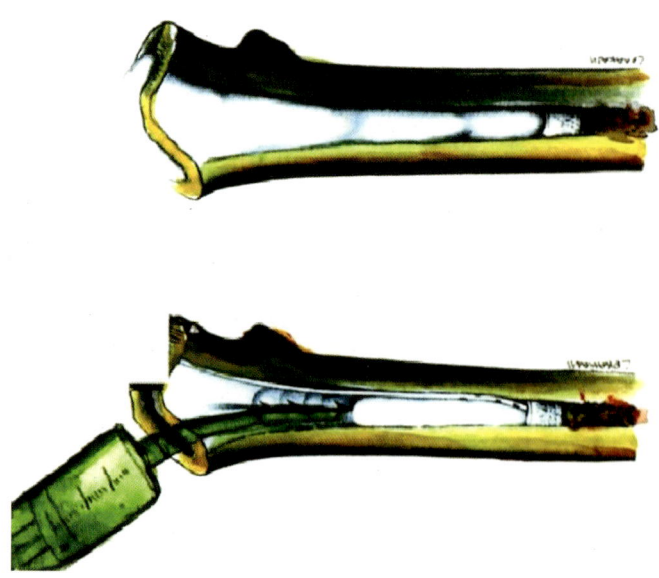

The aim is to produce a uniform two to three millimeter cement mantle all around the femoral component with a restriction to the cement being pushed way down into the femur.

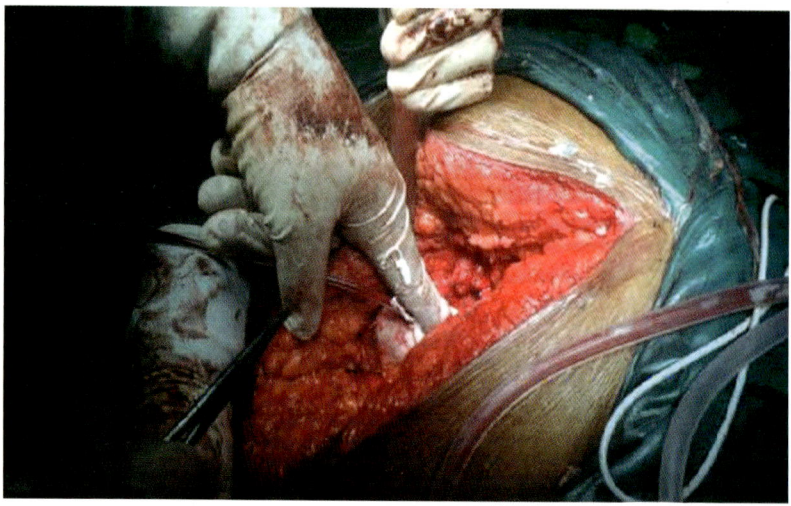

The femoral component is now inserted and pushed in right down till a perfect calcar seating is achieved. The correct version is also maintained.

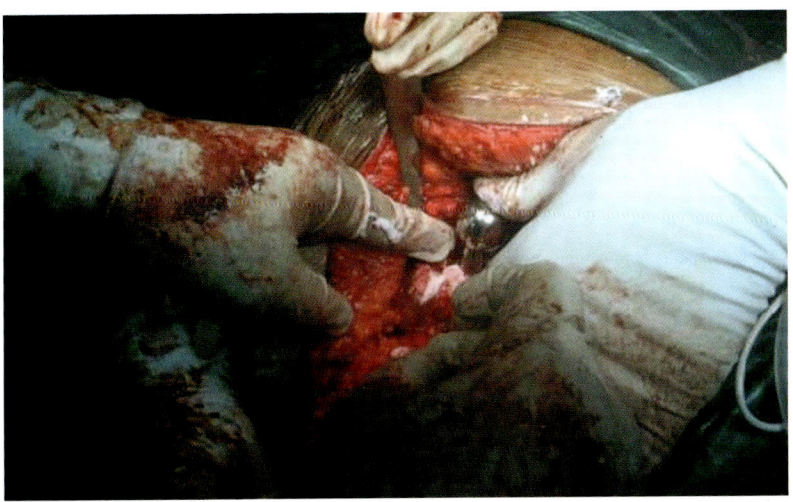

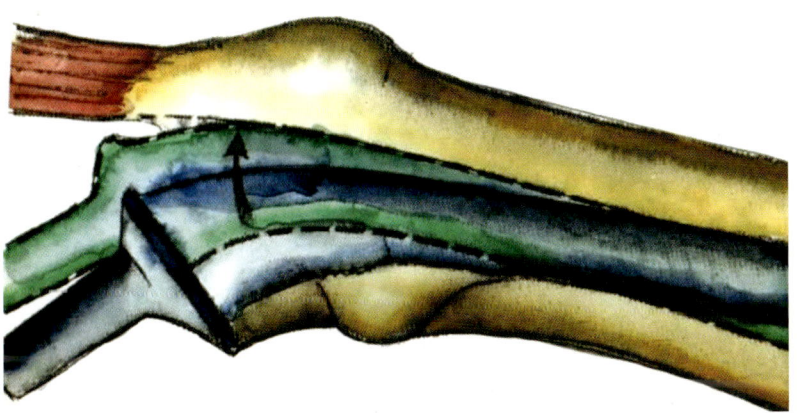

During insertion, the prosthesis is pushed backwards to ensure that the stem lies in a neutral to valgus orientation. Varus stems tend to fail in medium to long term and this orientation should be avoided.

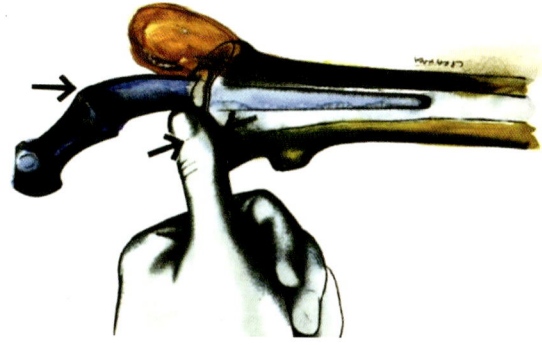

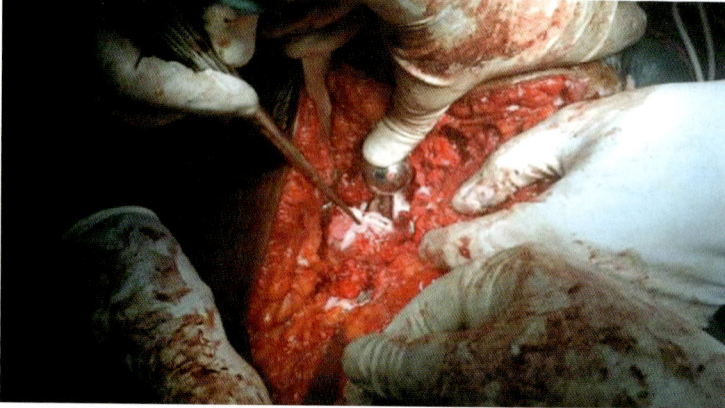

Sustained pressure is applied on the head as all excess cement is removed. No hammering should be done as it weakens the cement mantle considerably.

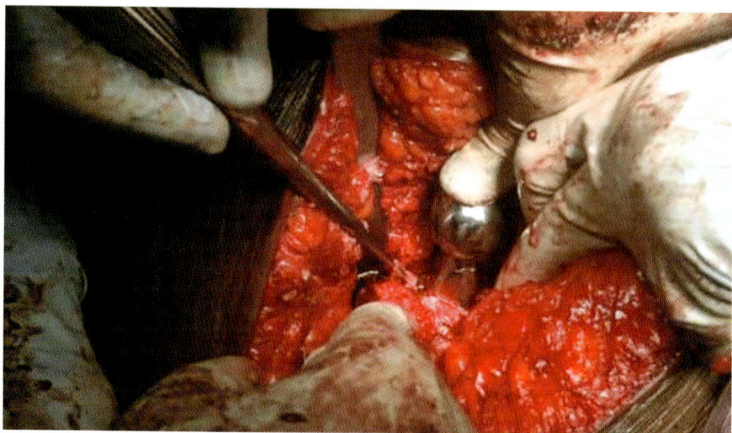

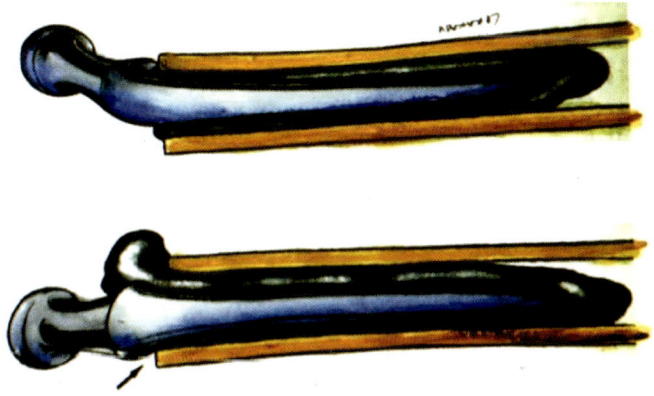

The key is to have no breaks or gaps in the cement mantle, ensure that it extends well beyond the tip of the prosthesis, and sufficient quantity surrounds the prosthesis uniformly all around it.

Gentle sustained manual push and continuous pressure on the femoral head with the impactor is the key to a successful long term outcome. The instrument impactor is a misnomer, because it is not advisable to hammer or impact the prosthesis.

Cement is not glue but more like space filler. Uniformity of the substance is the key to have a stable mantle resulting in long term success.

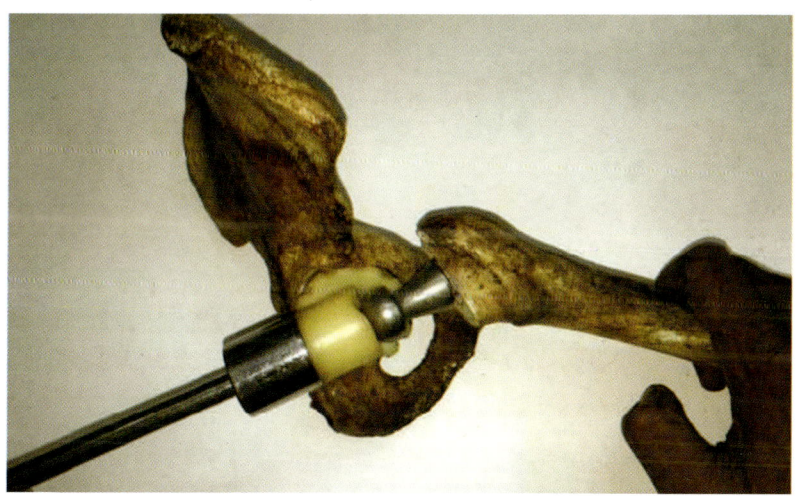

After it sets, all excess cement is removed and the hip is reduced. A head pusher assists the assistants efforts to reduce the hip with the thigh as the lever arm.

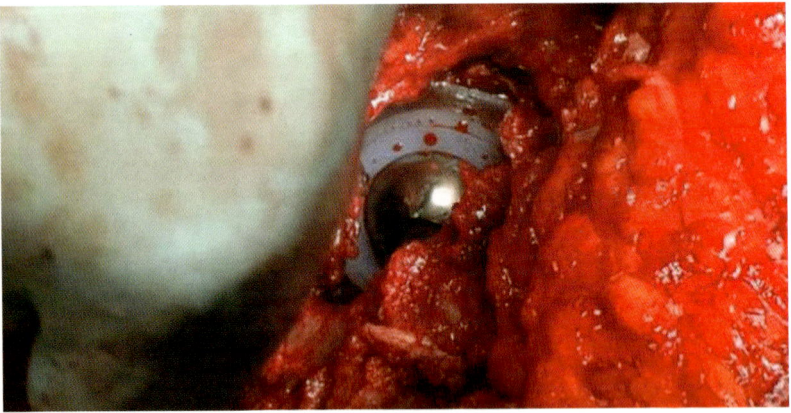

The hip joint is washed thoroughly with saline and all loose bits of cement are removed.

A digital palpation into the area is done to ensure that no excess cement is present.

The hip is put through full range of movements and should be wholly stable, especially in adduction, flexion, internal rotation.

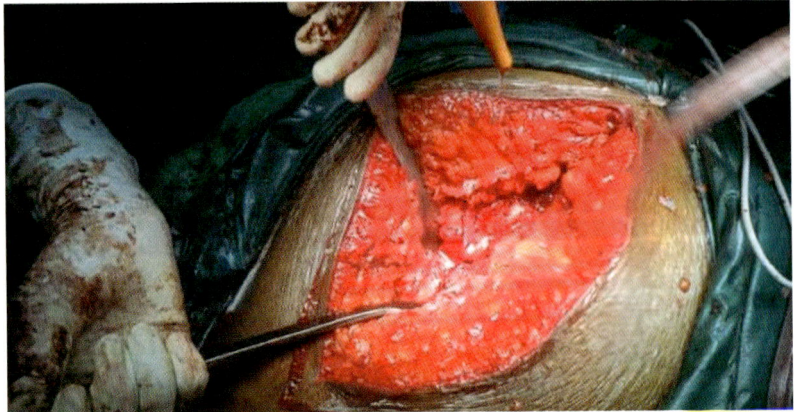

The short lateral rotators are reattached to the stubs left behind earlier. Keeping the hip in external rotation facilitates reattachment of the short rotators.

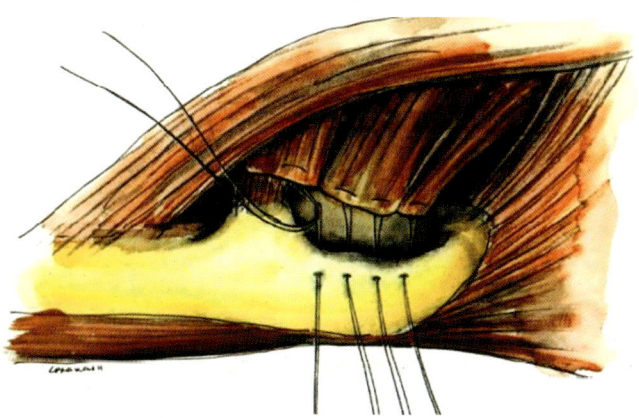

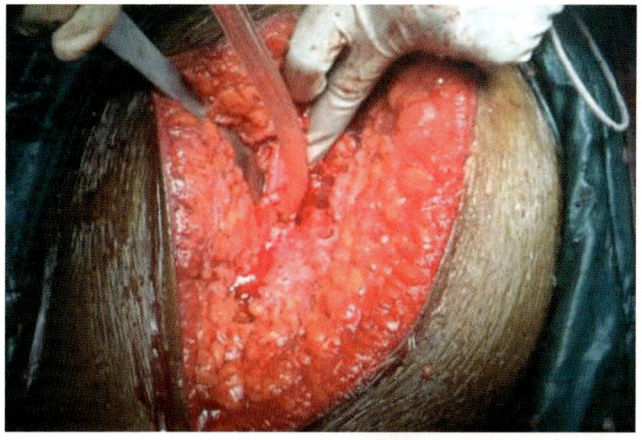

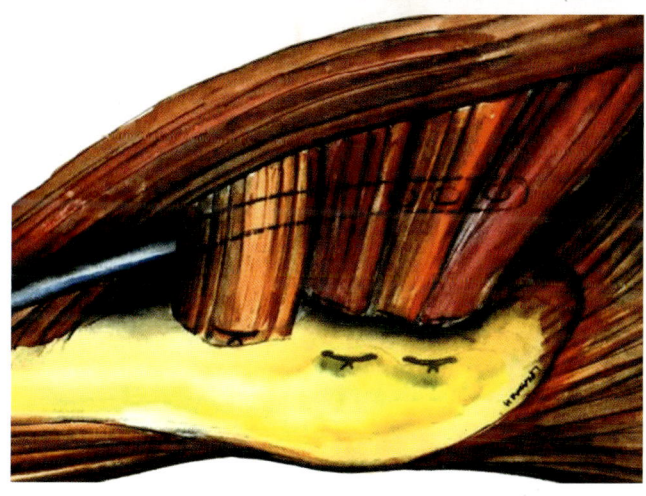

A suction drain is inserted, and the tip is placed under the short rotators to drain the hip directly.

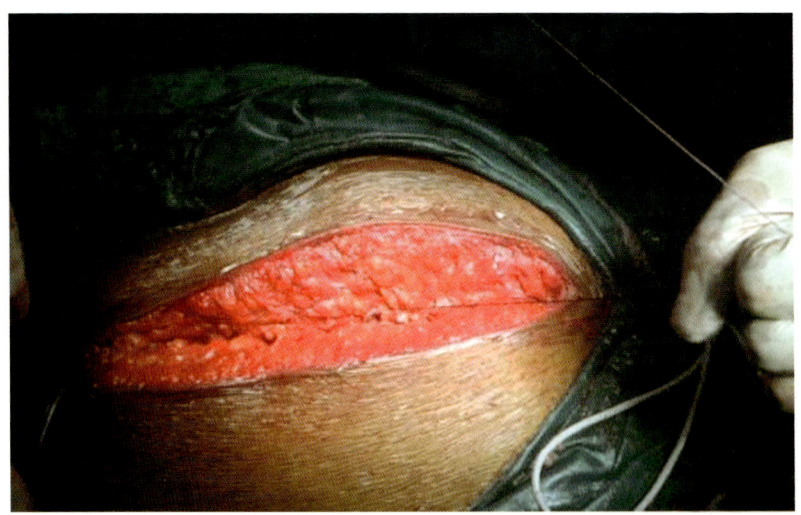

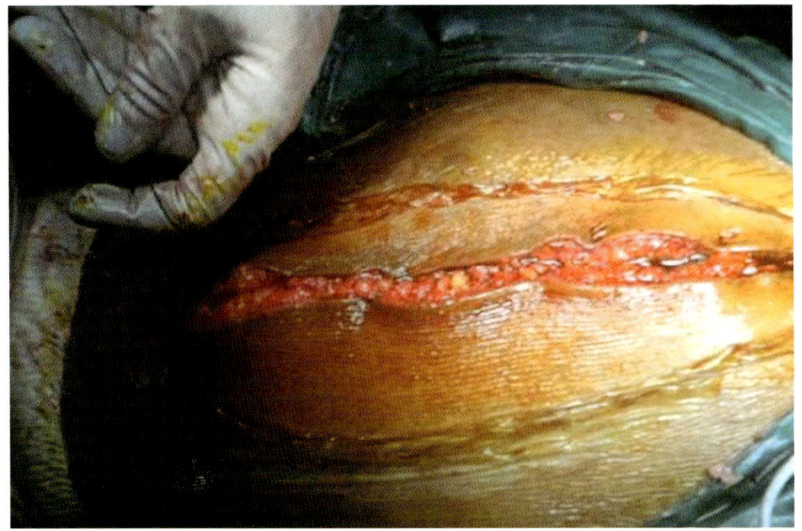

The wound is closed in layers
Use of staplers eases skin closure. An adhesive bandage seals the wound.

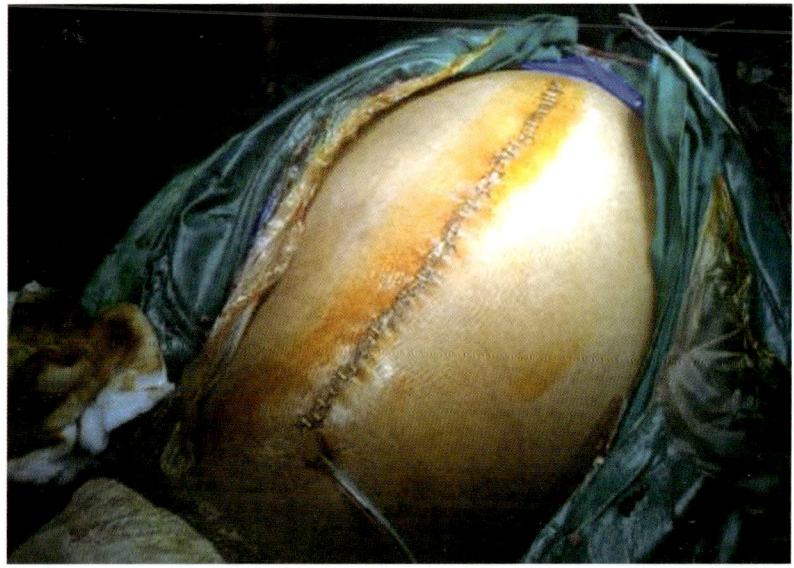

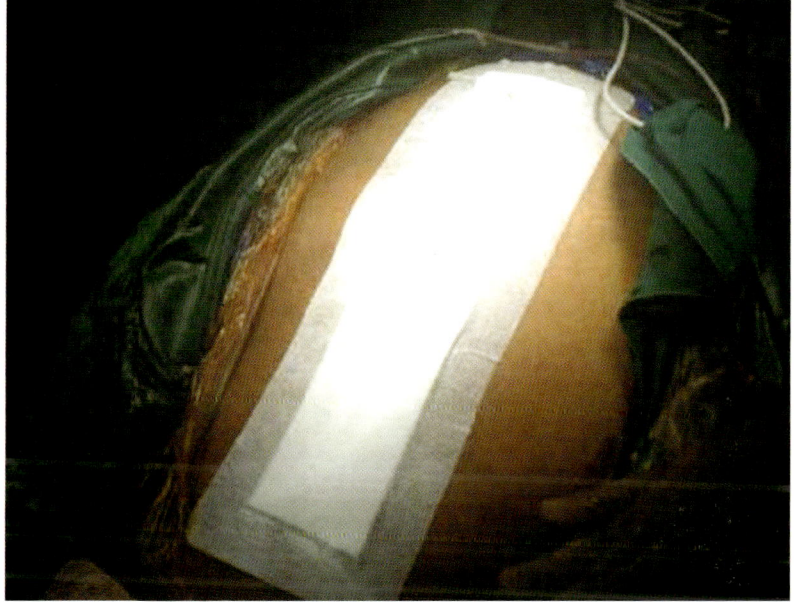

Pad and bandage are now applied. In this case the operated hip is brought out to its normal length because of the exact positioning of the cup and stem.

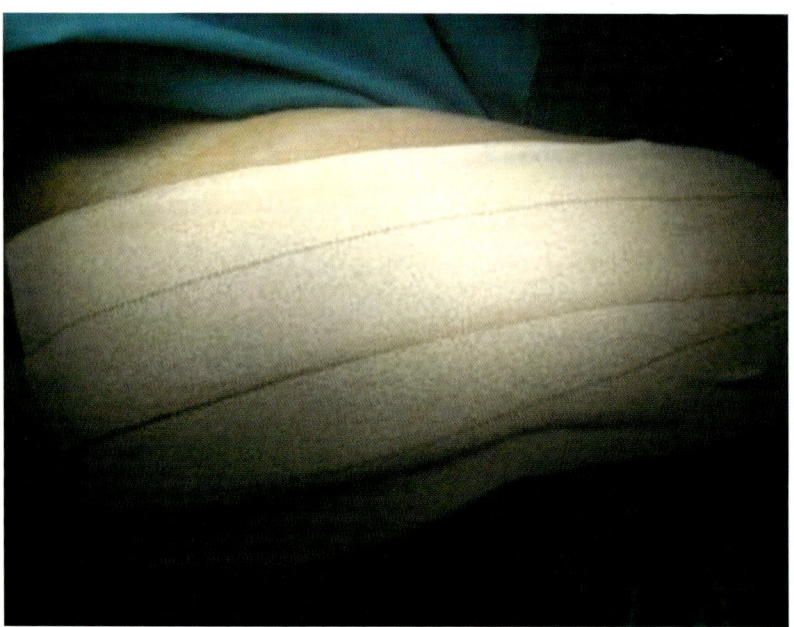

The operated limb is now three cm longer because the acetabulum has been brought out to its correct inferior position resulting in the normal placement of the hip.

As usual the patients drains are removed in a day and she walks with a walker on the next day. This is only possible with a cemented hip.

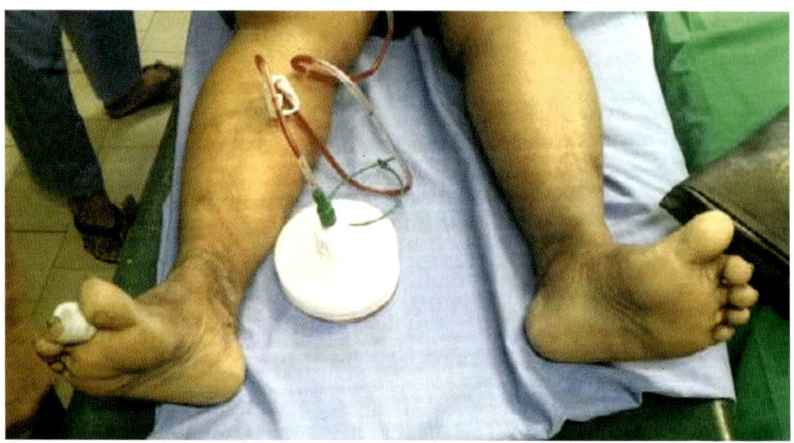

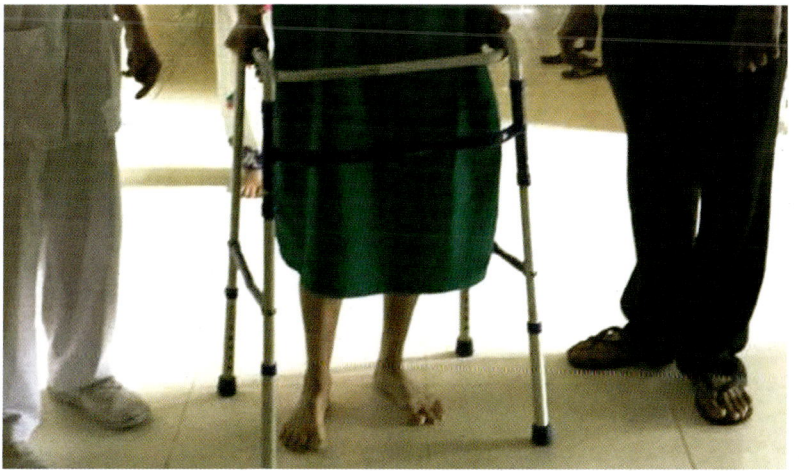

8

Cementless Hip Replacement

CEMENTLESS HIP

The approach depends on the surgeon's choice, and I use a posterior-lateral modified Müller's approach described here.

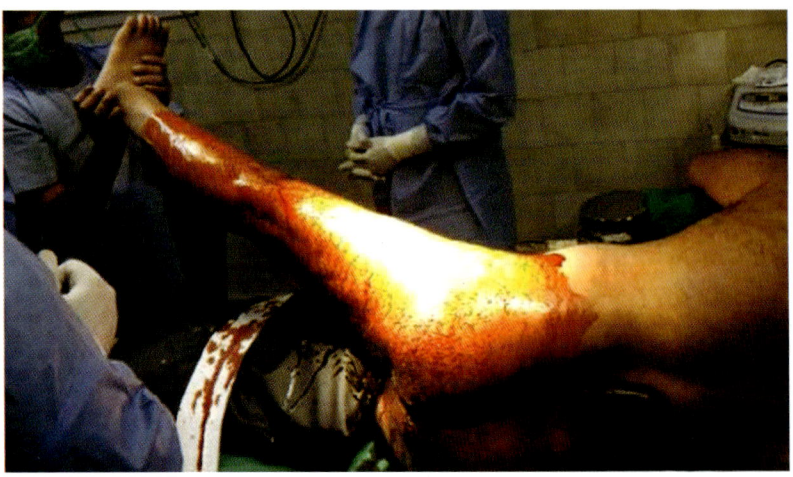

The surgery is performed under regional or general anesthesia. An epidural anesthesia with the catheter left in situ will provide continuous post-operative analgesia for two days.

The patient is placed dead lateral and strapped to the table with back supports and front restraints.

A pillow is placed between the legs and taped to the operation table to render the patient immobile.

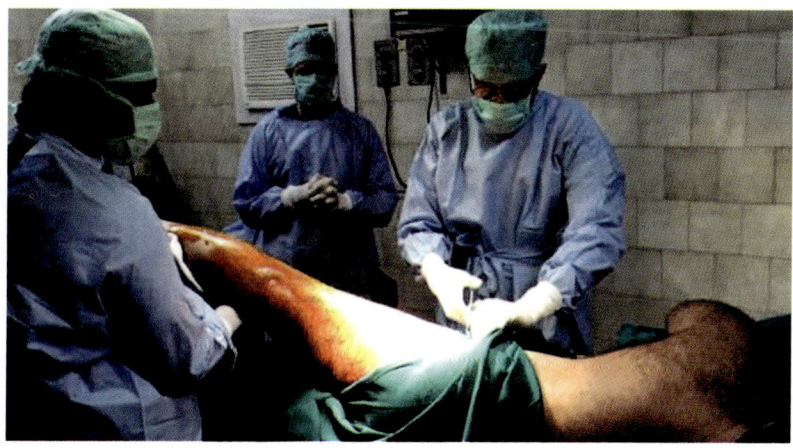

A pelvis rigidly immobile in lateral position is the key to a precise plcementy of the acetabular component.

The incision is dead lateral over trochanteric flare extending six to eight centimeters proximally and distally.

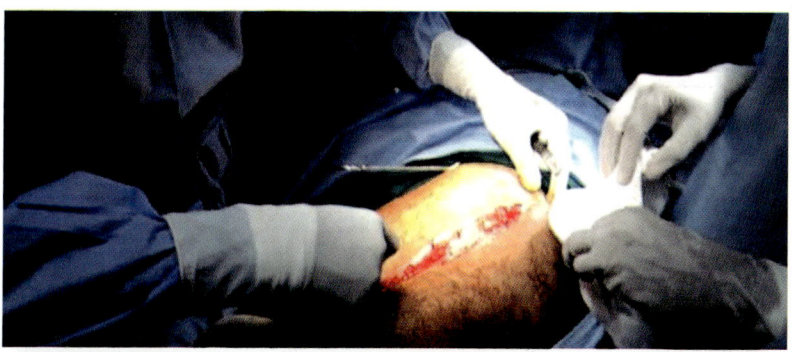

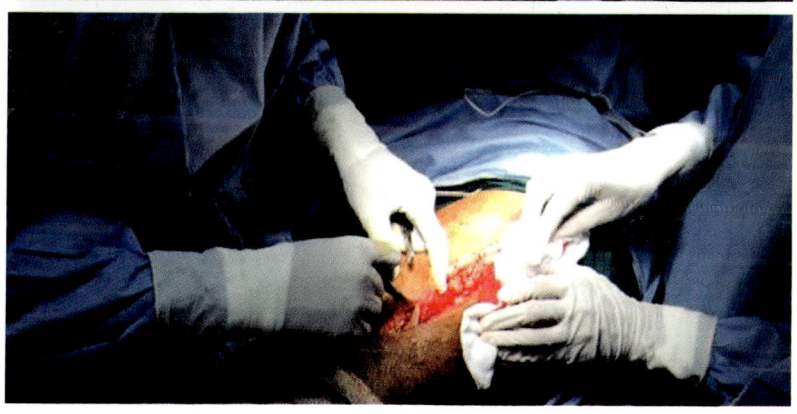

The subcutaneous tissue and fat is cut in the line of the skin incision.

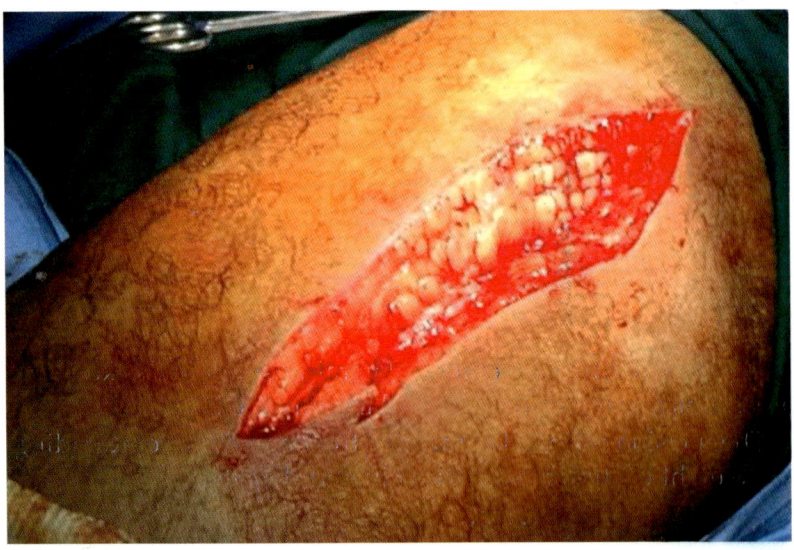

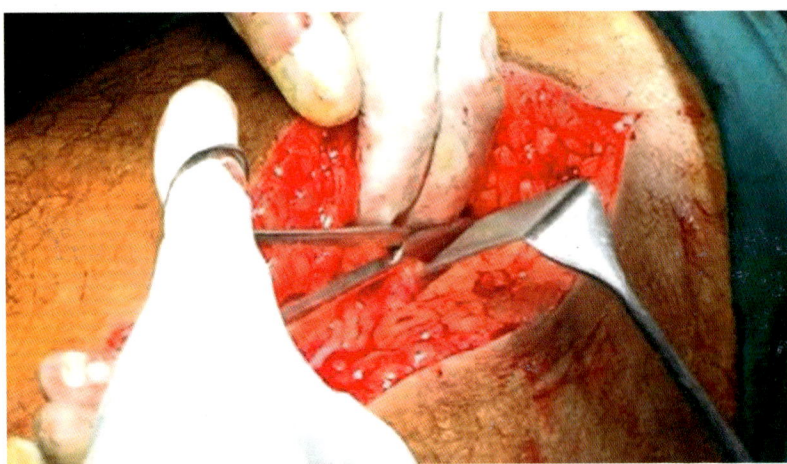

In the distal part of the incison the Tensor Fascia Lata is cut in line of skin incision, while proximally, the fibres of the Gluteus Maximus and Medius are split to expose the small lateral rotators of the hip.

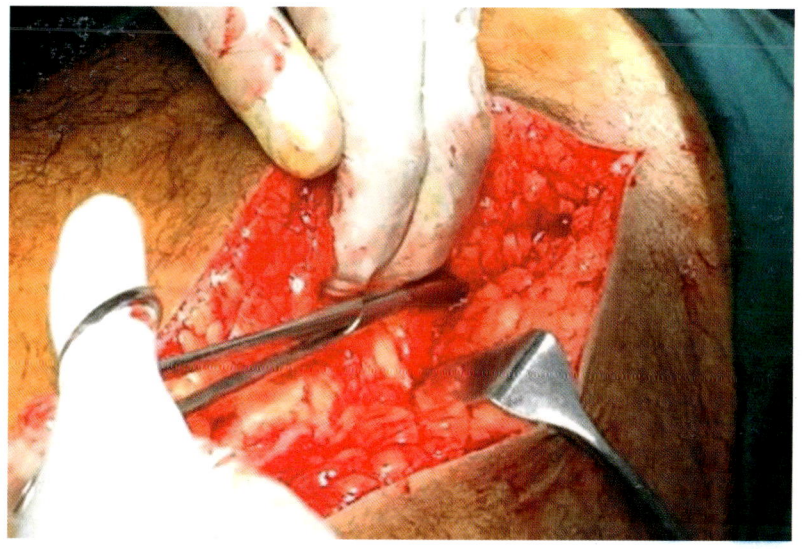

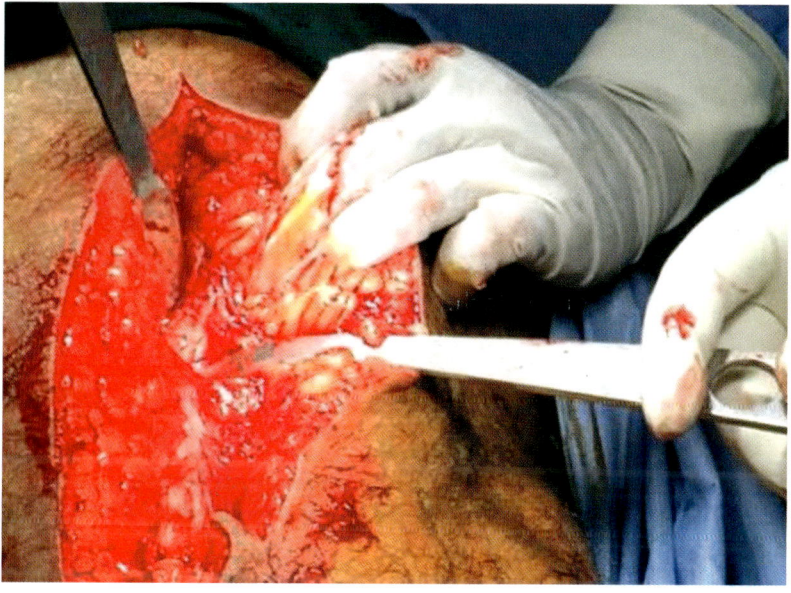

The short lateral rotators; Quadratus Femoris, inferior gamellous, superior gamellous, and piriformis are identified and stay sutures applied.

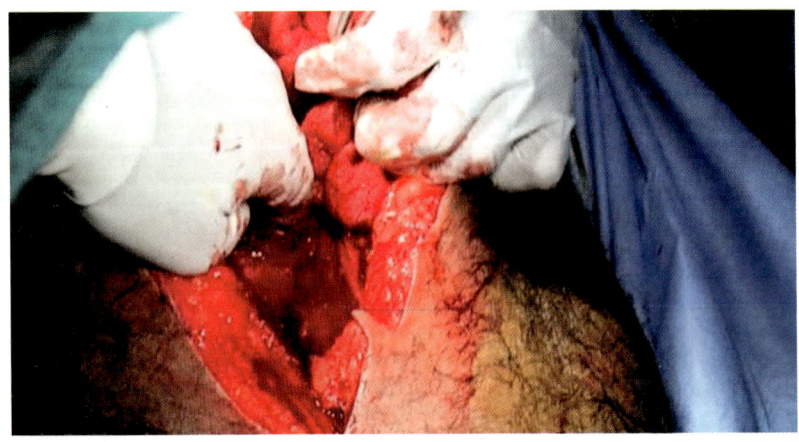

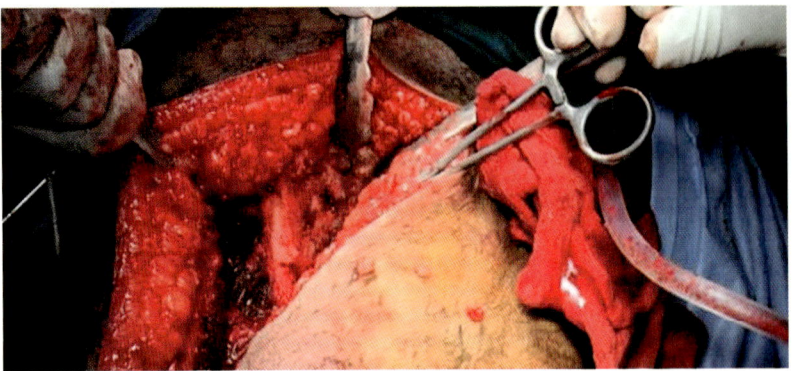

The assistant internally rotates the hip using the flexed knee as a liver arm to tighten the short rotators, which are cut leaving adequate stubs for reattachment.

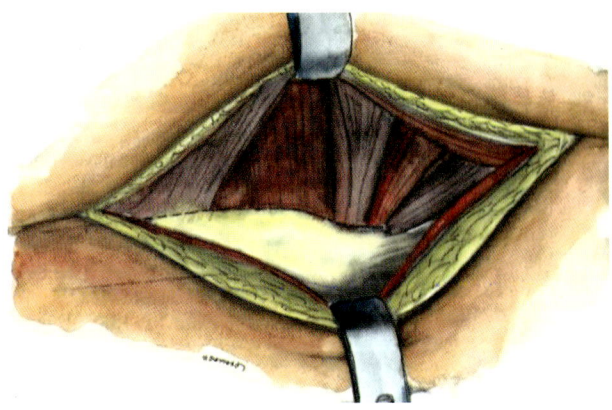

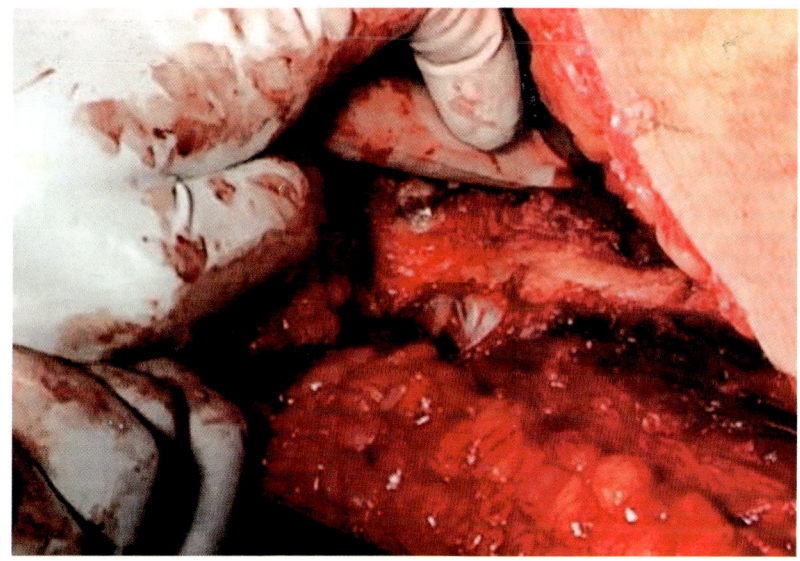

The short lateral rotators except the superior most part of piriformis are now cut with a diathermy, retracted aside and the hip capsule is exposed.

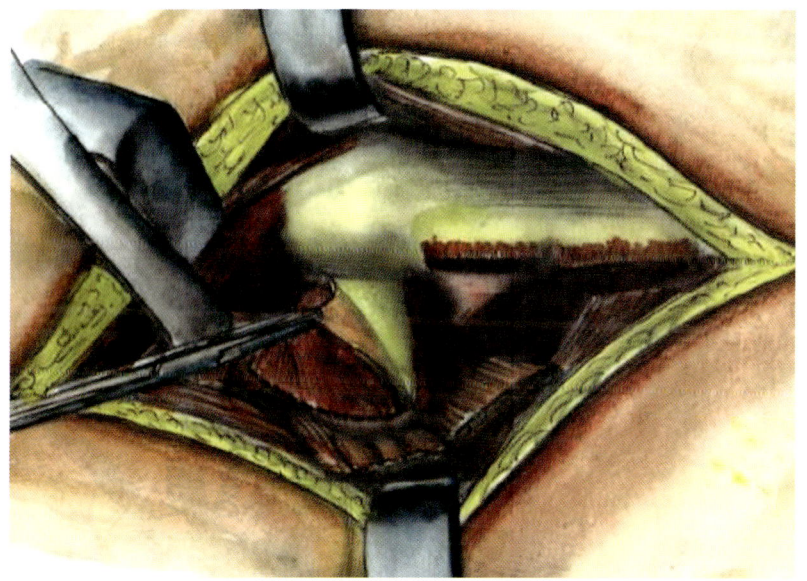

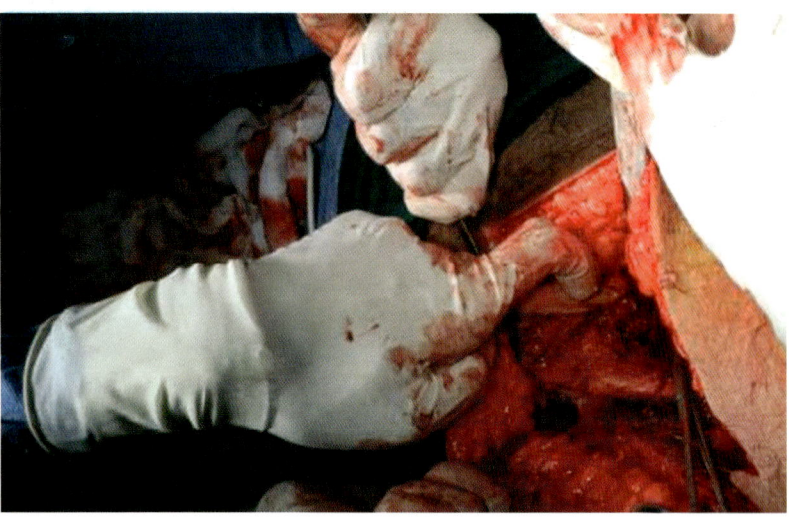

An incision in the capsule, exposes the femoral head. The assistant gradually internally rotates the head, making it more uncovered from the socket.

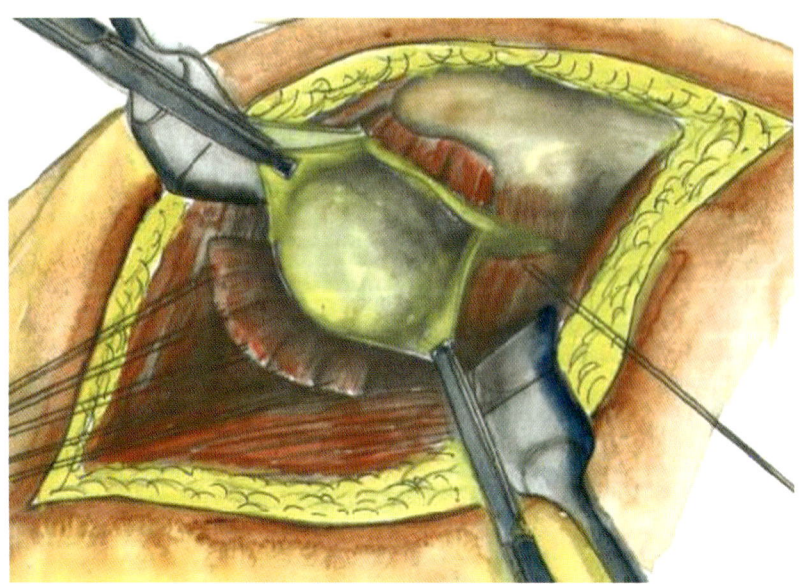

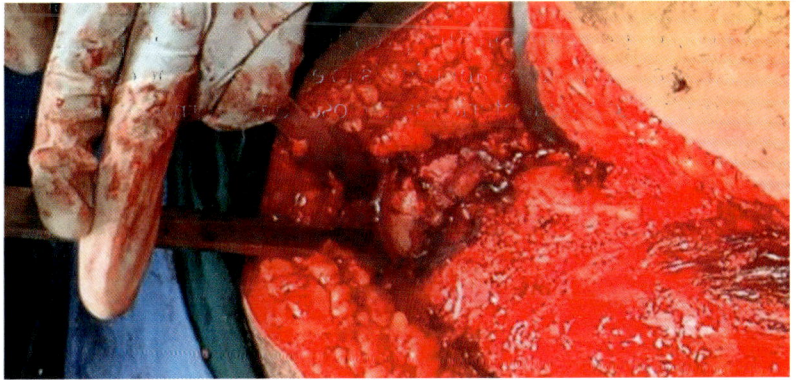

Gentle rocking movements dislocate the head. The neck is visualized and homman retractors are placed above and belof to expose its circumference.

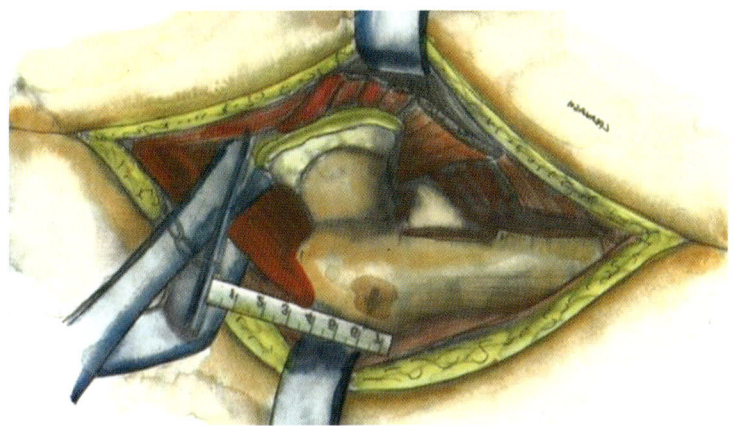

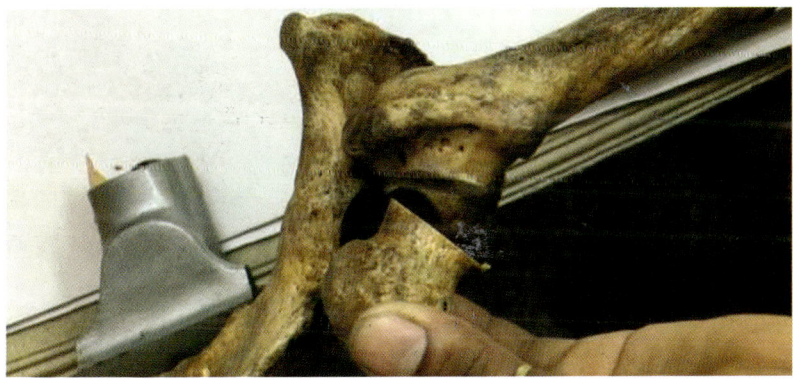

The neck is now cut at a 35 to 45 degree angle in the correct version, depending on the prosthesis used. Templates are available and an important trick is to ensure that the cut extends way back into trochanteric fossa close to piriformis insertion.

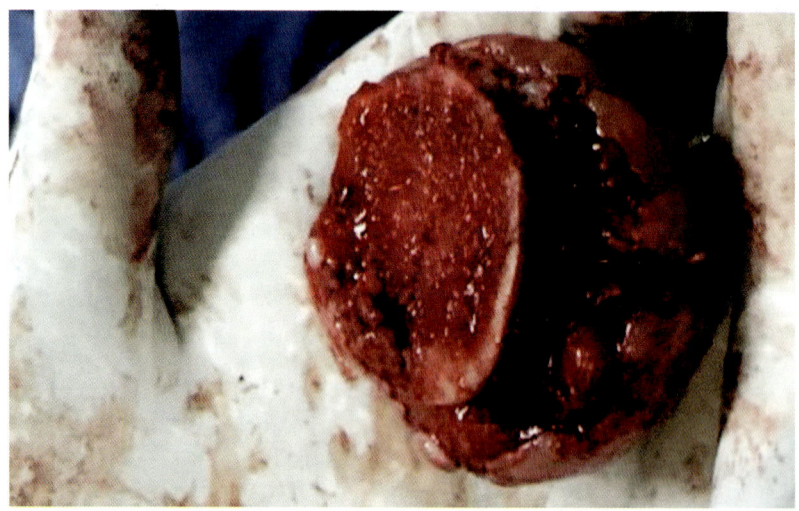

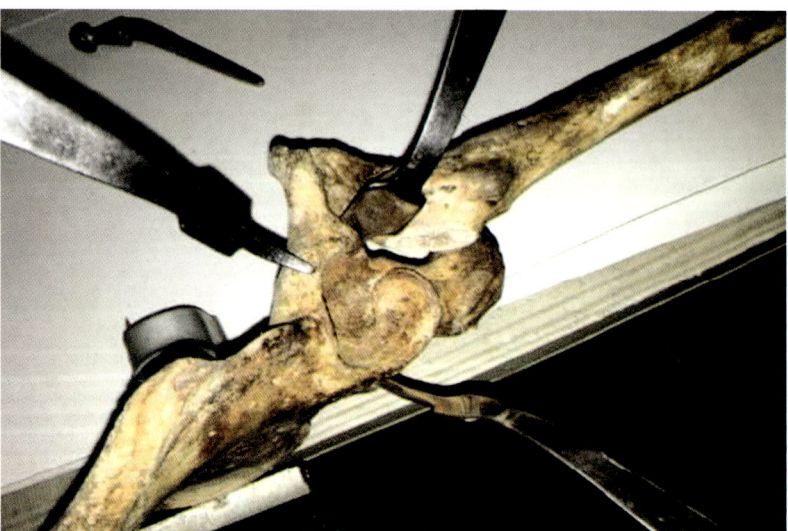

Judicious placement of three Homman retractors gives a 360 degree exposure to the acetabular cavity.

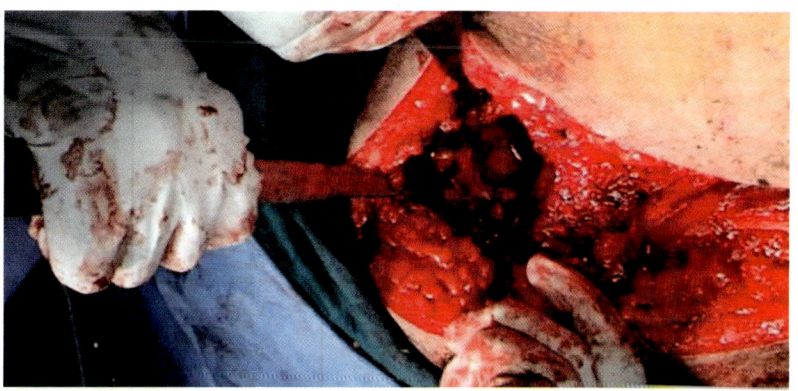

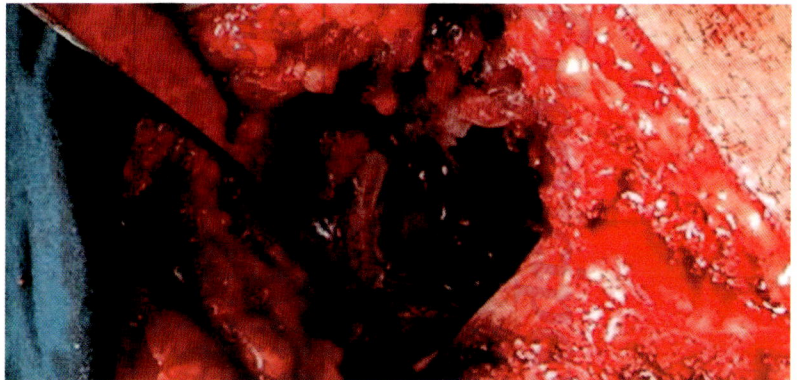

Capsule overhanging the acetabulum is cut, and a reamer is used to grate the remaining cartilage out of the socket.

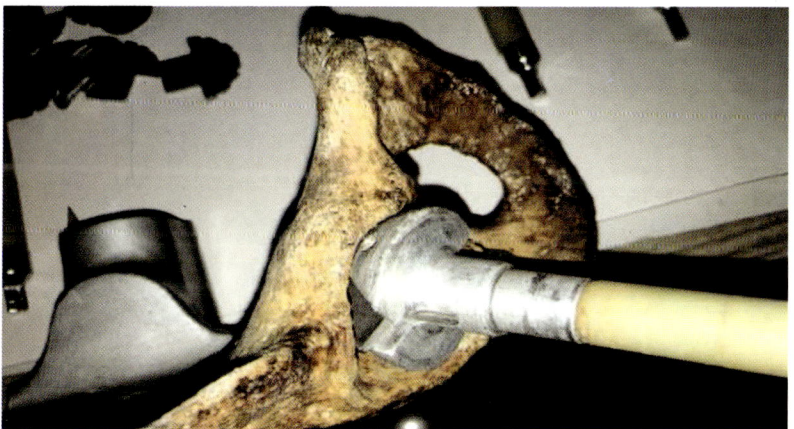

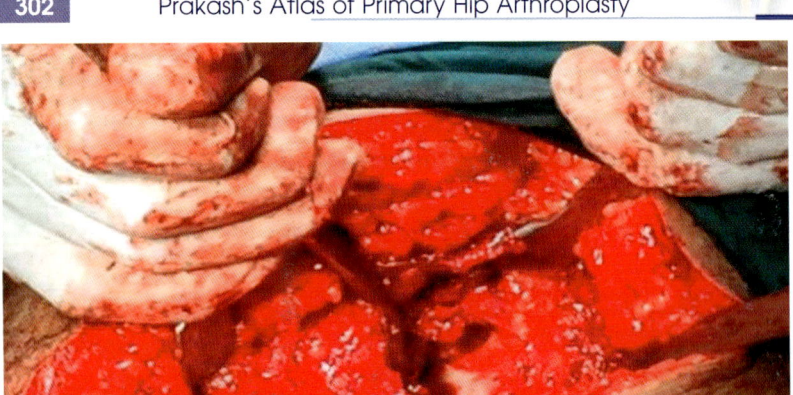

This step can also be done manually with a special instrument. I use an instrument designed by me; The Prakash cheese grater.

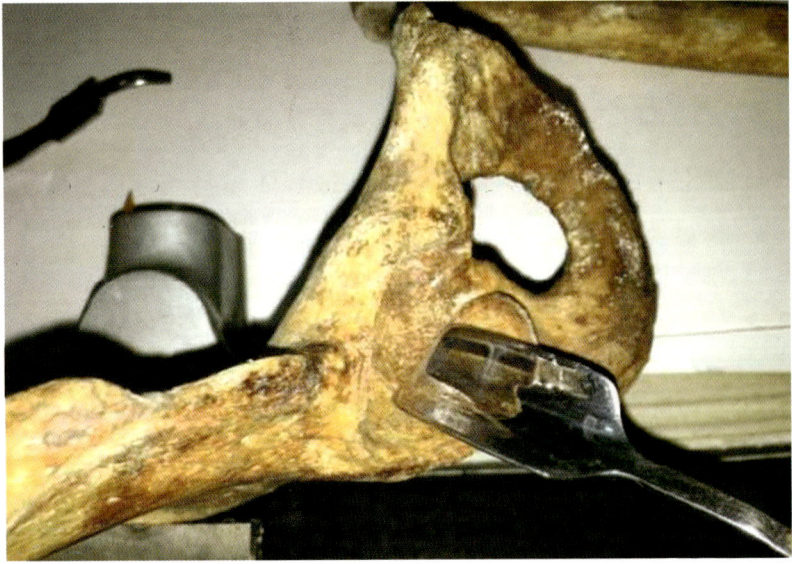

The acetabulum is reamed with progressive larger reamers. The trick in cementless hips is to ream the hard acetabular chondral bone right up to bleeding cancellous areas.

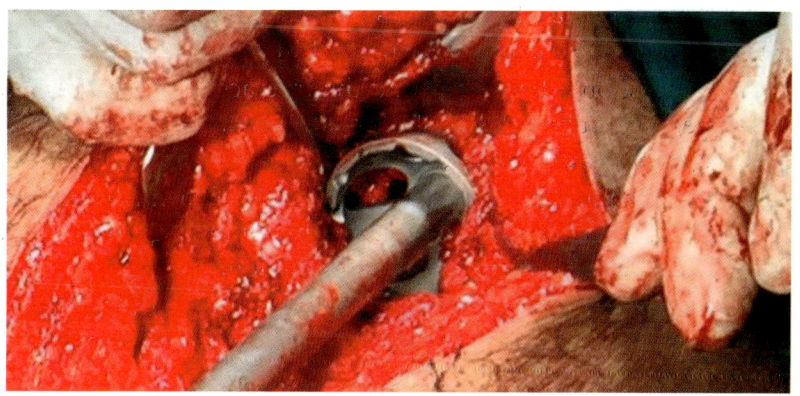

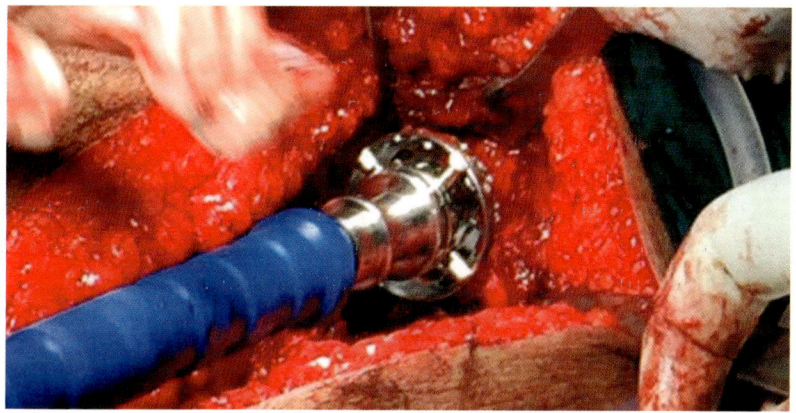

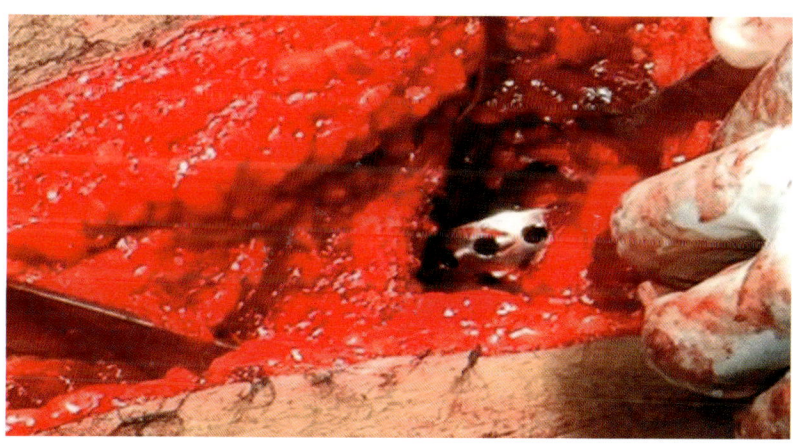

The sequence and directions of reaming is of paramount importance for the exact placement of the cup.

The cup should be placed into the true acetabulum as far as possible, especially in dysplastic hips with shallow false acetabuli and superiorly subluxating hips.

Reaming should be up to the correct depth. Too much reaming will cause the acetabular wall to become egg shell thin. Inadequate reaming will cause poor fixation.

The teardrio of the fovea has to be identified at the inferior aspect of the acetabular socket and this is the central point around which the acetabular rearming happens.

A decent pericapsular release is done to ensure proper seating of the acetabular reamer.

The smallest acetabular remur should be used first and reaming should be begun in the inferior aspect.

The reamer should be directed in such a manner that its outer rim eventually will stay uniformally concentric around the true acetabular margins.

The reamer should be directed forty five degrees to the long axis of the body and be in fifteen to twnty degrees anteversion to provide more coverage posteriorly than anteriorly.

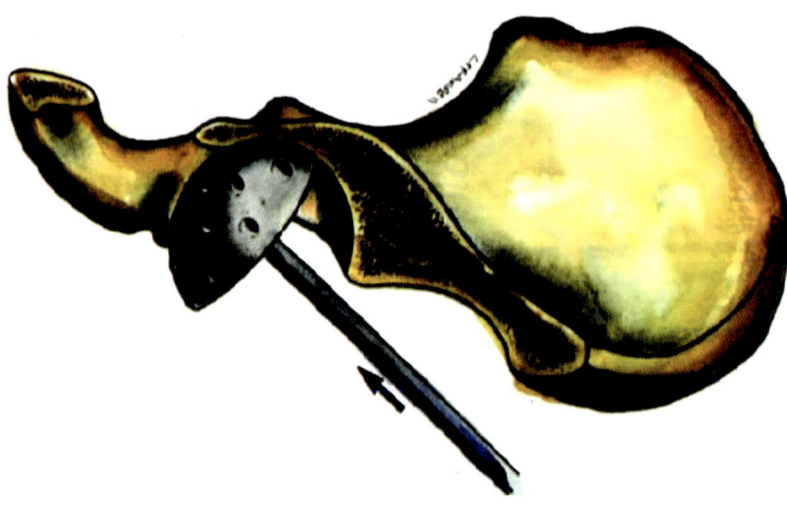

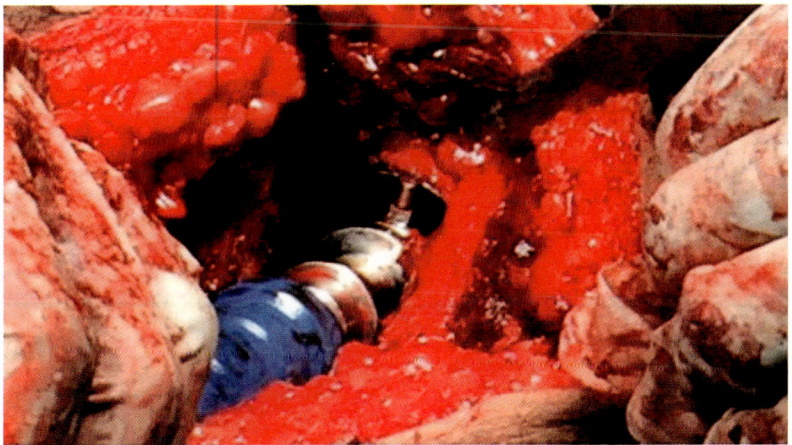

Larger reamers are then used to expand the cavity until fresh bleeding cancellous bone is visuaslised.

The acetabulam is thoroughly washed and cleared of all bone debris. Additional soft tissue exicion or capsular releases are done if needed.

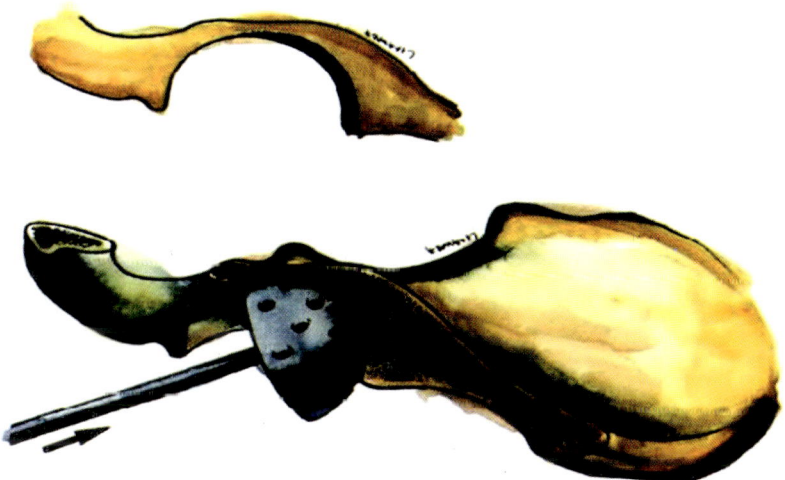

The acetabular positioning guide is now placed in position and two things are checked. It should fit correctly around the

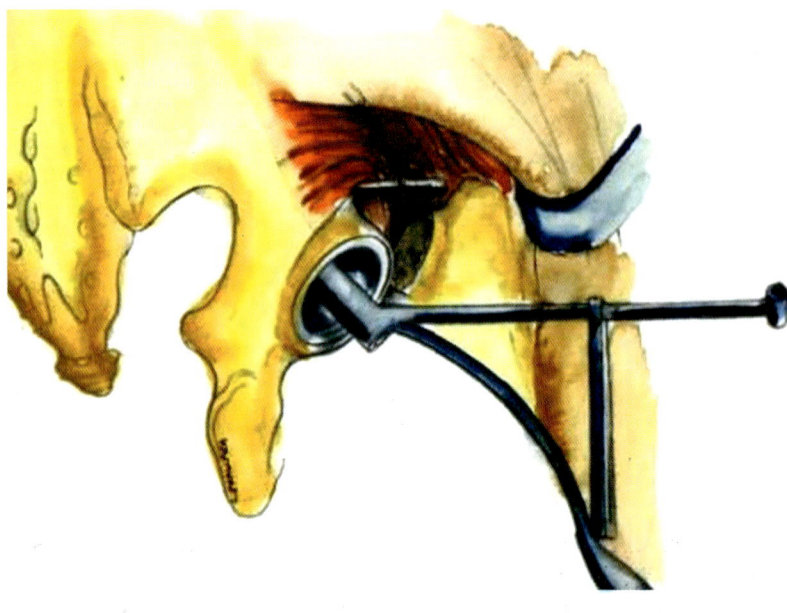

acetabular rim, and the directional guide should point towards 45 degrees position with a fifteen degree inclination.

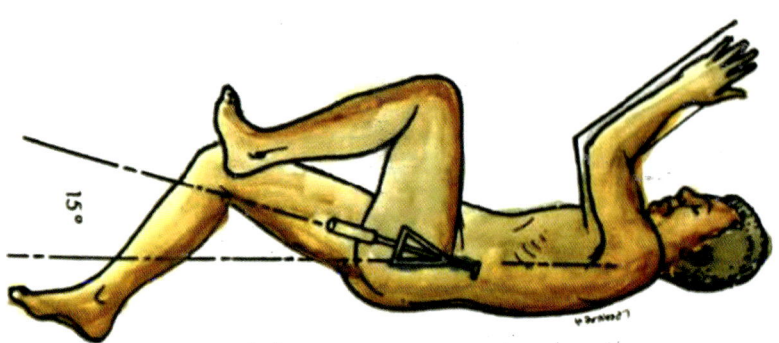

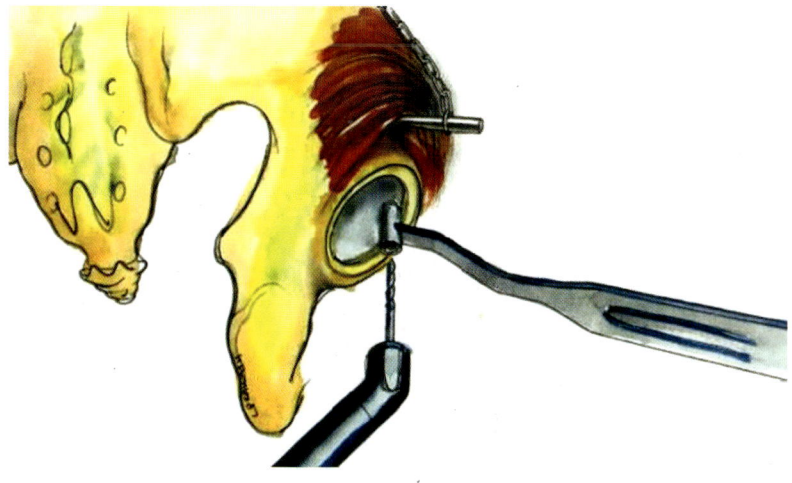

Using a drill guide and a flexible screw driver, appropriate sized cancellous screws are drilled into the roof of the acetabulum.

It is important to know the areas of the pelvis which will accommodate the screw and the approximate length to which these can be accommodated.

The cementless cups work by osteointegration by a circumfrential compaction. The screws only compress the cup

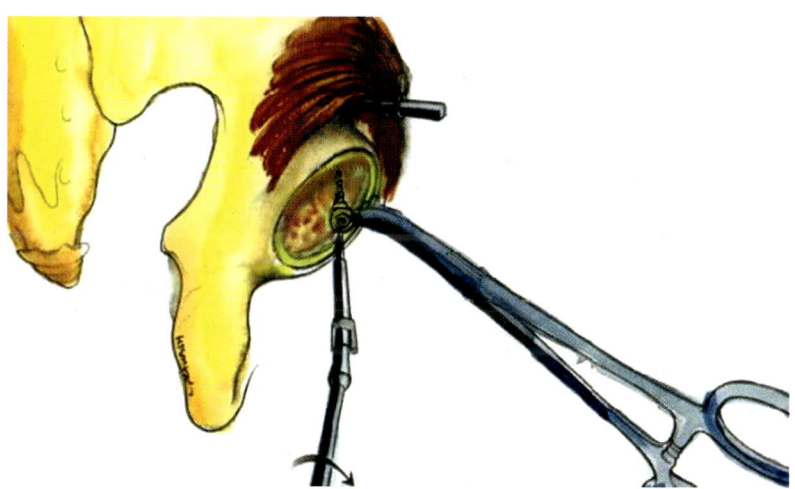

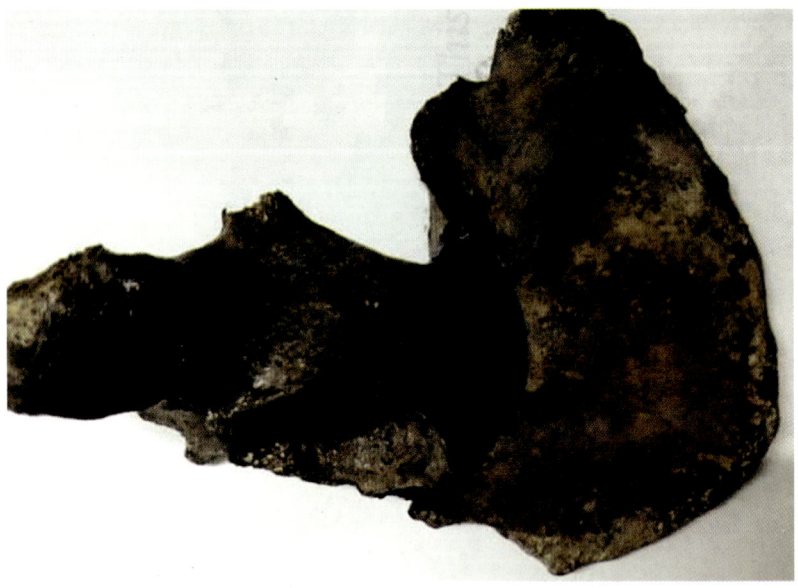

shell to the cancellous bone, and impart rotational stability until bone-metal interface is bonded by ingrowing into the porous coating or hydroxyappatite.

The screws should be placed in the posteriosuperior quadrant of the acetabulum.

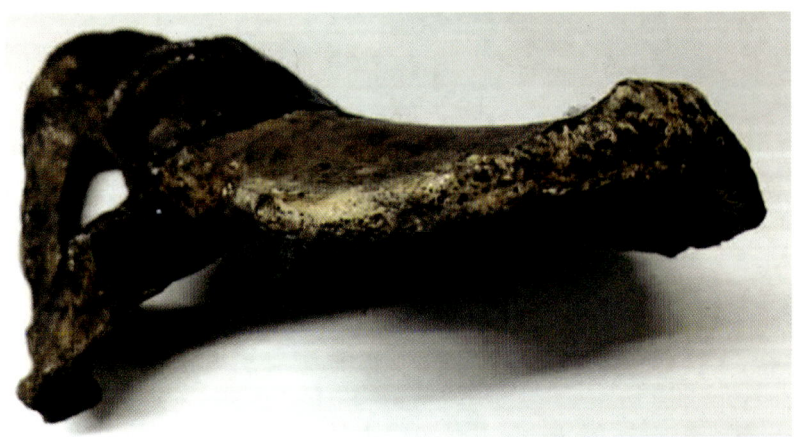

The screw direction should be posteriosuperior quadrant towards the sciatic notch.

Measurements with a depth gage will ensure that the screws don't poke into the pelvis.

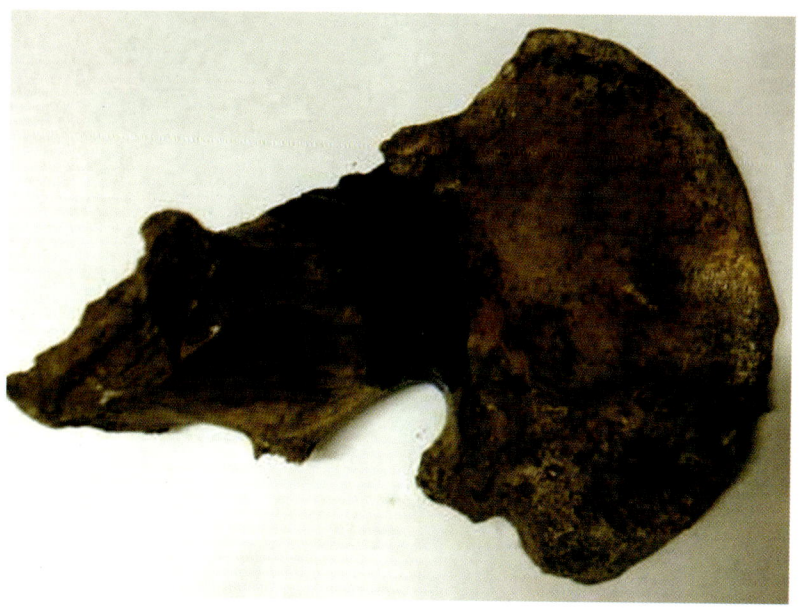

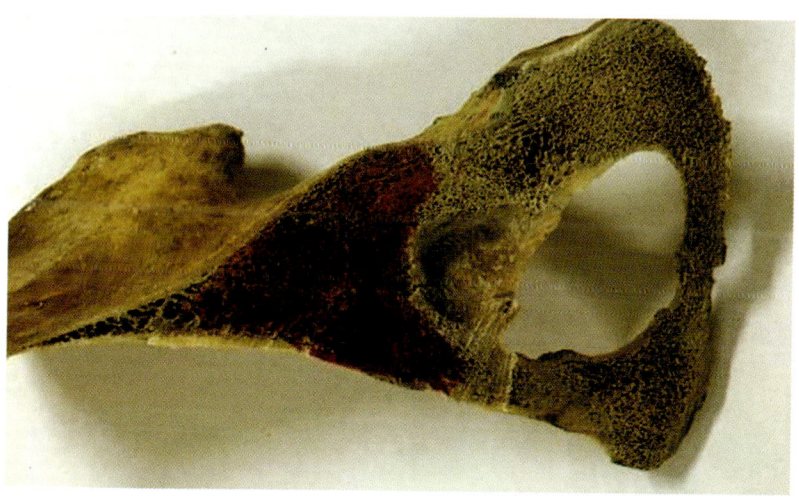

The cross section of a hemi pelvis shows the areas with good cancellous bone, into which the shell anchorage screws are inserted.

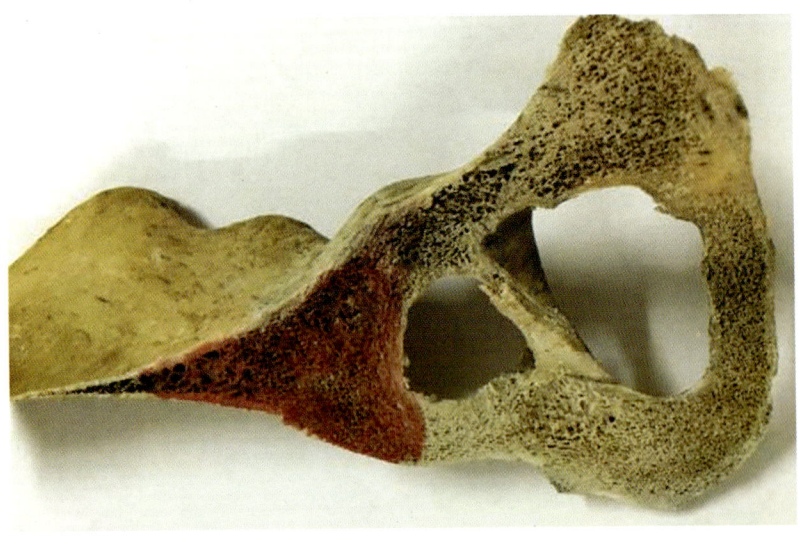

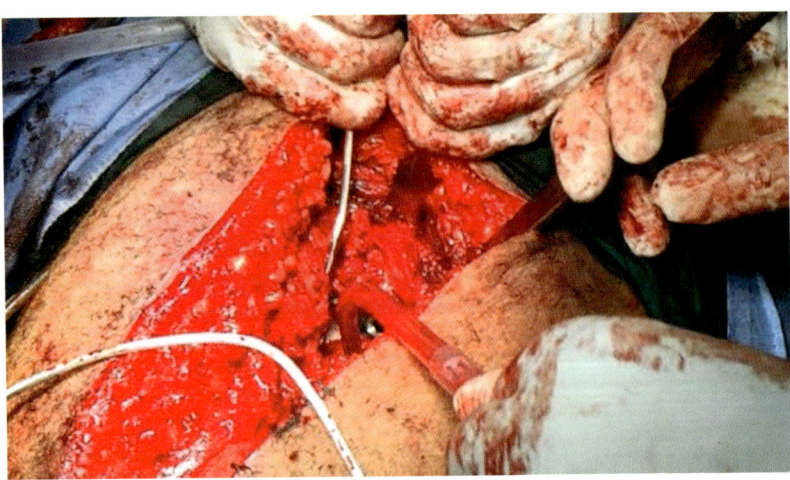

Flexible drill shafts, and screw drivers ensure that the screw is inserted in the correct direction.

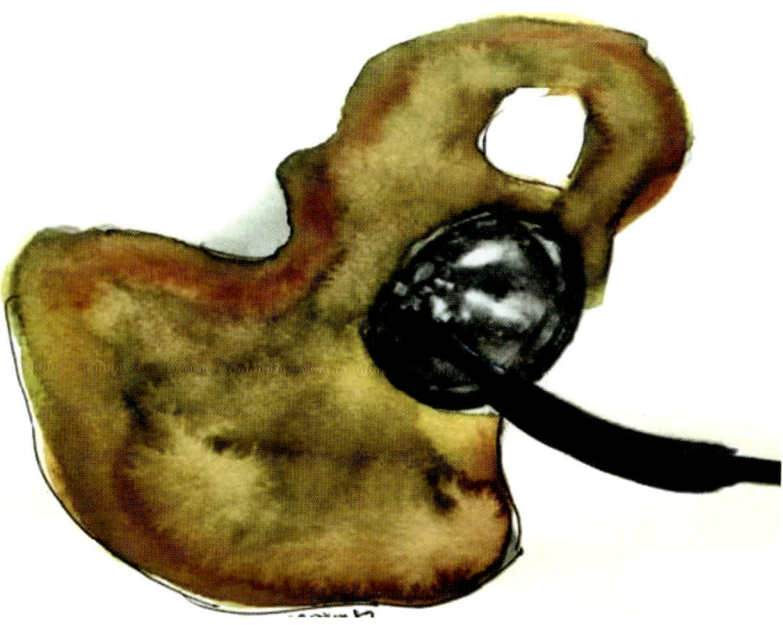

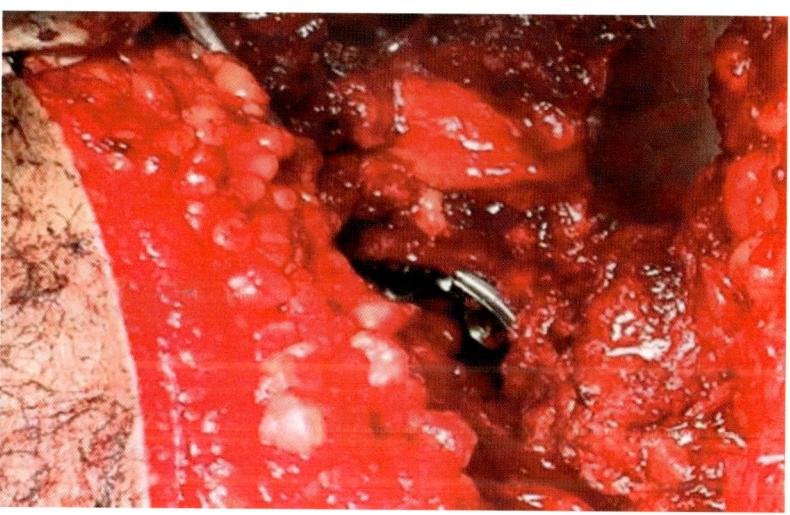

The screw heads must be deep sunk into the shell to allow for proper seating of the HDPE liner.

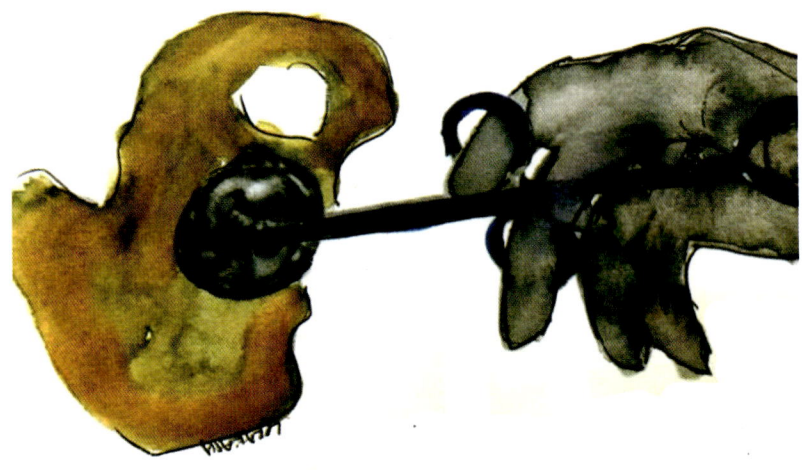

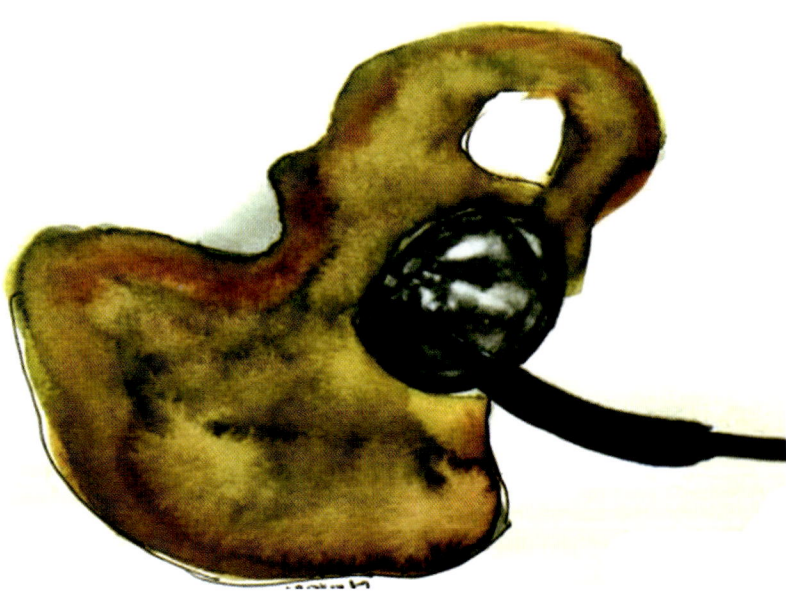

After the shell is screwed, the surgeon must ensure that the rim seats circumfrentially all around the acetabular borders and that the component doesn't stand proud in any direction.

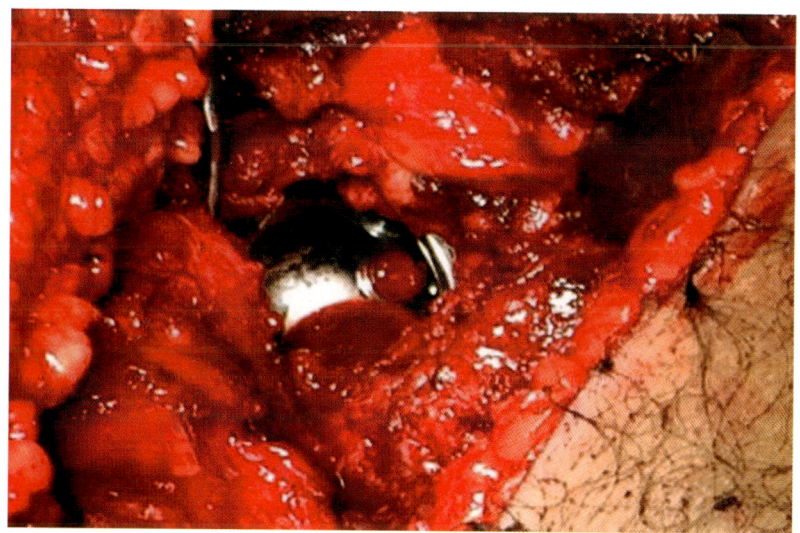

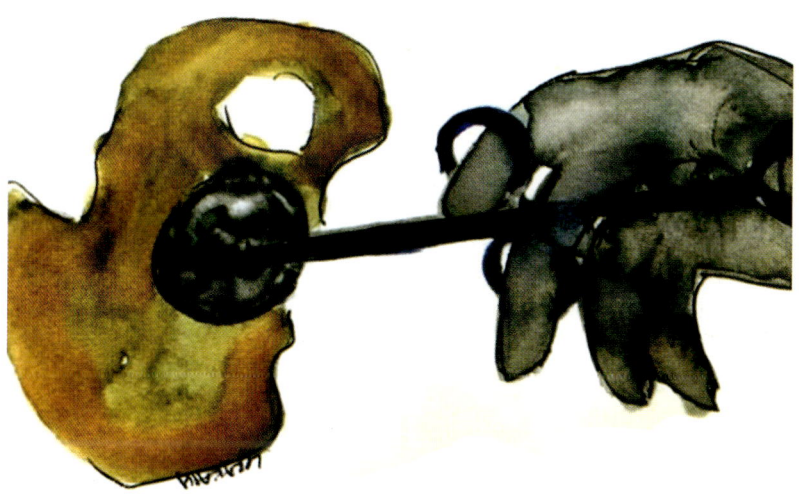

Judicious placement of Homman retractors ensures that the acetabulum is visualized properly.

Using an artery forceps, the edge of the cup is shaken slightly to ensure that it does not rock.

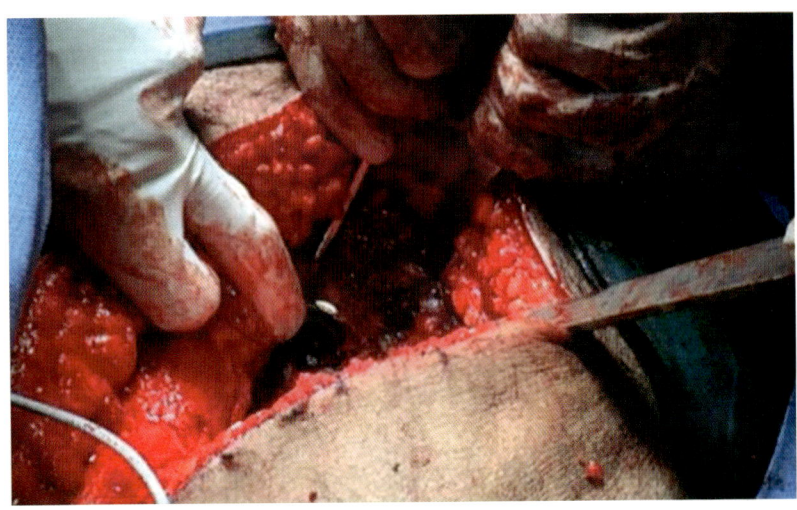

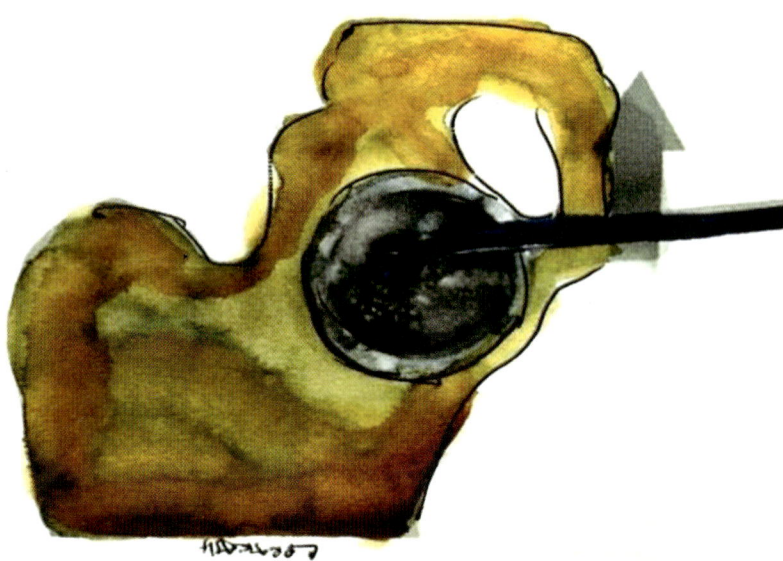

Additional screws are now inserted, ensuring that they are directed towards the sciatic notch in the posteriosuperior quadrant.

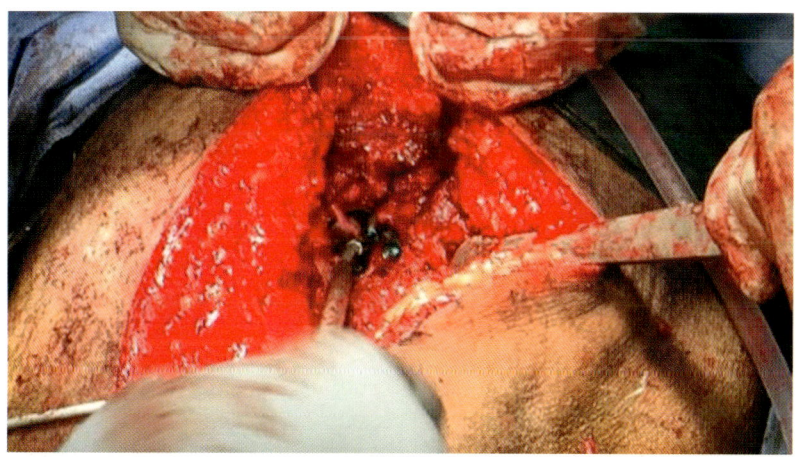

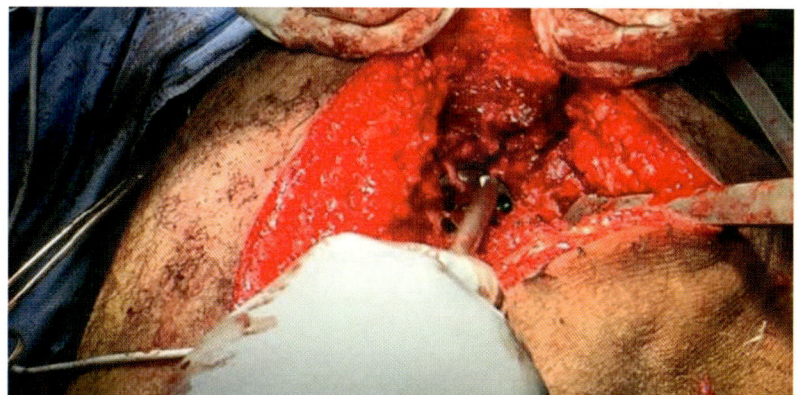

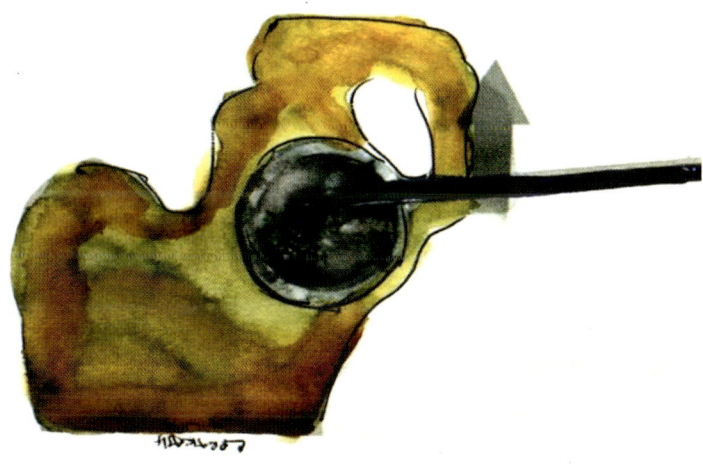

The approptiate screws are now tightened. The shell is checked for stability. Additional tightening of a screw or two may be needed.

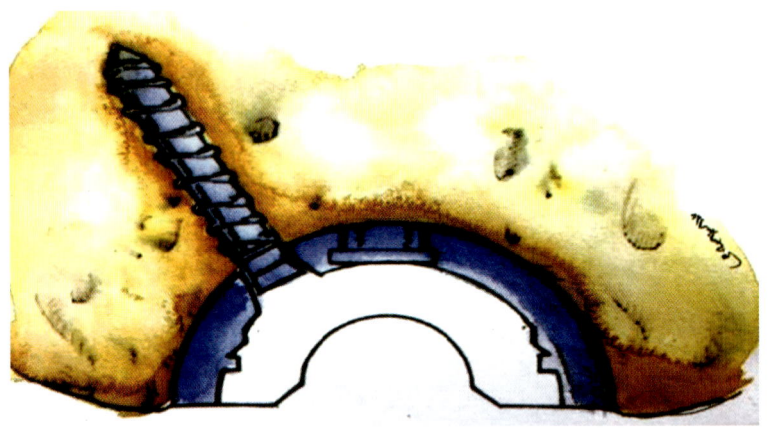

Long term results of cementless cups depend upon 1, Precise placement of the shell.

1. Precise placement of the shell.
2. Proper reaming to ensure a good contact between the porous outer implant surface and healthy bleeding cancellous bone areas.

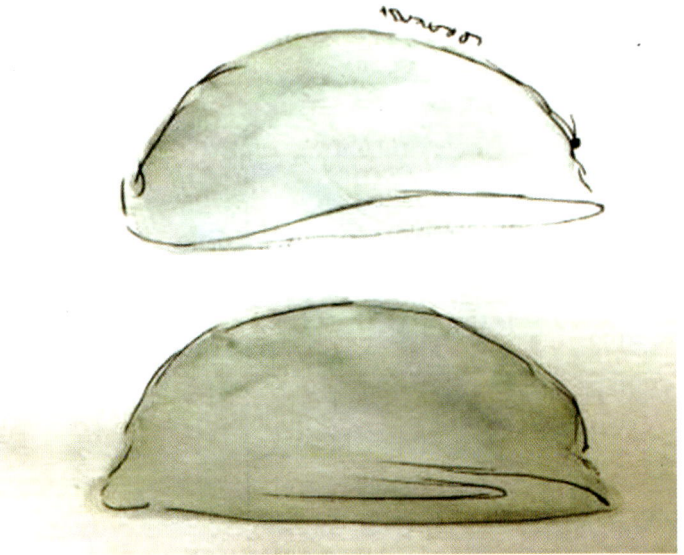

3. Placement of the cancellous screws in the right direction and quadrant.

4. Tightening of the screws to ensure that no projections remain.

5. Tighter the fitting of the metal acetabular shell, earlier the weight bearing can be commenced.

Acetabular liner shells are available in two designs, standard and long posterior wall.

The long posterior wall gives an additional fifteen degree protection posteriorly and should be used as a routine choice.

If the acetabular orientation necessitates the fixation of the metal shell with a posterior overhang producing a posterior impingement with a long posterior wall cup, then a standard cup is used. Use of standard cups is pretty selective and in less than 15% of the cases. Its routine use is not recommended.

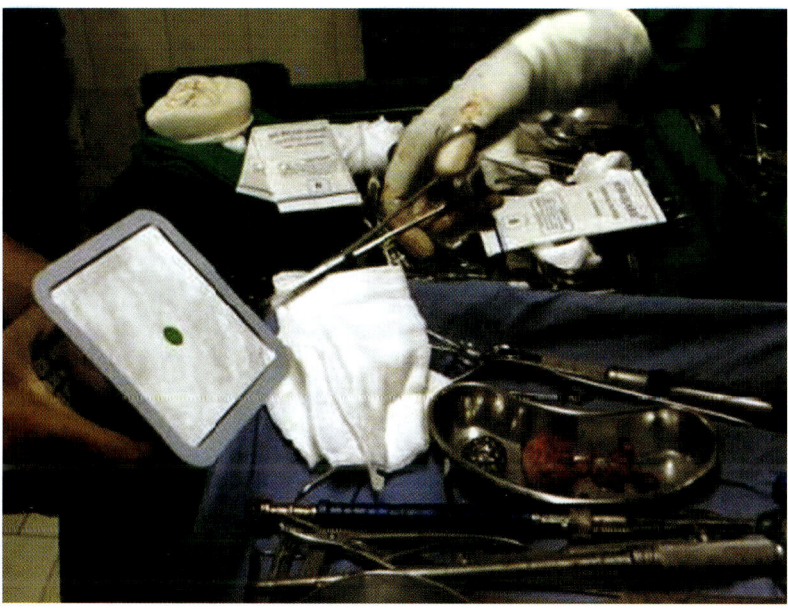

The correct sized HDPE liner is unpacked and hammered in the right orientation to produce a tight stable fit.

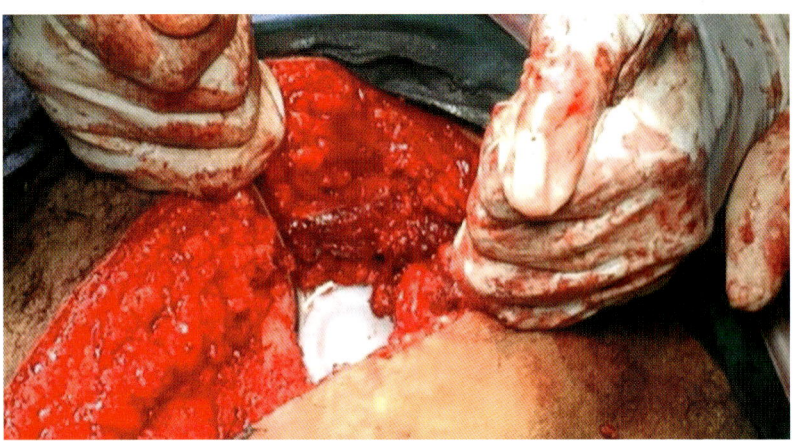

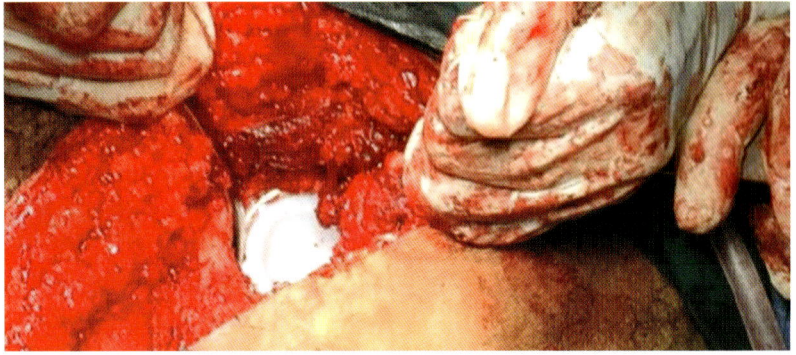

The long posterior wall should be oriented correctly before the insert is hammered in.

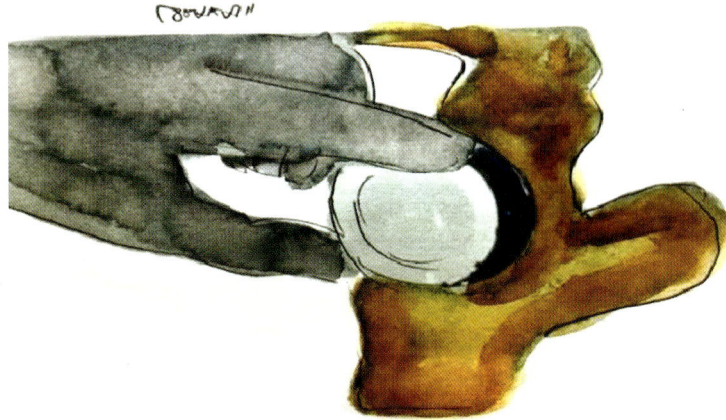

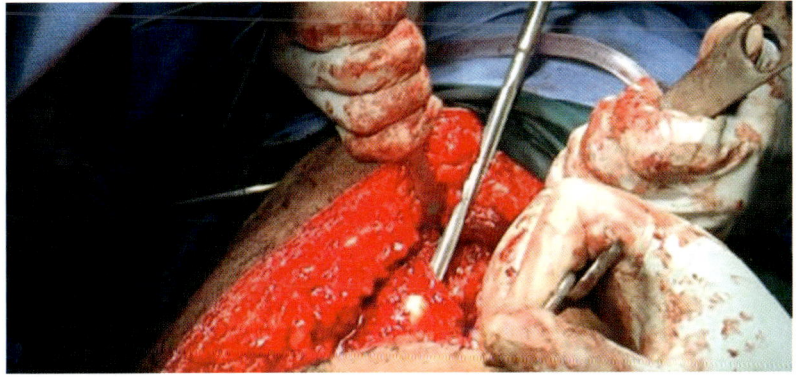

The femoral medullary preparation is the next step.

Using a broach, the medulla is opened from as far back in the trochanteric fossa as possible.

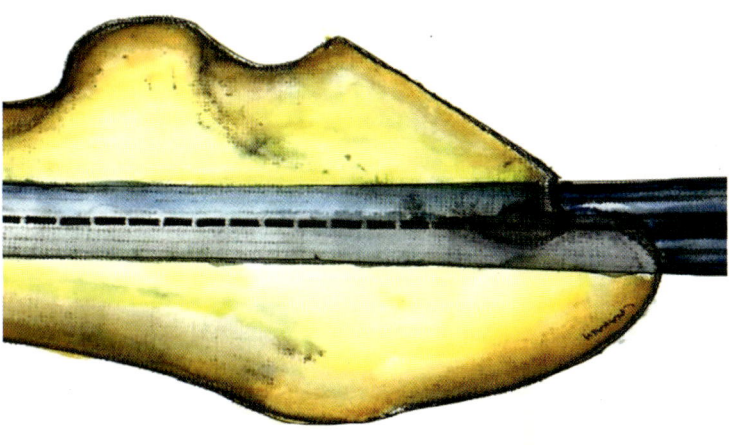

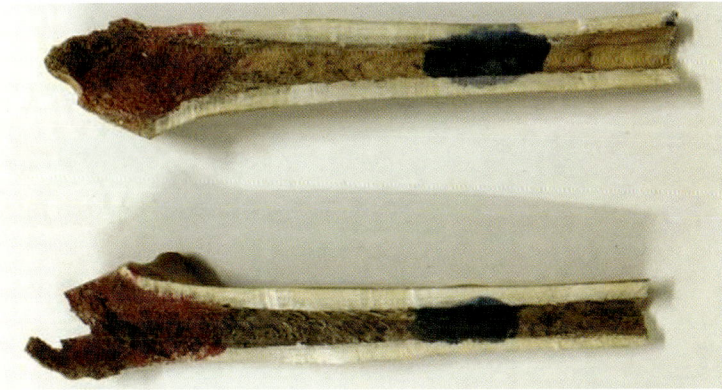

The broach should enter the trochanteric fossa popsteriorly close to the attachment of piriformis to avoid damage to the cortical wall.

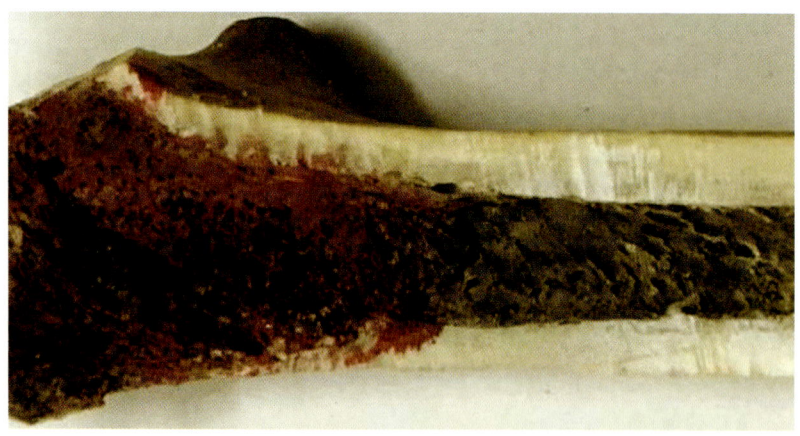

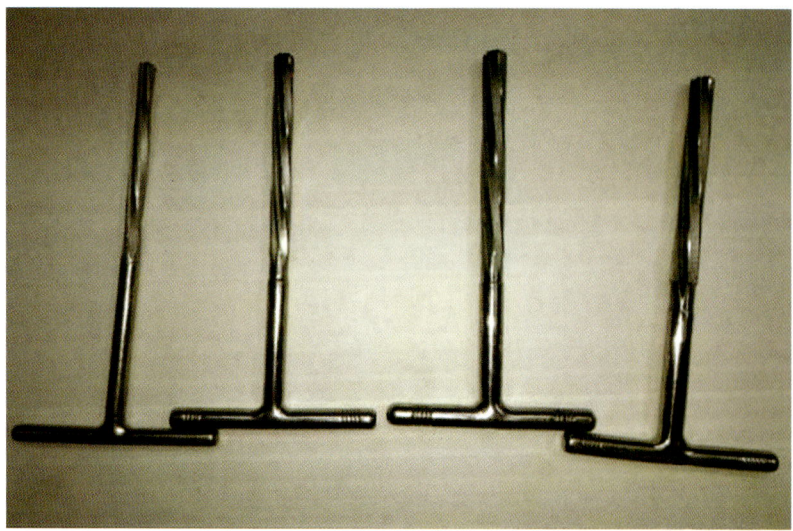

Different companies have their own broache designs. They all have sharp cutting edges. Shown above are the authors design of broaches.

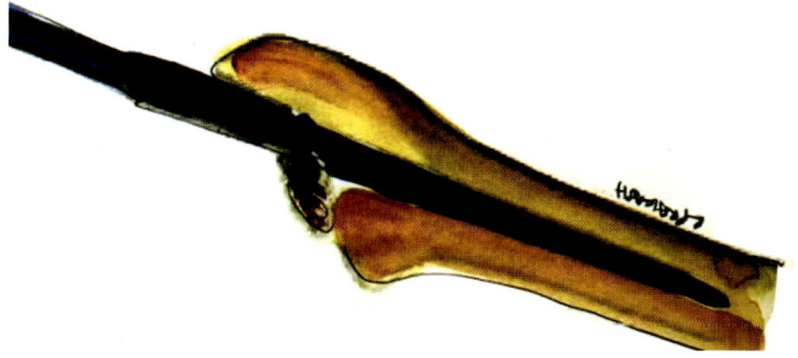

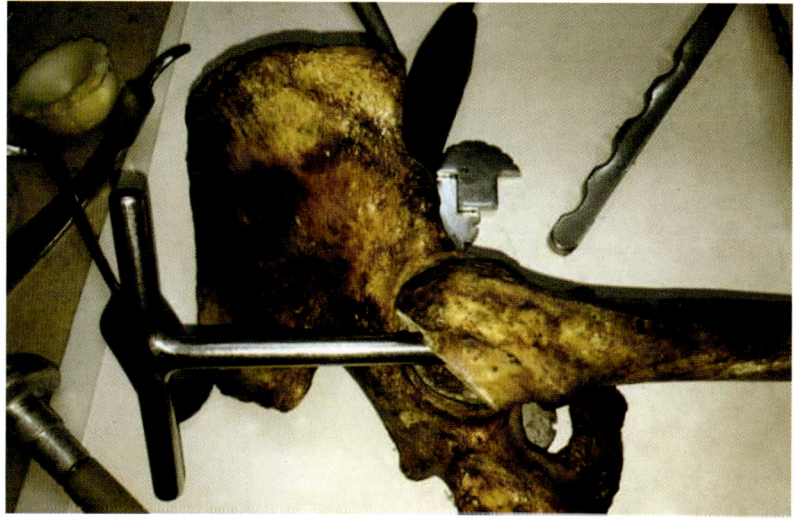

This stage of operation should be done by manual force, avoiding power tools to prevent breach of lateral cortex by power reaming.

A box chisel now cuts a wider opening for introduction of a femoral rasp.

This is a very important step, because the rotational orientation of this chisel is an important determining factor for the stability of the hip.

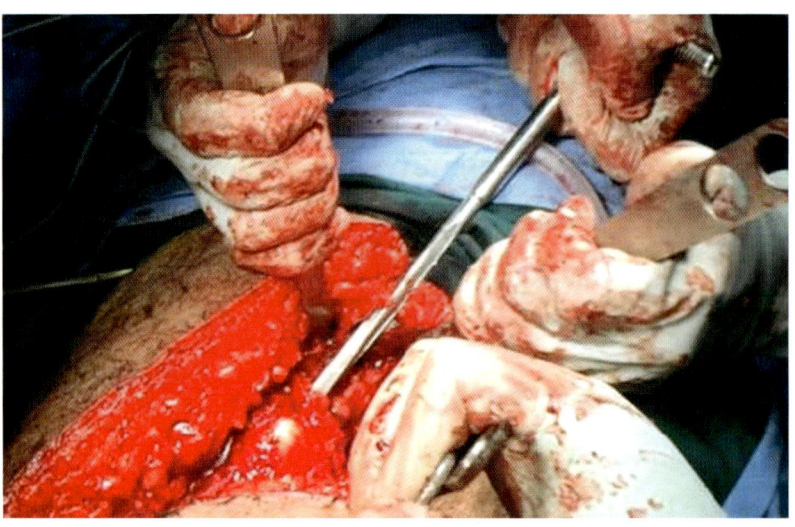

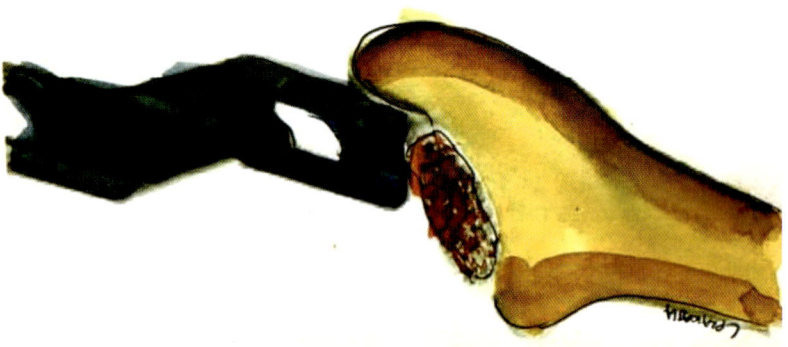

The head should be in fifteen degrees of anteversion for stability in flexion and internal rotation.

The best way to ensure this is to keep the stem orientation twisted about fifteen degrees away from the lesser trochanter.

Another method is to faithfully follow the rotational orientation of the neck and match it precisely. Some surgeons prefer this method because of the variation of the anteversion in the population.

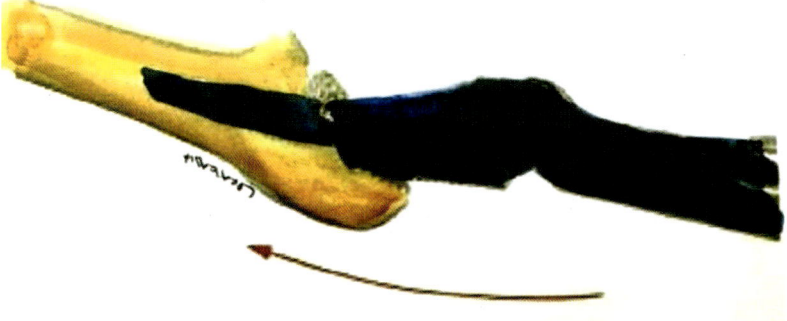

Femoral rasps are now used to broach the canal. Increasing rasp sizes are used to get the best fit.

The surgeon should aim for a global fit, rather that proximal or distal.

The rasp should exactly follow the version for stable neck.

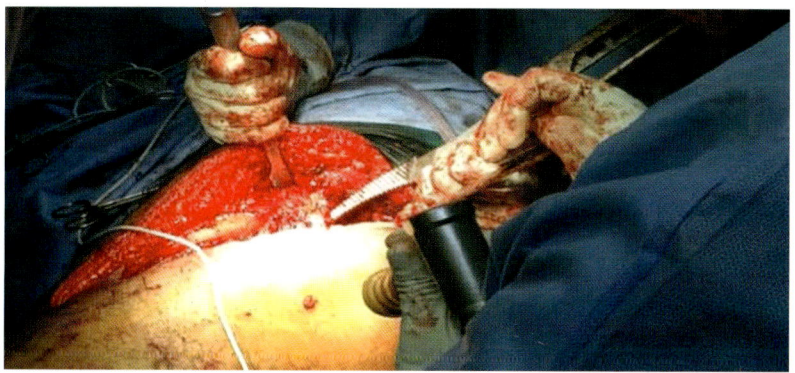

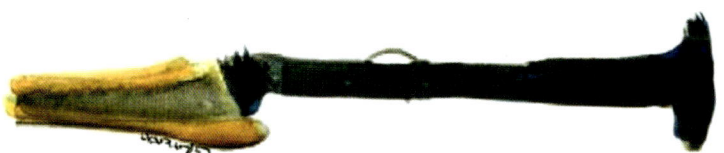

Care must be taken that the femoral shaft is not broken while using successively larger rasps.

The surgeon should strike a balance between the rasp size and femoral dimensions to ensure that the largest size that does not split the femur is used.

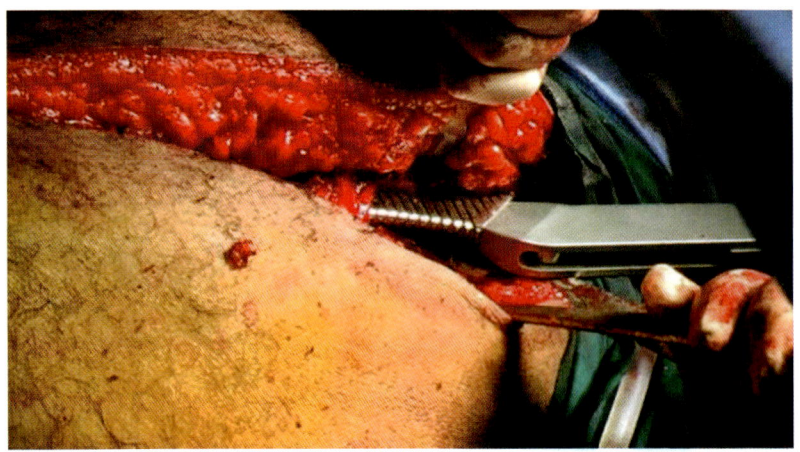

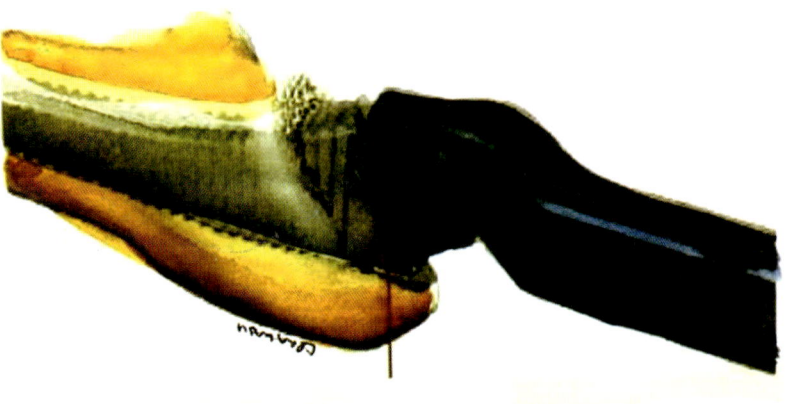

As shown in the operative photos, most of the current cementless instrumentation sets, have a combined rasp trial unit. The handle can be detached and the head – neck component easily added.

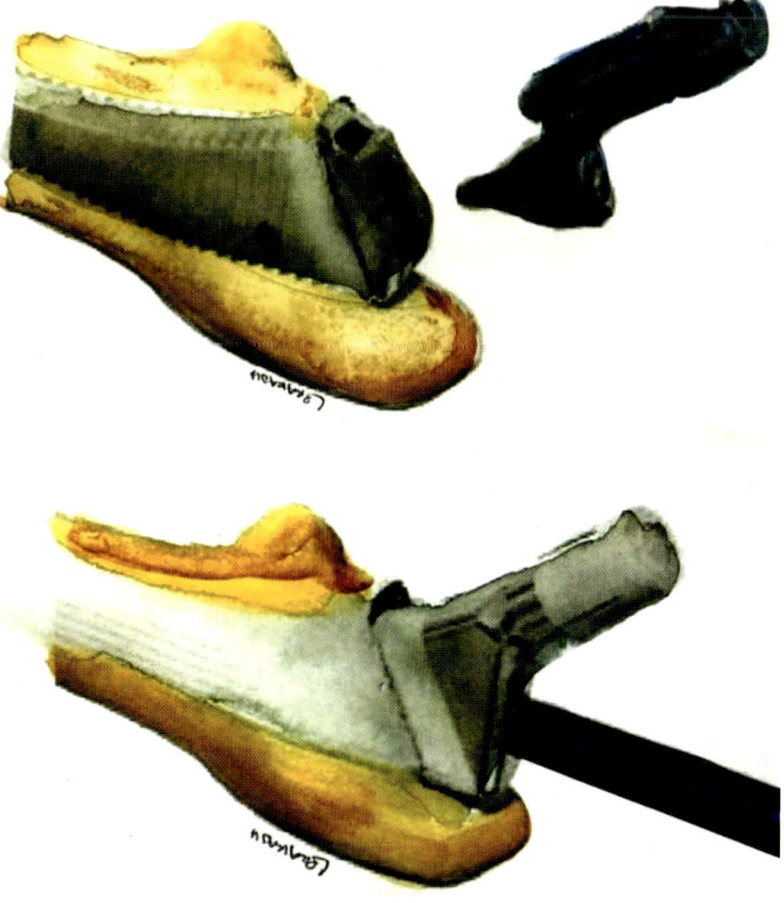

The actual implant is now hammered in taking care that the stem enters posteriorly and is in the correct orientation.

The ideal stem should be seated in valgus with the prosthesis tip touching the medial femur. Varus stems fail in a short while and need revision.

Most porous coated and hydroxy appatite plasma coated stems have upper markings; the level up to which they have to be hammered in. the surgeon must stick to this and errors in hammering in less are more forgivable by neck length adjustments at a later stage, than shattering the femur, needing additional procedures.

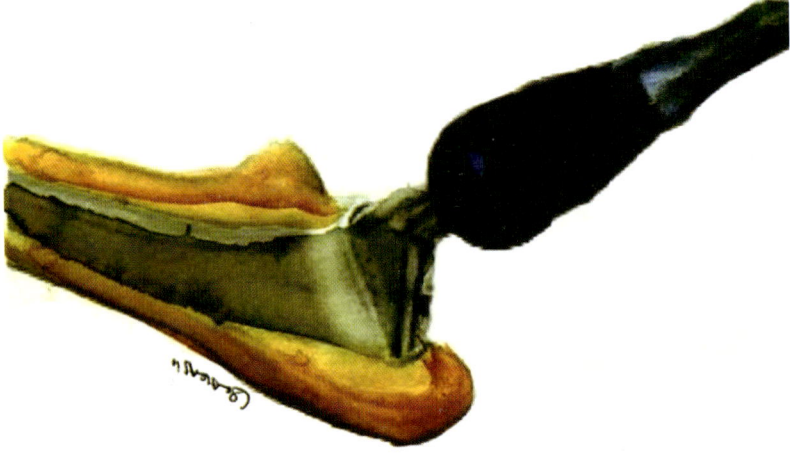

A rule of thumb for the correct prosthesis impactation level is to ensure that the middle of the neck is at the levl of greater trochanter. This can be checked with a scale or a k wire.

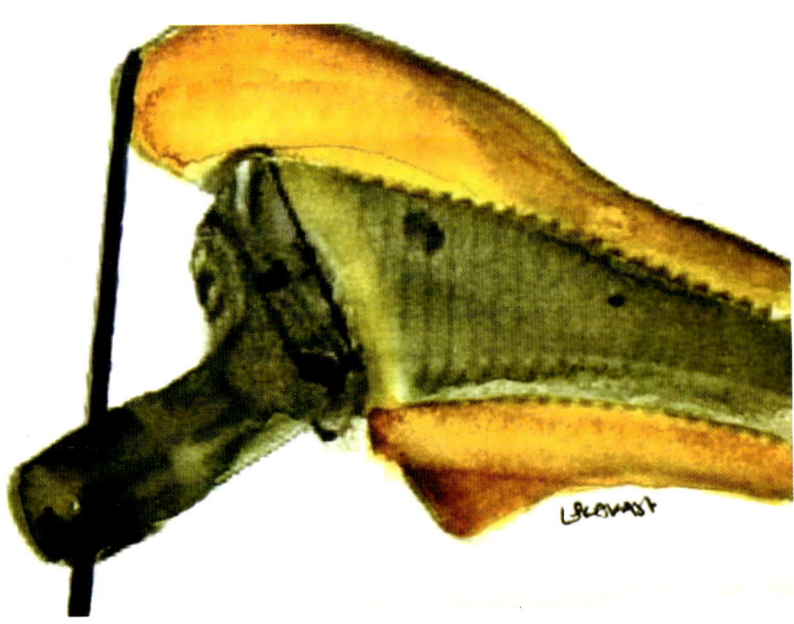

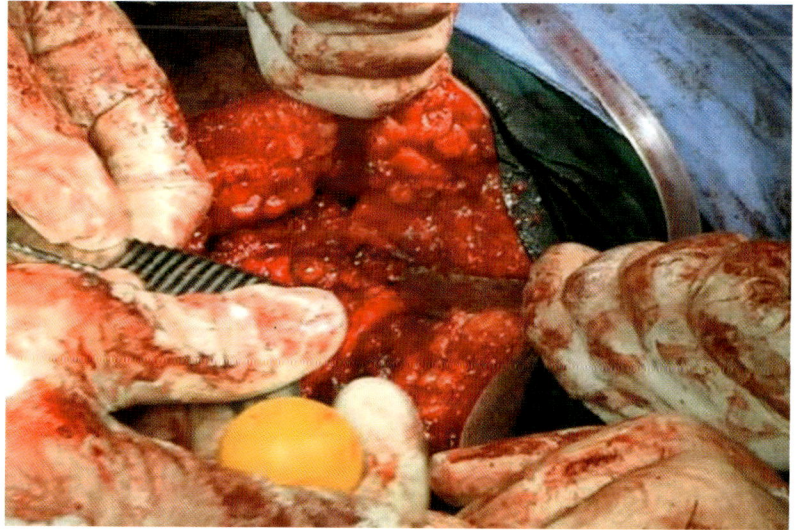

A trial head is snapped on to the rasp cum femoral trial. Heads are usually available with varying neck lengths.

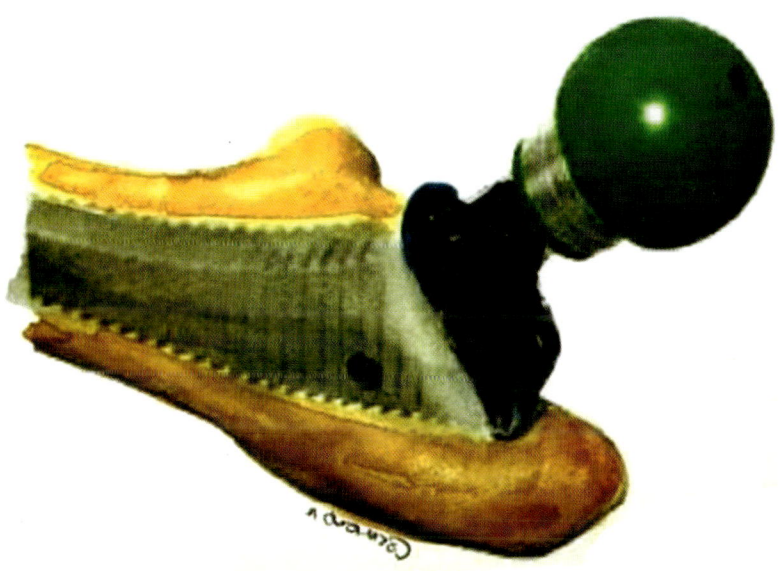

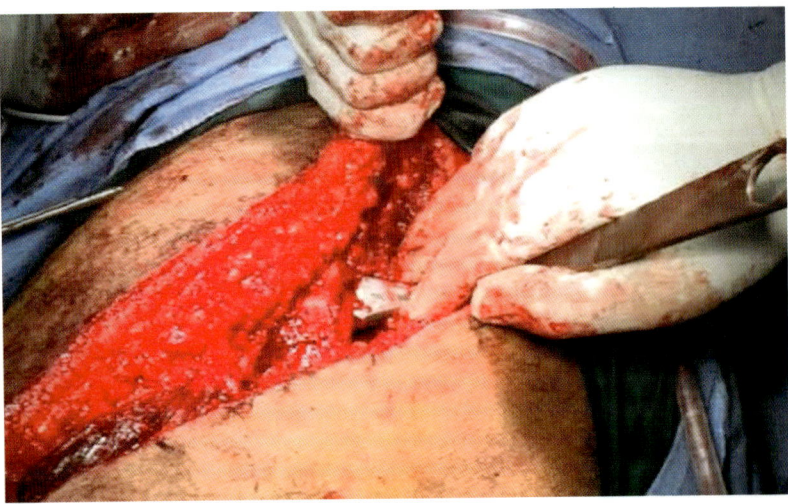

Older designs had just short medium and long necks, but newer cementless models have minus four to zero and from one to four plus sizes to fine tune the hip tension after reduction.

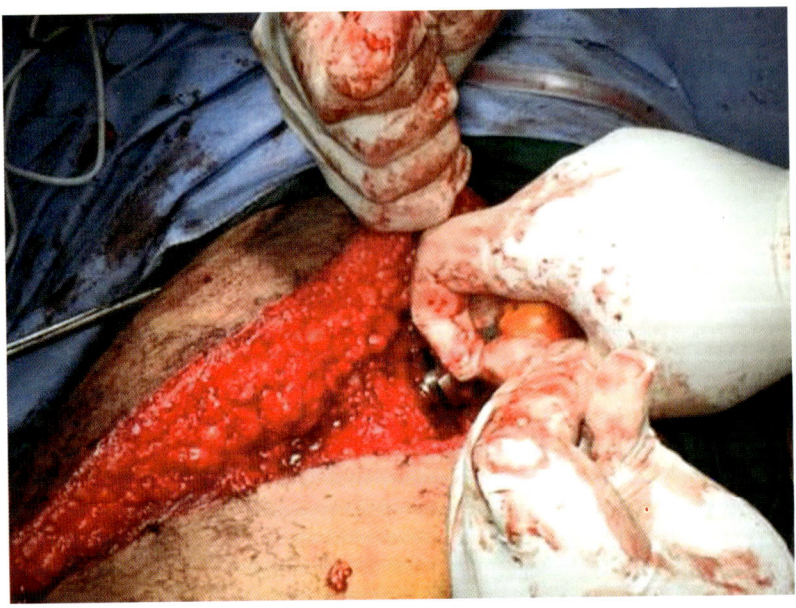

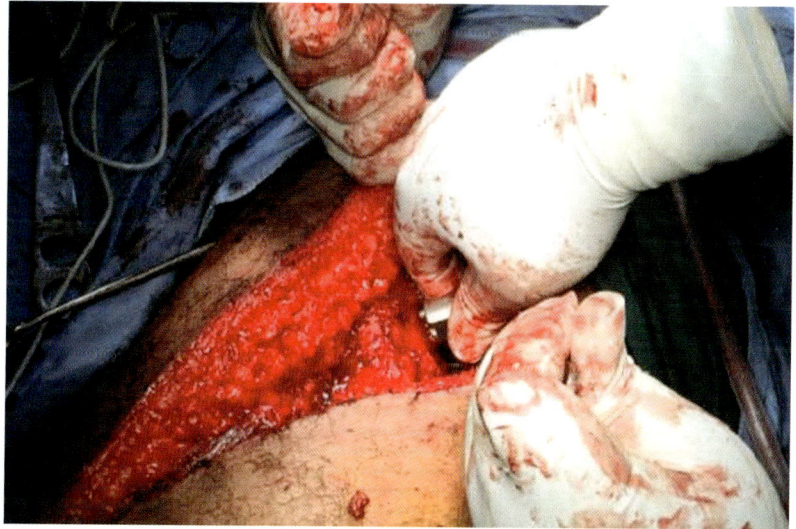

The hip is reduced after the appropriate head is inserted.

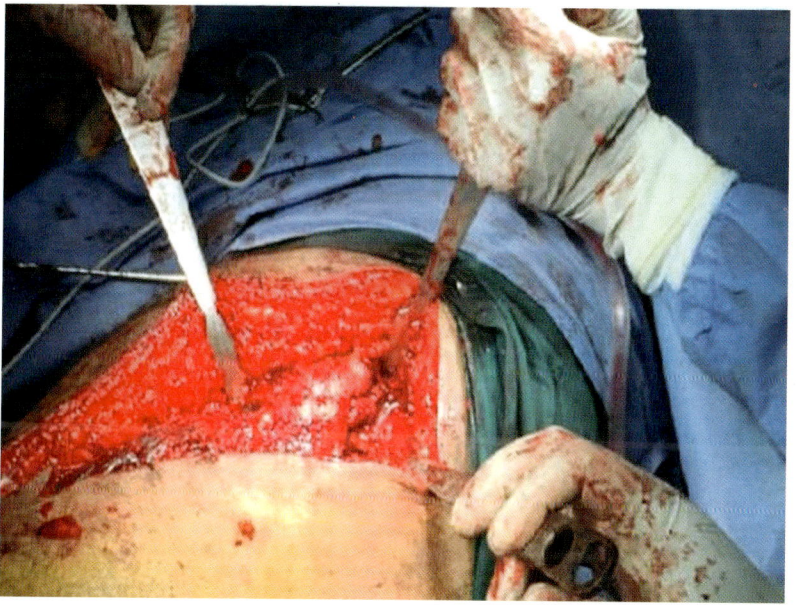

The instrumentation sets differ from company to company but the fundamental principles are the same.

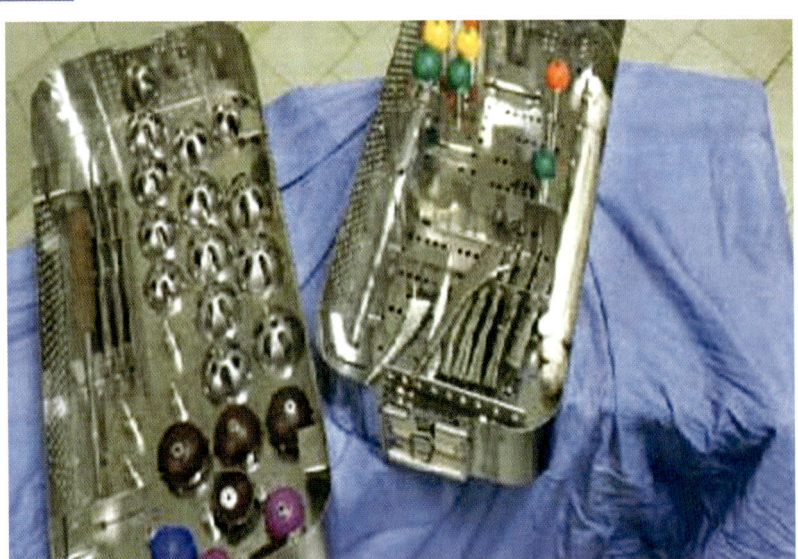

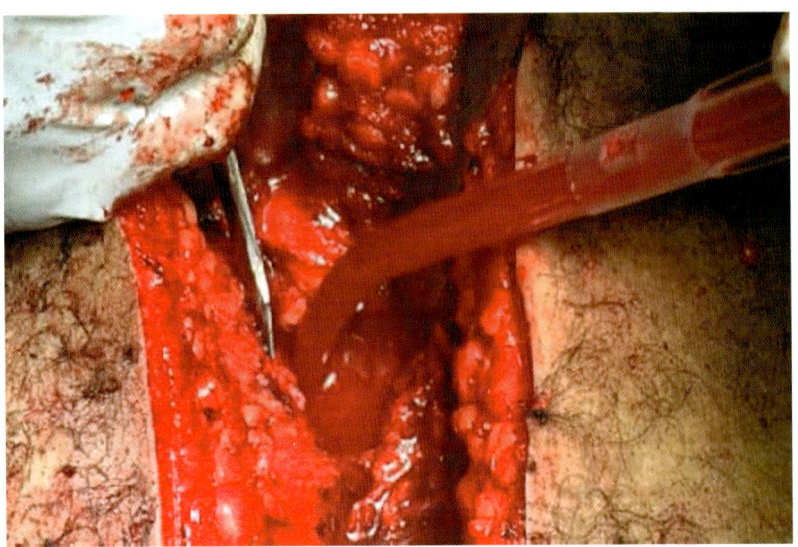

The joint is thoroughly washed with saline and the head coverage is checked once again.

The actual head is now snapped over the rasp-trial and another trial reduction of the hip is done.

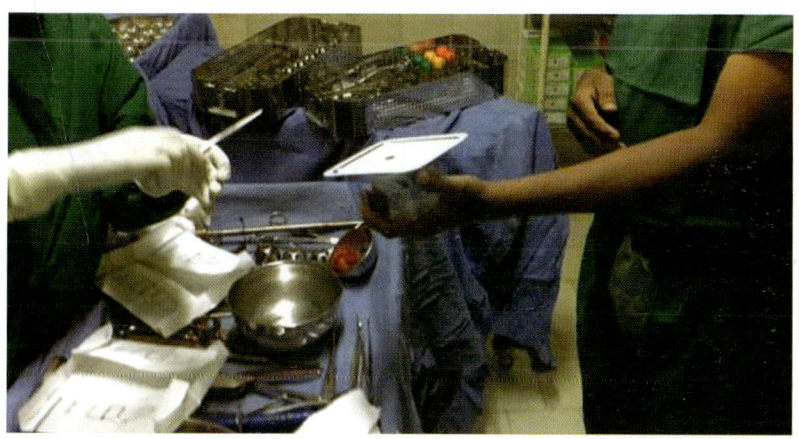

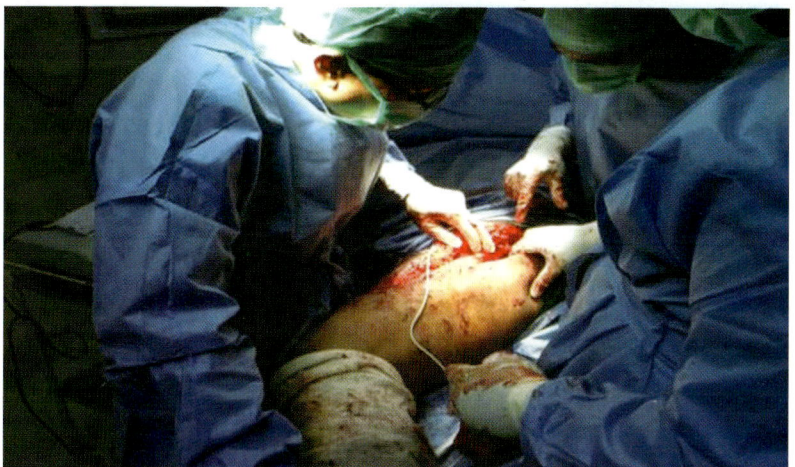

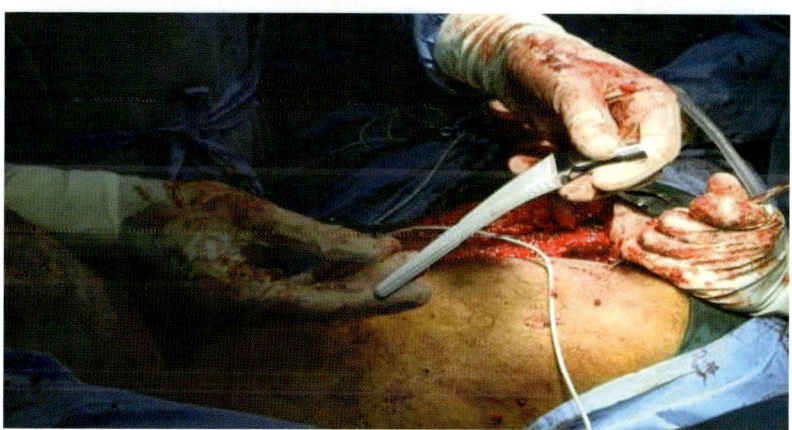

The actual femoral component is unpacked and hammered in.

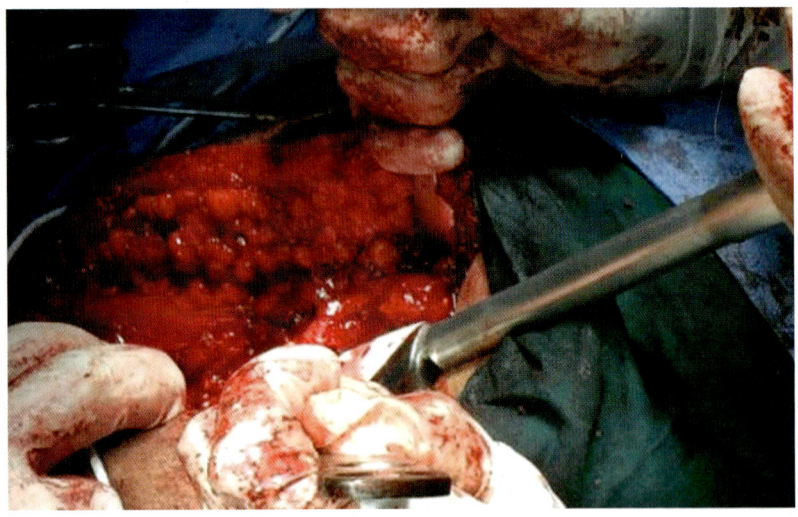

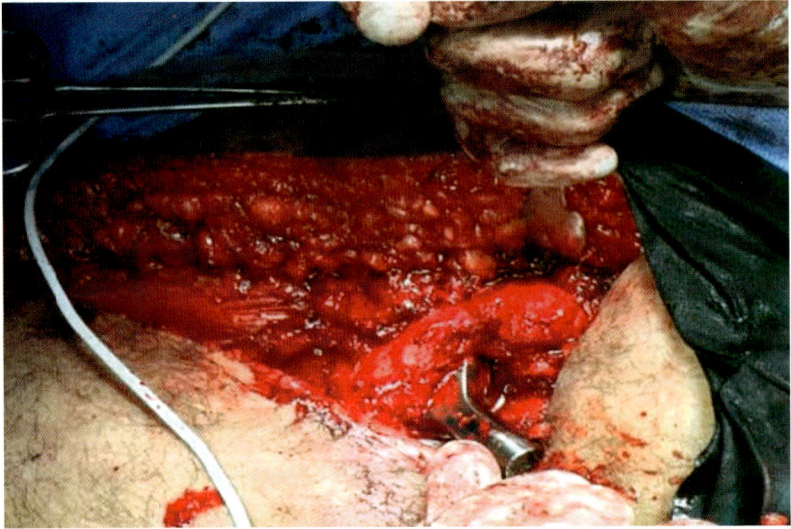

First reduction is attempted with a trial head. High end hips come in many neck lengths to ensure that the hip is perfectly balanced and neither tight nor loose after reduction.

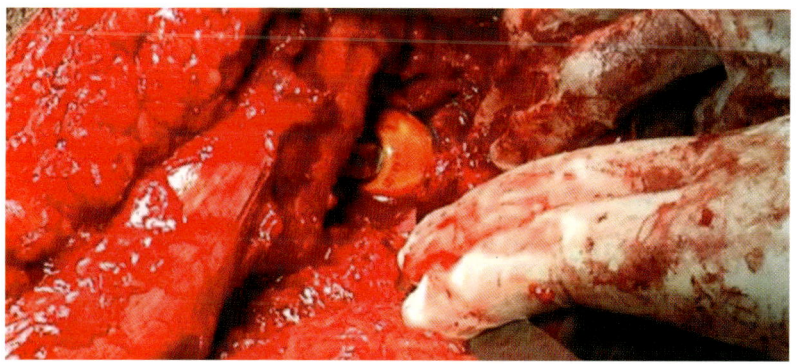

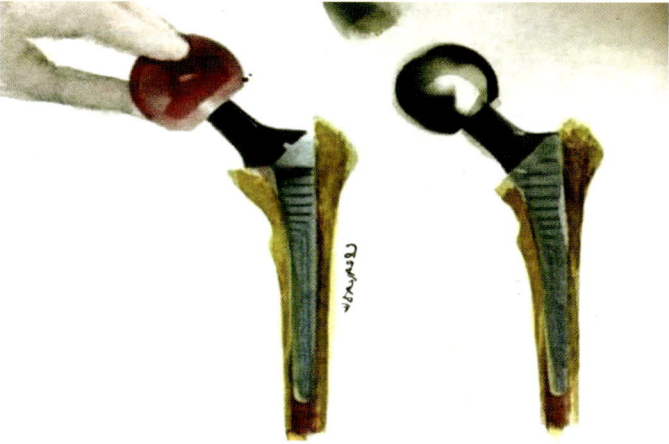

Different neck lengths come in different colours. The correct size is now opened.

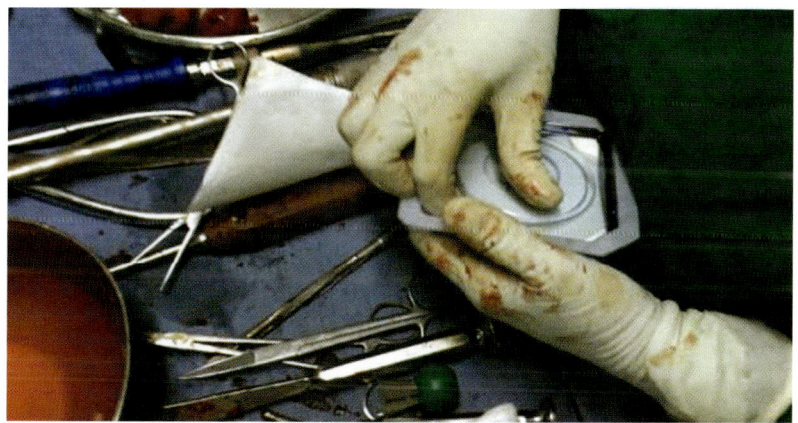

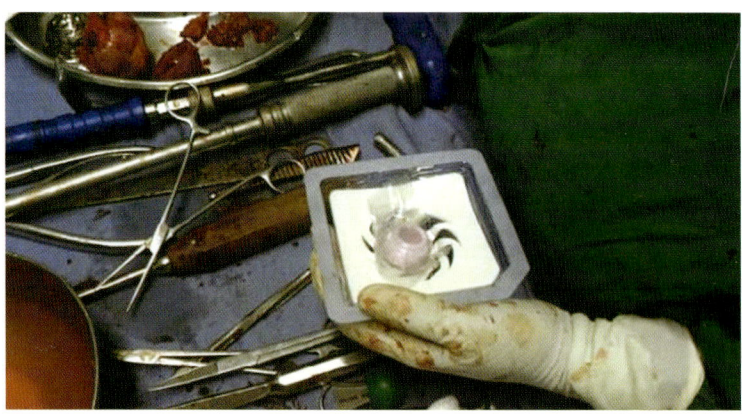

In this case a ceramic head is being used. It is tapped over the neck stub.

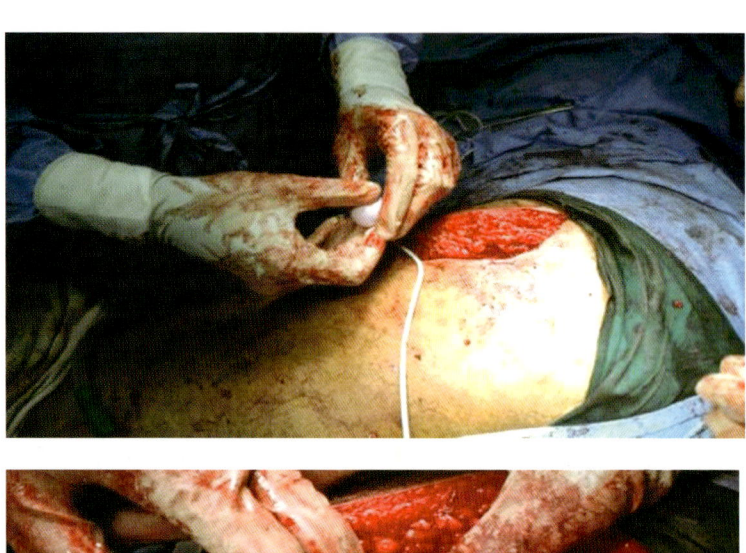

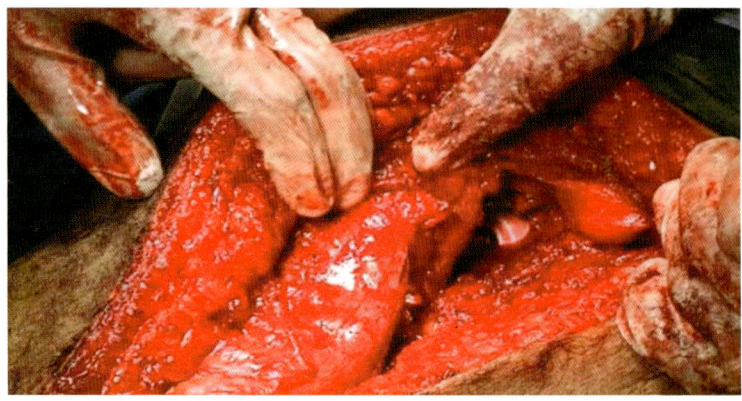

If the cuts and orientation have been correct, the hip should be stable in all directions.

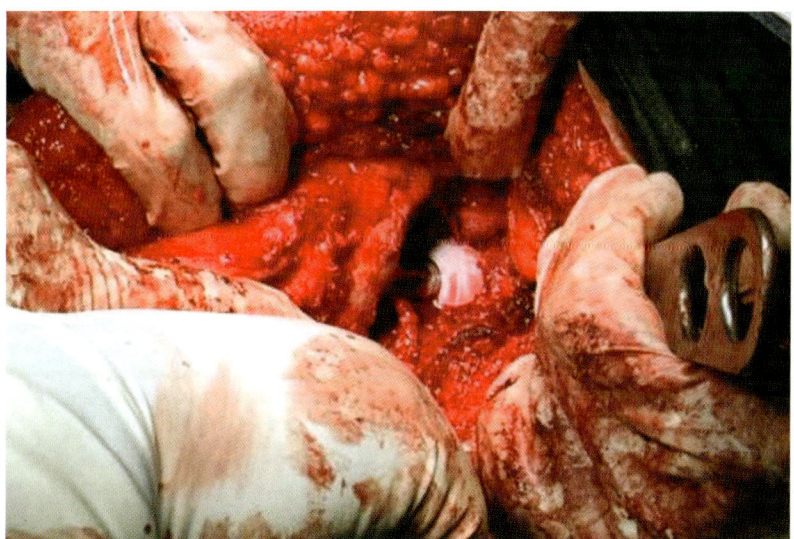

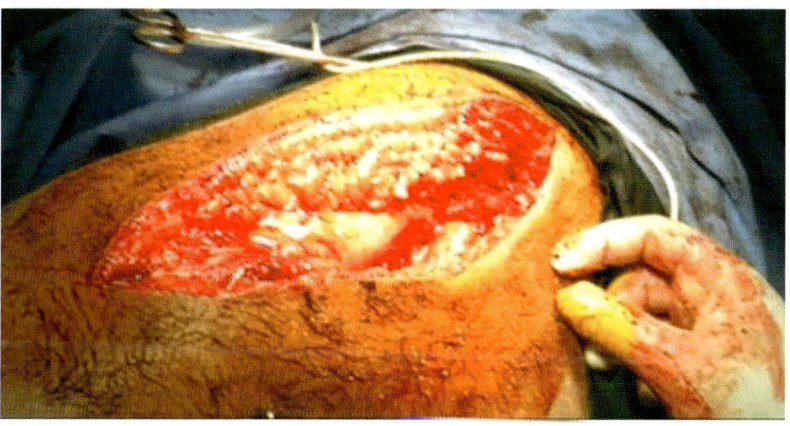

The small lateral rotators are now reattached using the stay sutures left behind earlier. It may not be possible to suture parts of piriformis and lower parts of quadrates Femoris, but this does not matter.

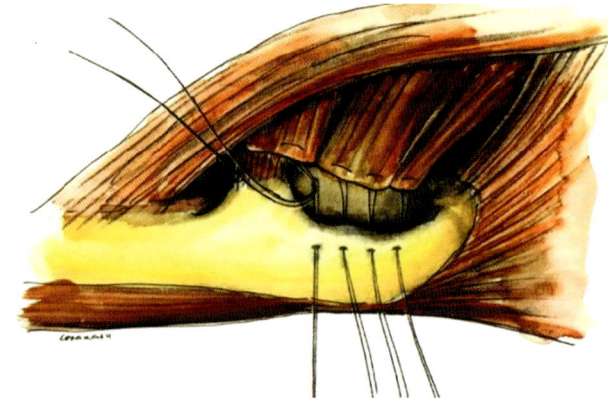

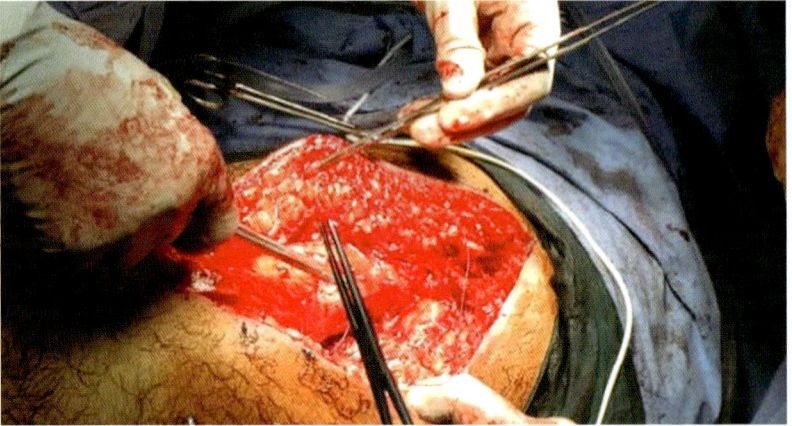

The deeper tissues are closed with absorbable sutures. The author uses continuous sutures.

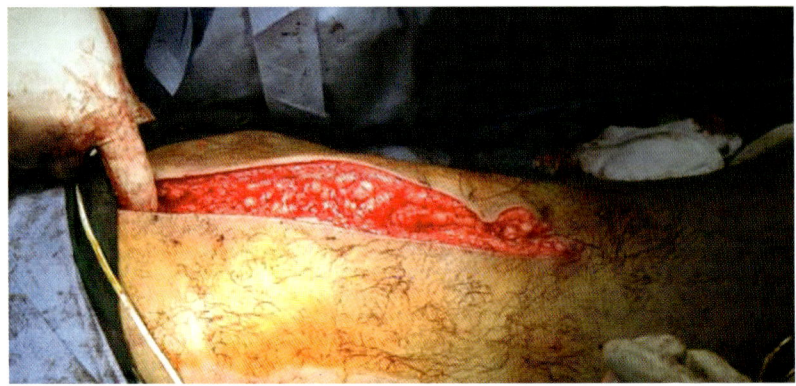

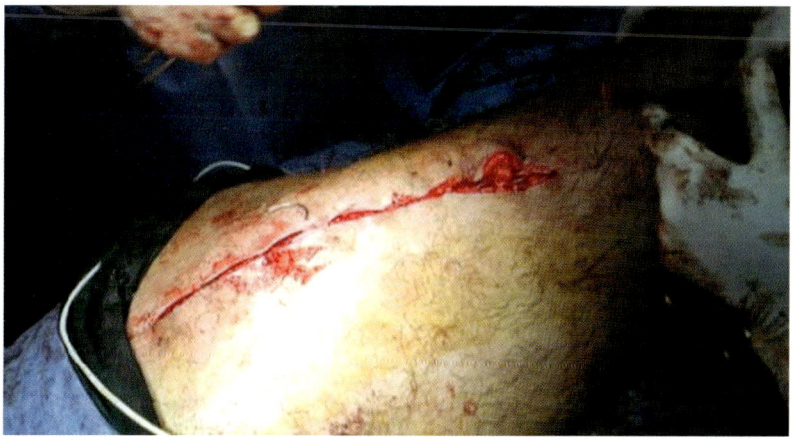

Good skin approximation by subcutaneous sutures will ensure that the final skin stapling would be easy and result in a clean scar.

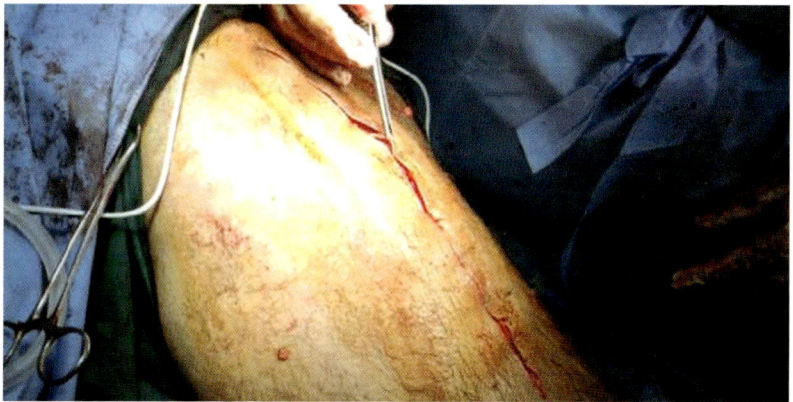

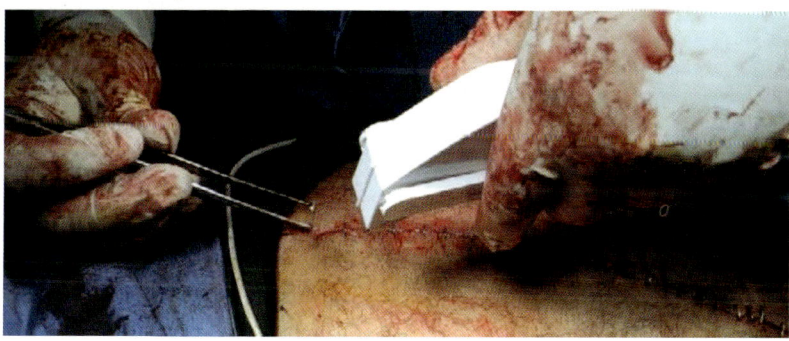

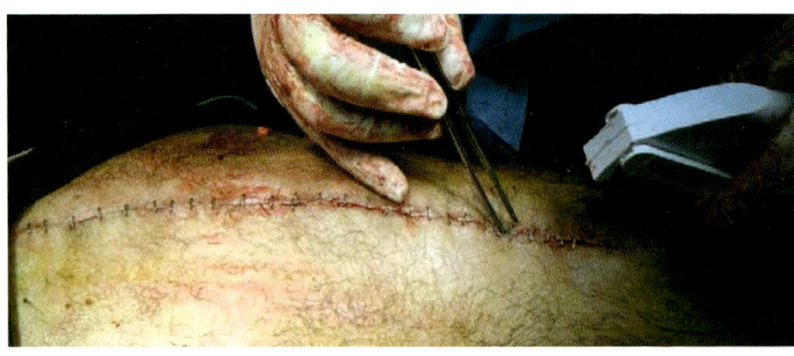

The skin is stapled.

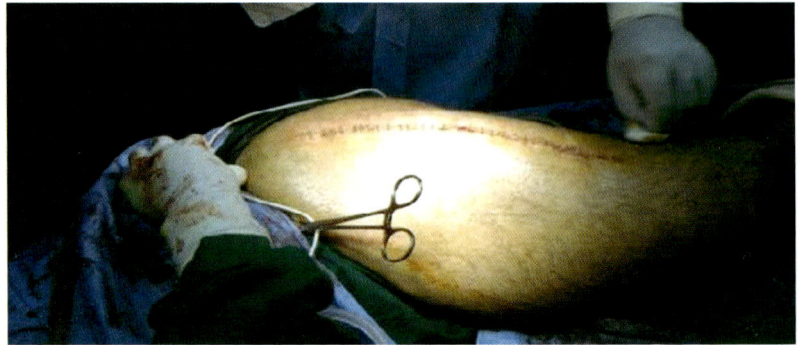

9

Clinical Examples

A well done cemented hip lasts at least 25 years comfortably as is seen in the above patient.

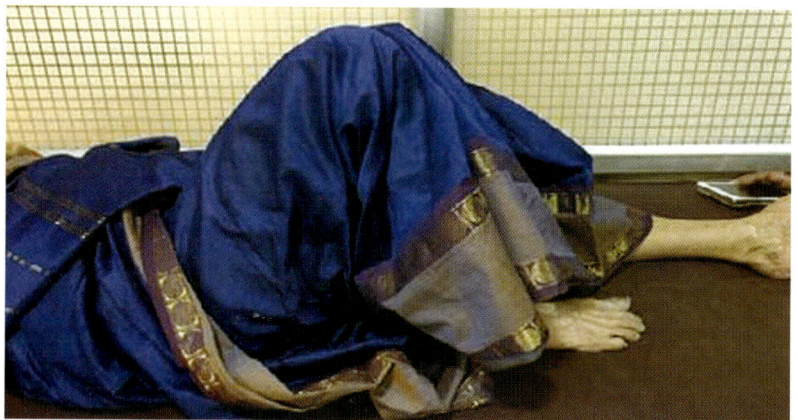

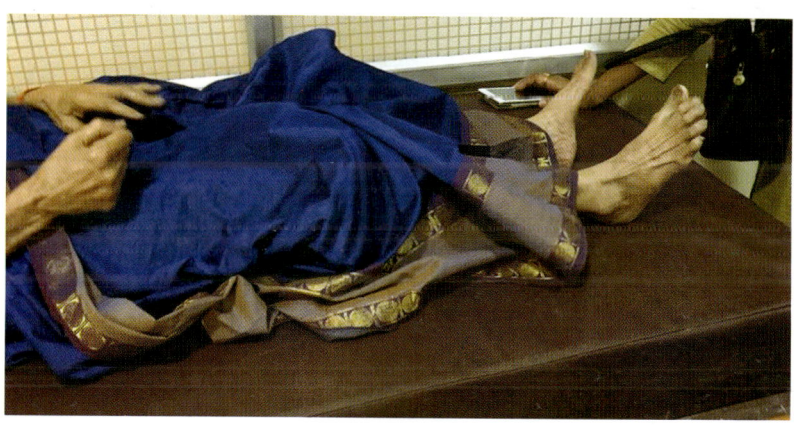

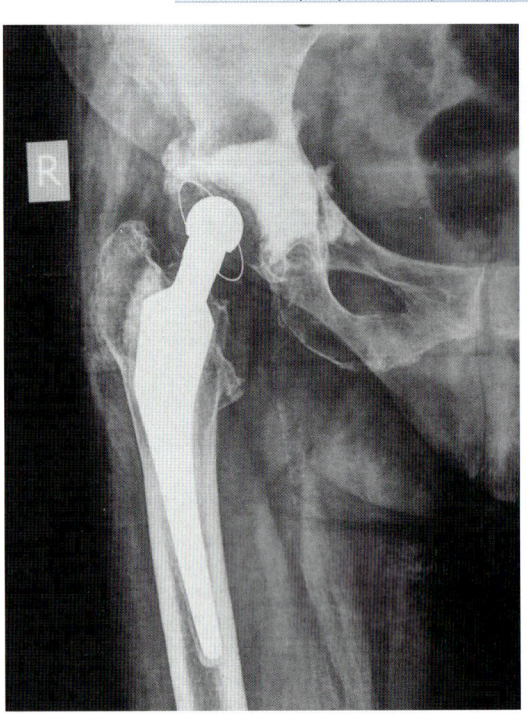

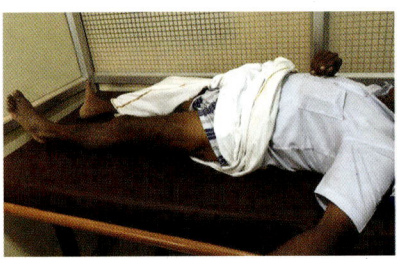
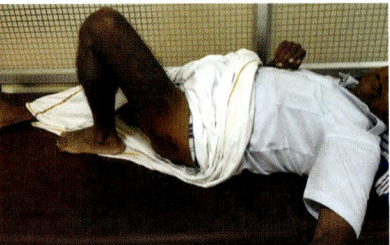

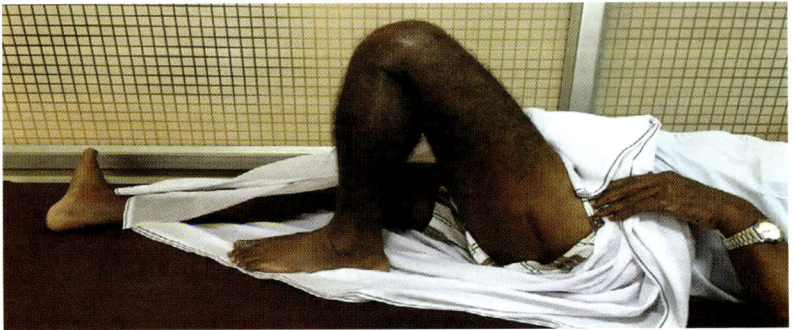

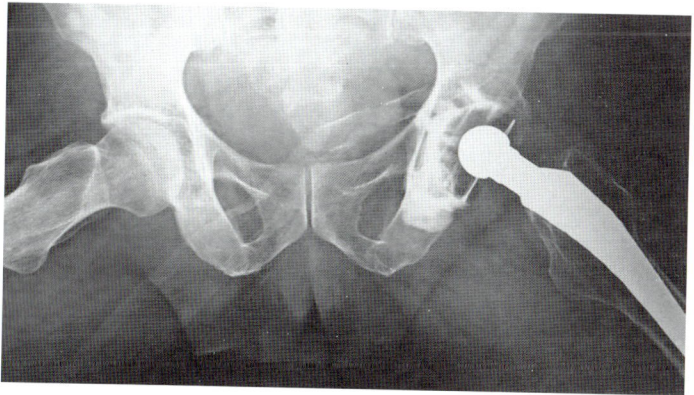

Properly done, Cemented hips usually last twentufive years, before the plastic debris from the cup wear begins to cause osteolysis and gradual loosening.

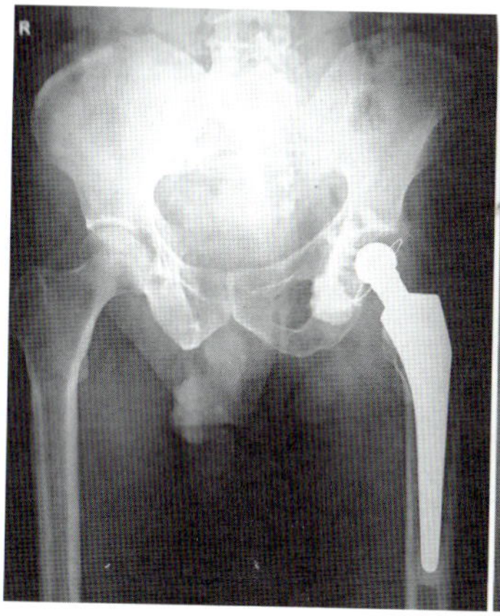

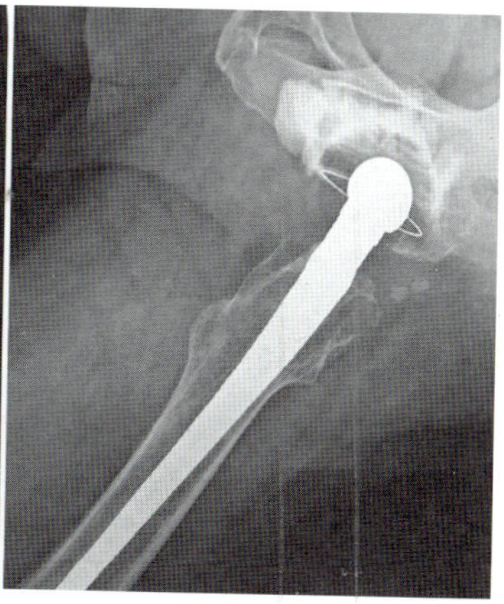

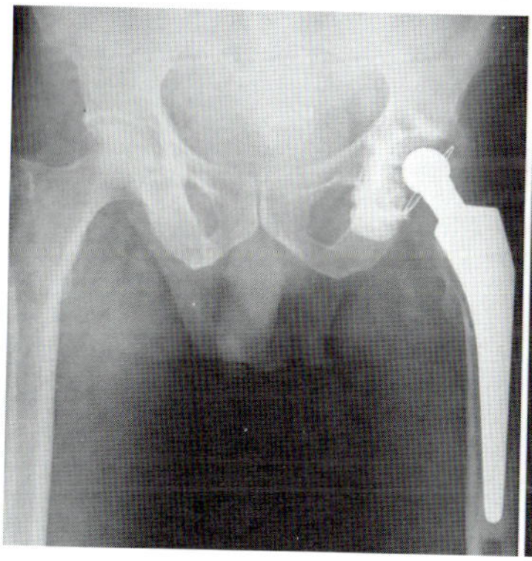

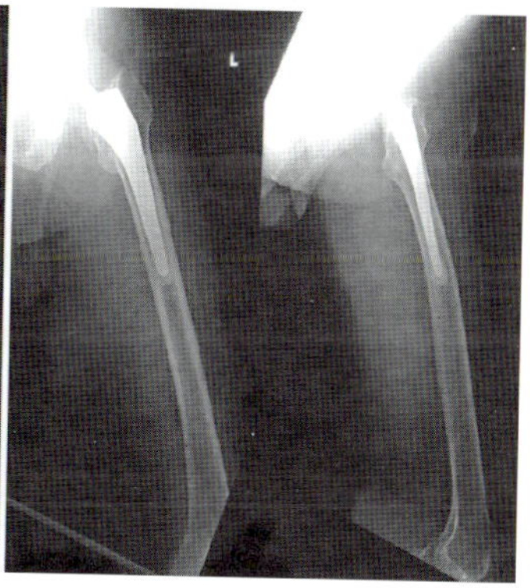

This cemented hip, operated twenty six years ago, is still going strong and the patient is totally asymptomatic, though we can begin appreaciating the osteolysis in the trochanteric area indicating that the loosening has begun. The superior plastic wear 4 can also be appreciated in the twentysix year old picture.

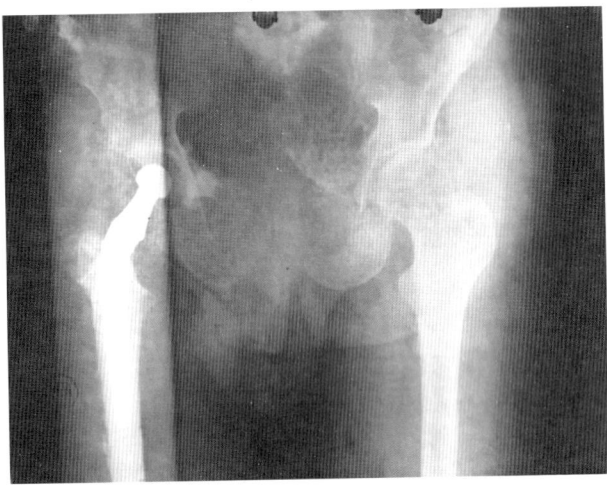

These X-rays show the natural history of a cemented total hip replacement. Above is the immediate post operative radiograph.

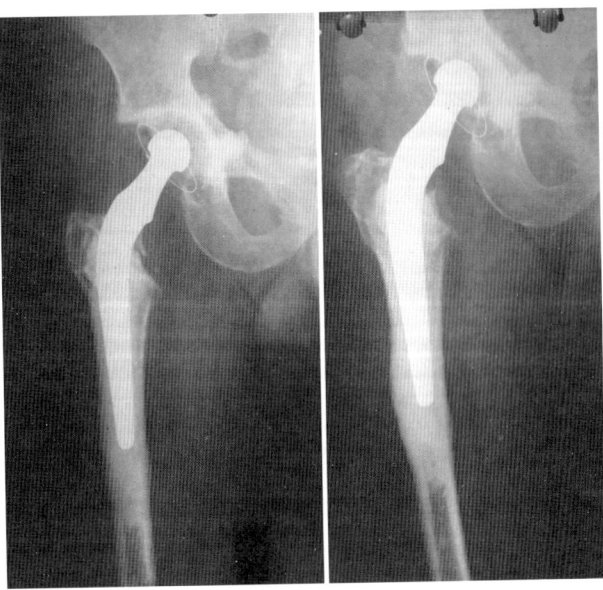

Follow up of five and ten years. There is hardly any acetabular wear and the stem is well cemented.

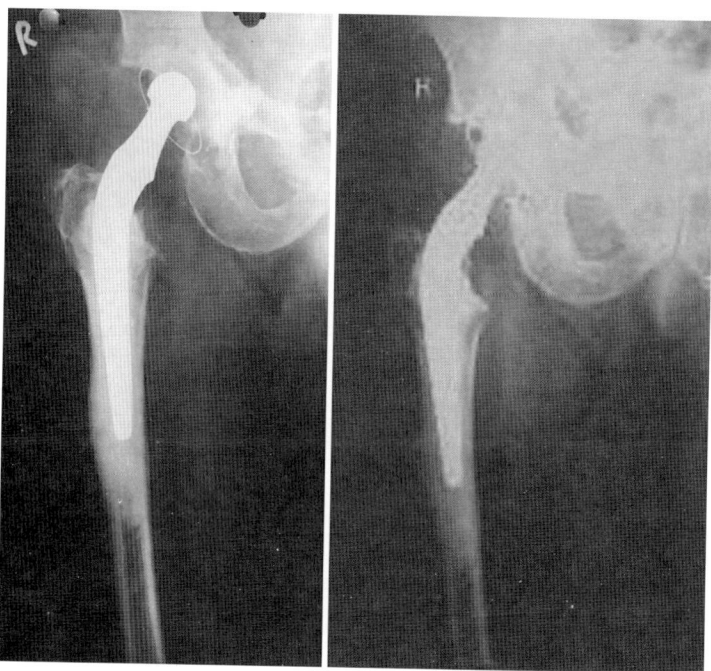

At fifteen and twenty years, we can see the beginnings of HDPE wear, and the gradually apparent difference between the superior and inferior walls of the acetabular cup.

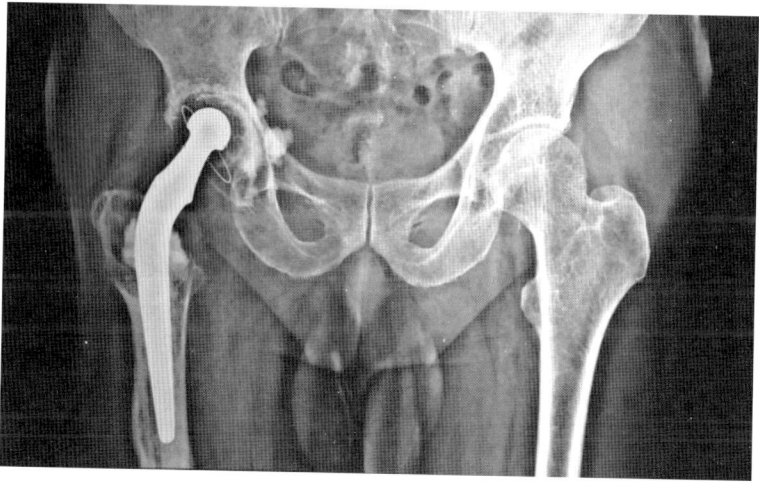

At twenty five years, asymptomatic loosening has begun. This is due to the plastic wear debris trickling down and producing a fibrous layer between the cement and bone. Lucent lines can be seen both in acetabular and femoral cement/bone interfaces.

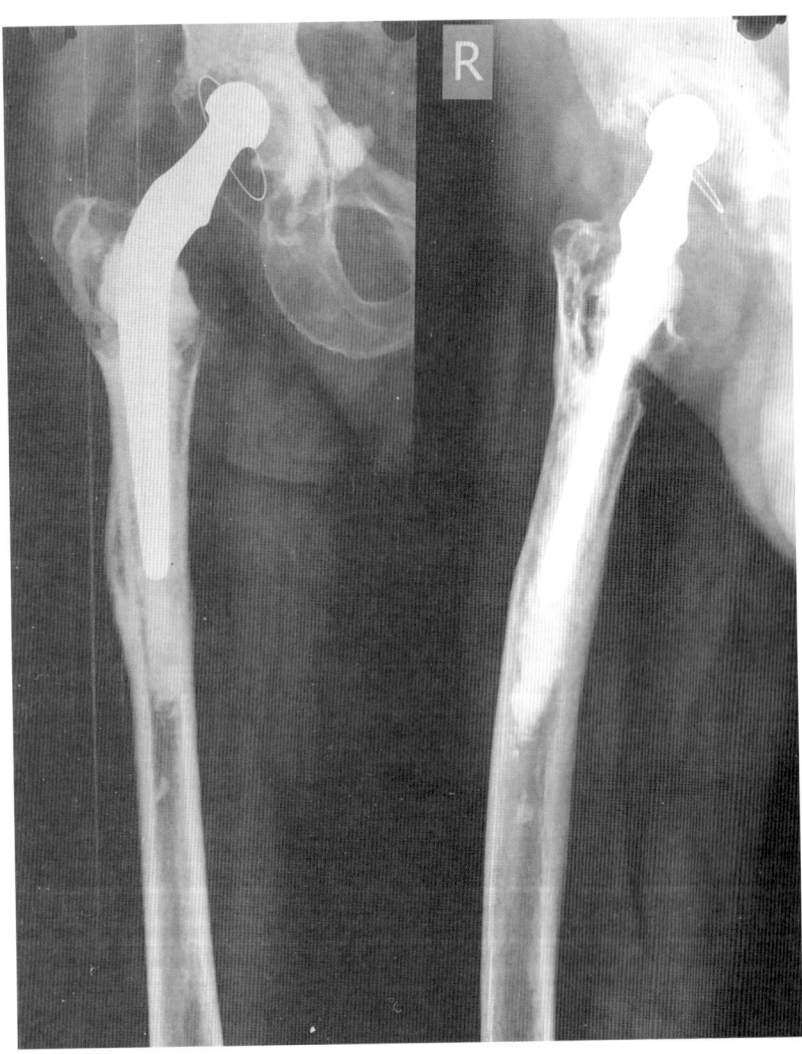

X-ray at 27 years when he was taken up for revision. He underwent a revision with another cemented hip and is doing well.

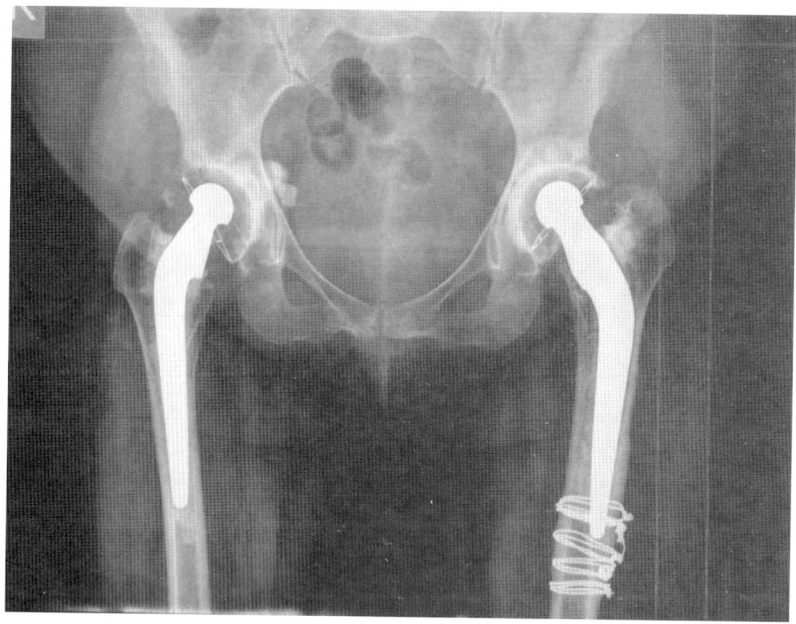

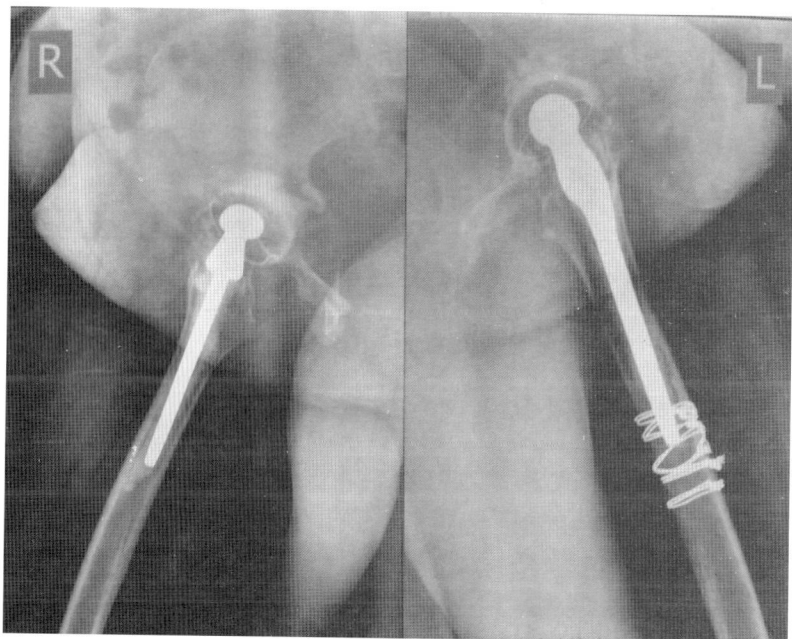

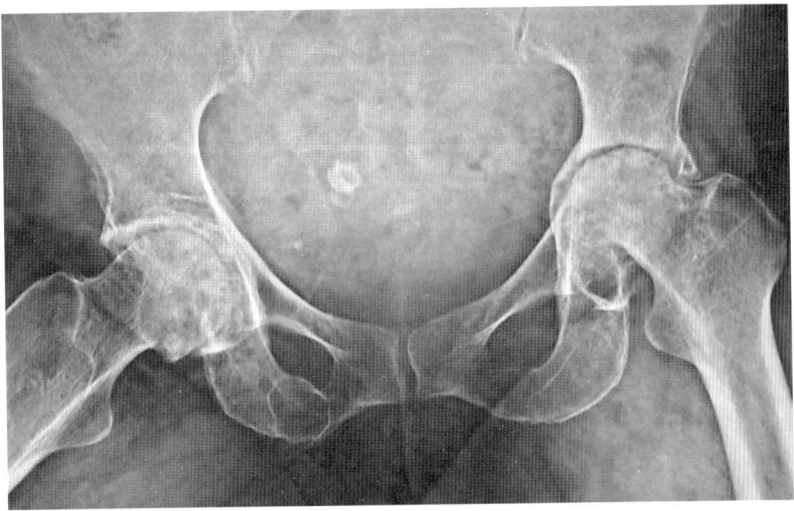

Bilateral steroid induced avascular necrosis treated with simultaneous cementless replacements. See the well seated cups, grafts between cups and acetabulam and the neutral tight fit prosthesis.

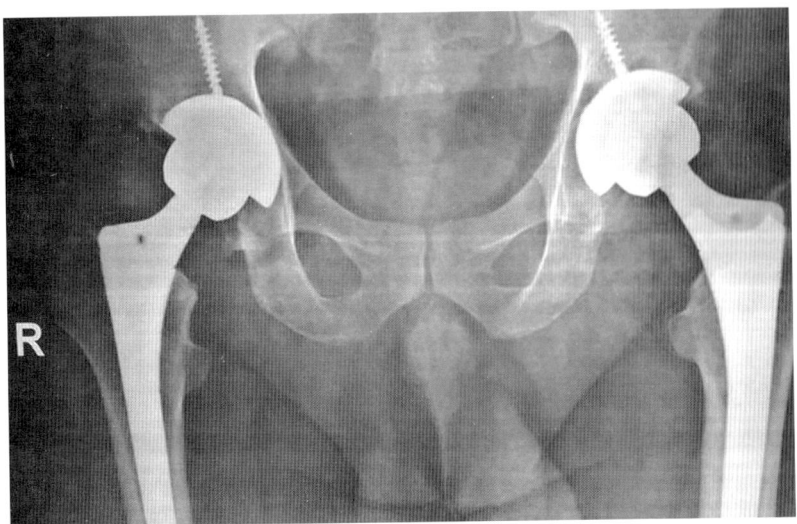

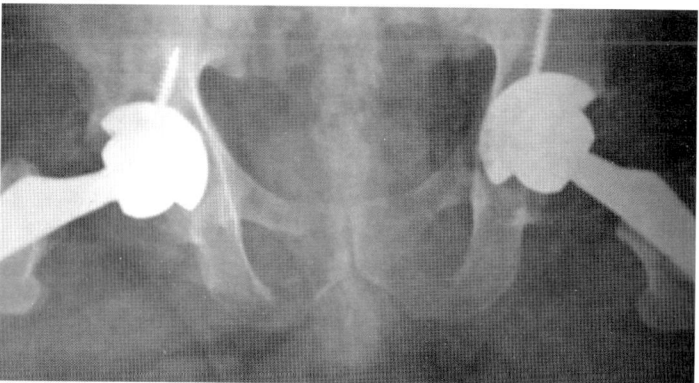

The case described in the previous page, followed up to six years. Excellent functional outcome and good integration of the cup and stem with bone.

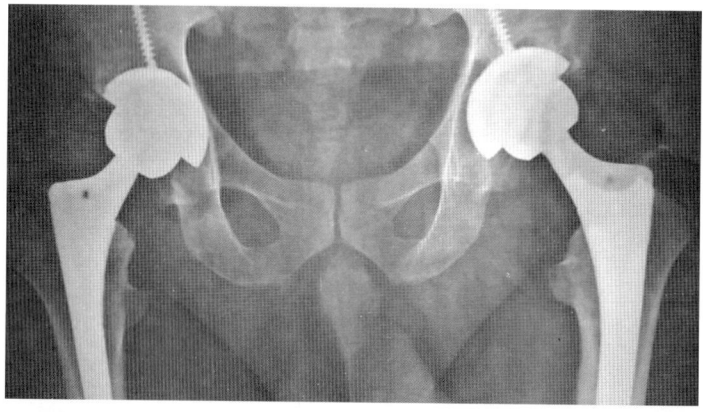

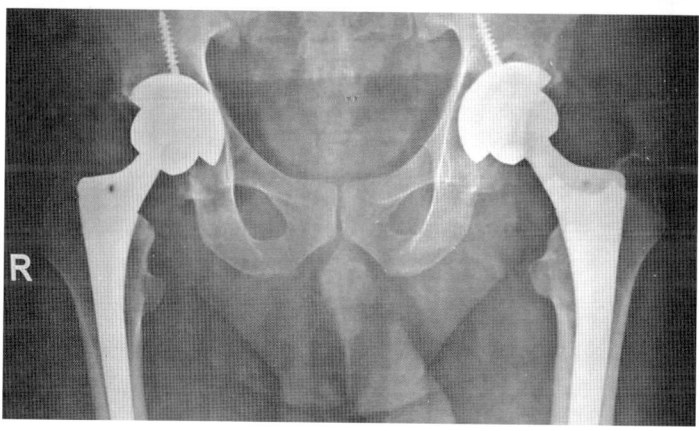

X-rays of the same patient after twelve years showing satisfactory component position and no evidence of loosening. Components placed anatomically with correct orientation last almost a quarter of century without problems.

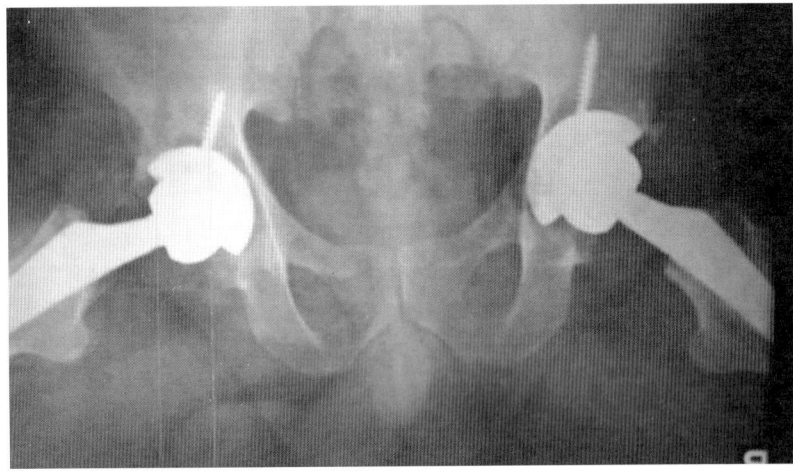

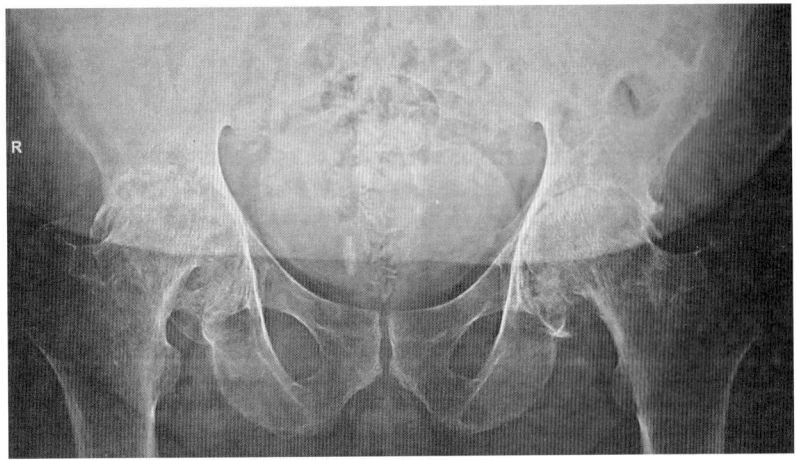

Progressive alcohol induced avascular necrosis in a fifty year old patient, rather obese, who was taken up for sequential bilateral hip replacements.

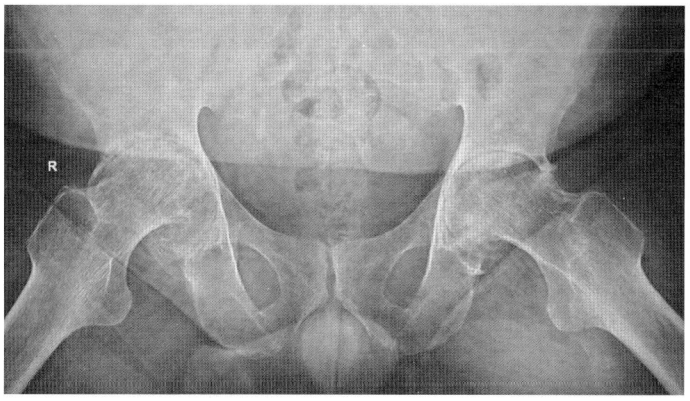

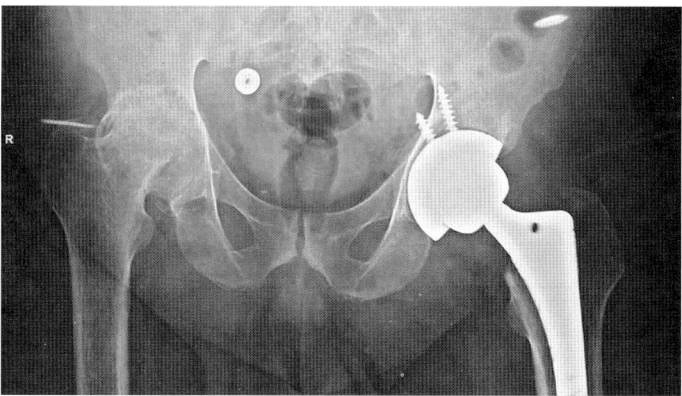

The left hip was operated first followed by the right hip.

The right acetabular cup is seated a little deep but has decent circumfrential fit.

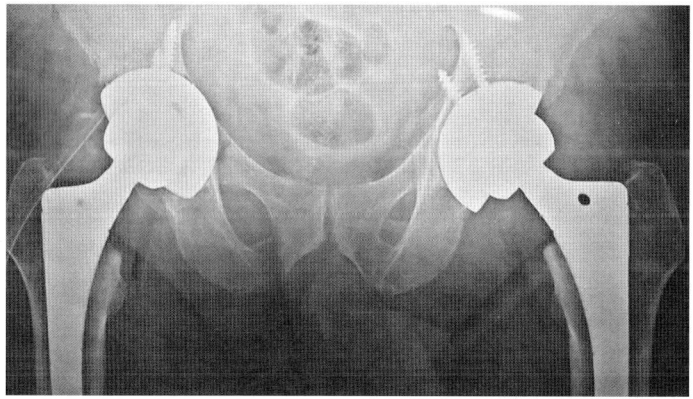

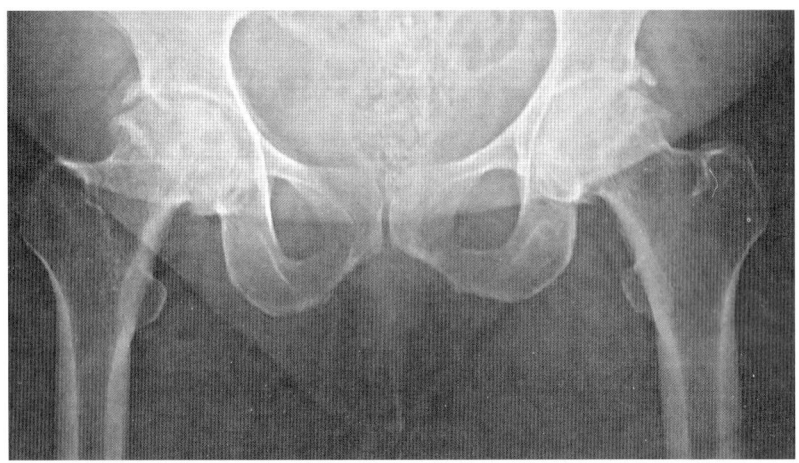

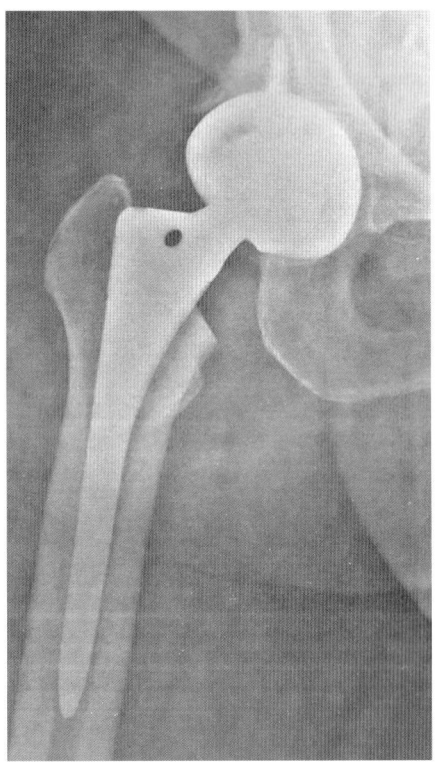

Another cementless hip replaced in a case of a 43 year old patient with idiopathic avascular necrosis with secondary osteoarthrosis.

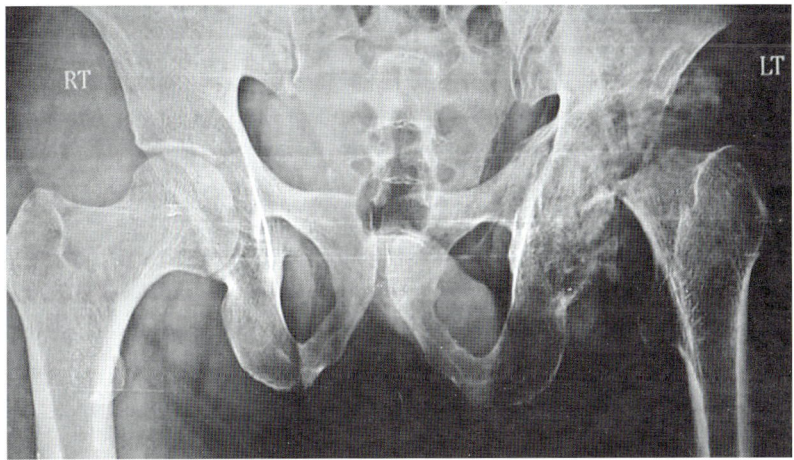

A case of old tuberculosis of the hip with massive destruction and damage to the joint. The acetabulum has deformed superiorly, and the head is high riding

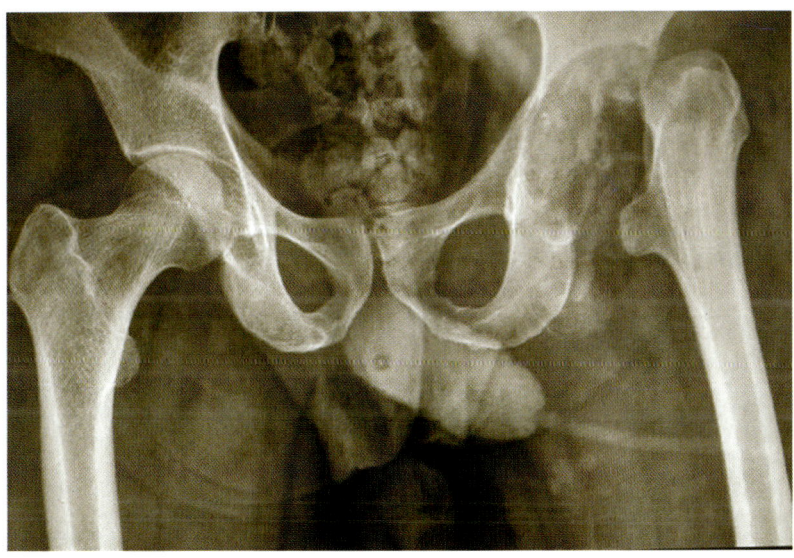

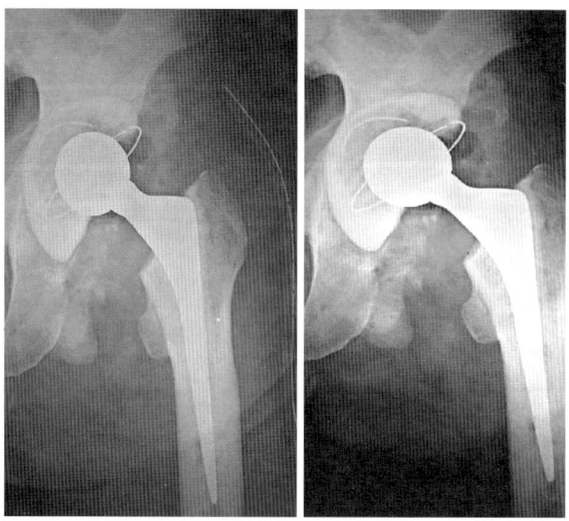

Immidiate post op and three years later. Patient is asymptomatic with excellent clinical results.

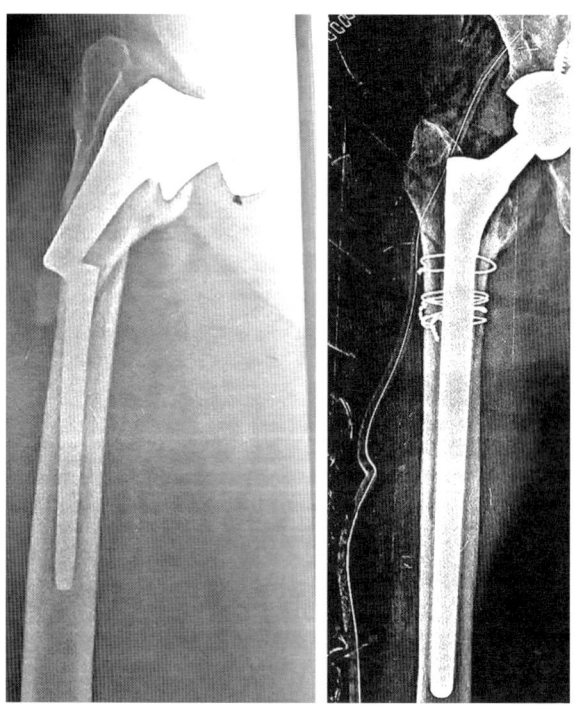

A broken bipolar hip converted to a distal fit cementless hip with correct seating of the components.

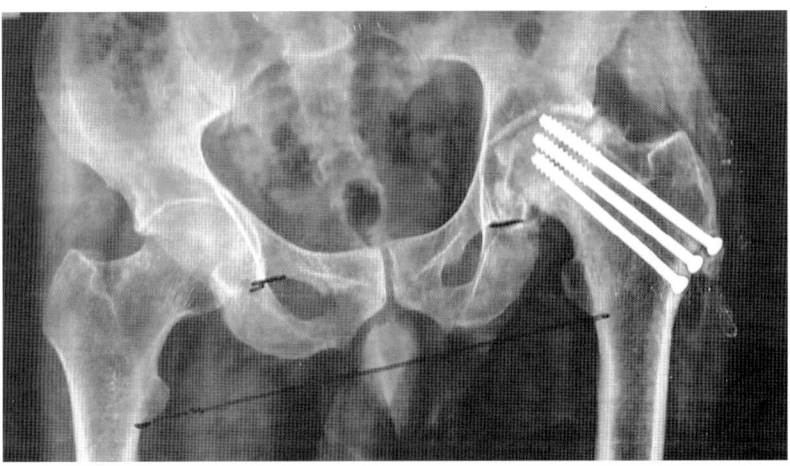

A porous coated stem and cup in a case of a 58 year old with post traumatic avascular necrosis of the femoral head.

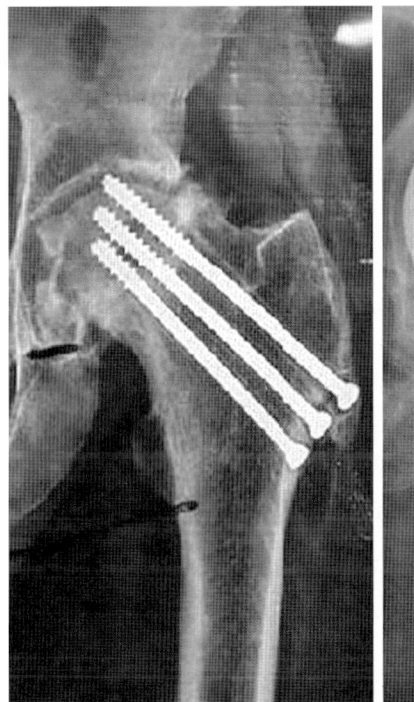 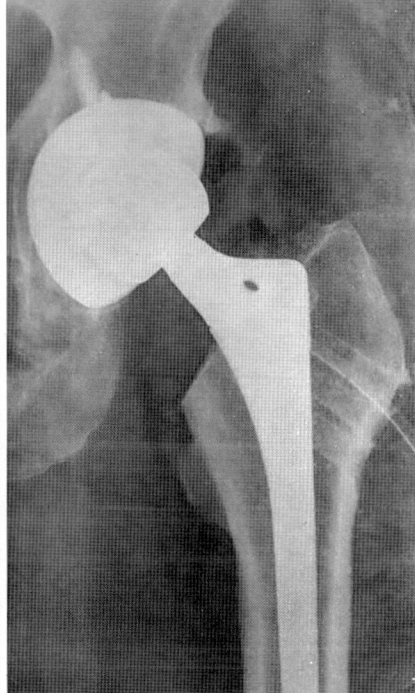

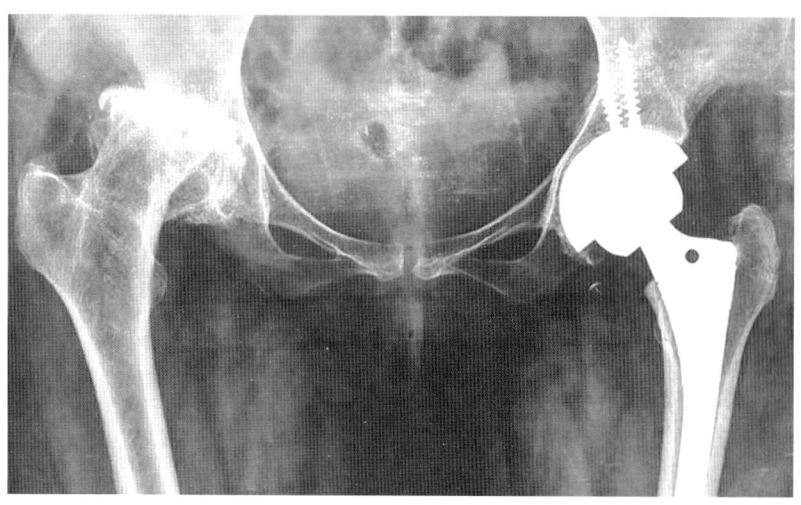

Bilateral Avascular necrosis treated with a staged bilateral cementless hip replacements.

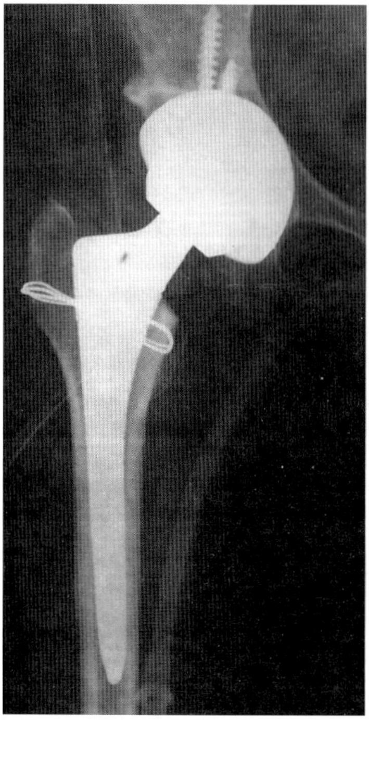

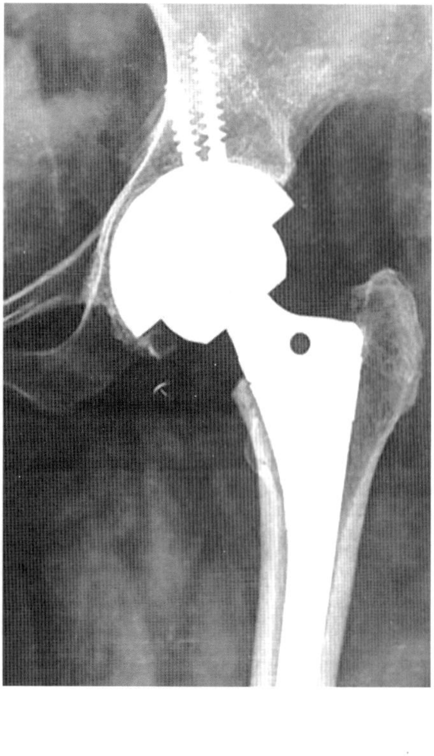

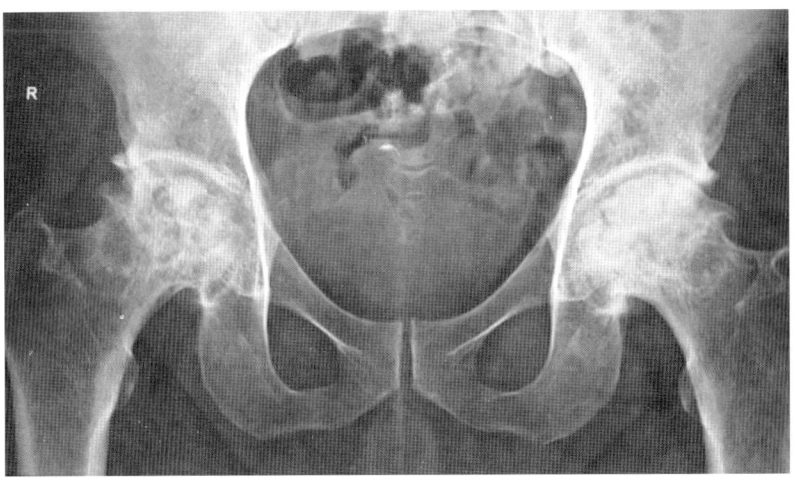

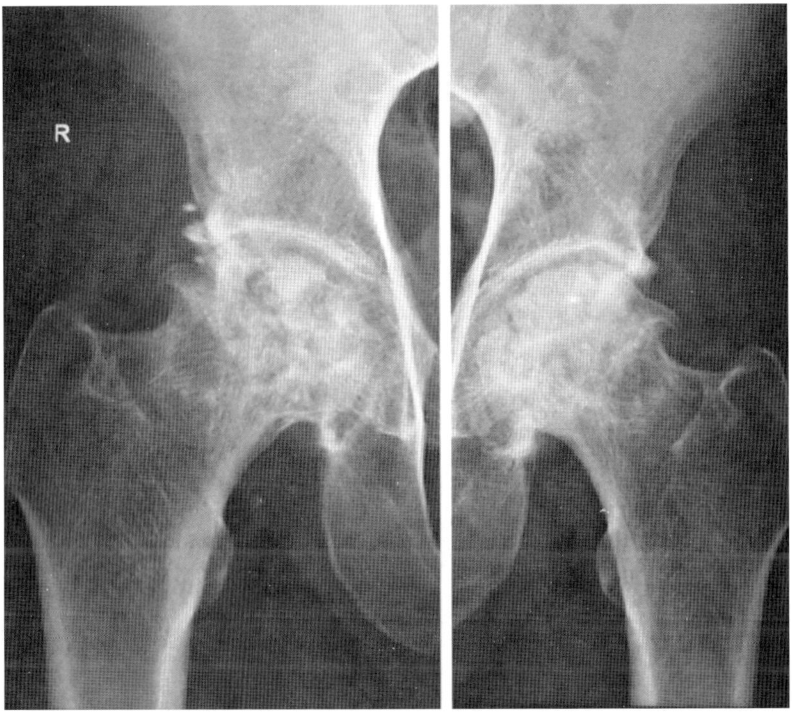

A case of bilateral rheumatoid arthritis with severe destruction of both hip joints.

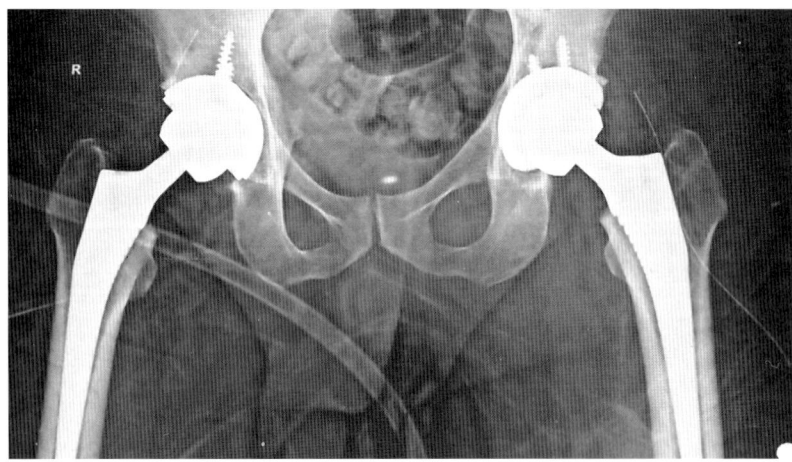

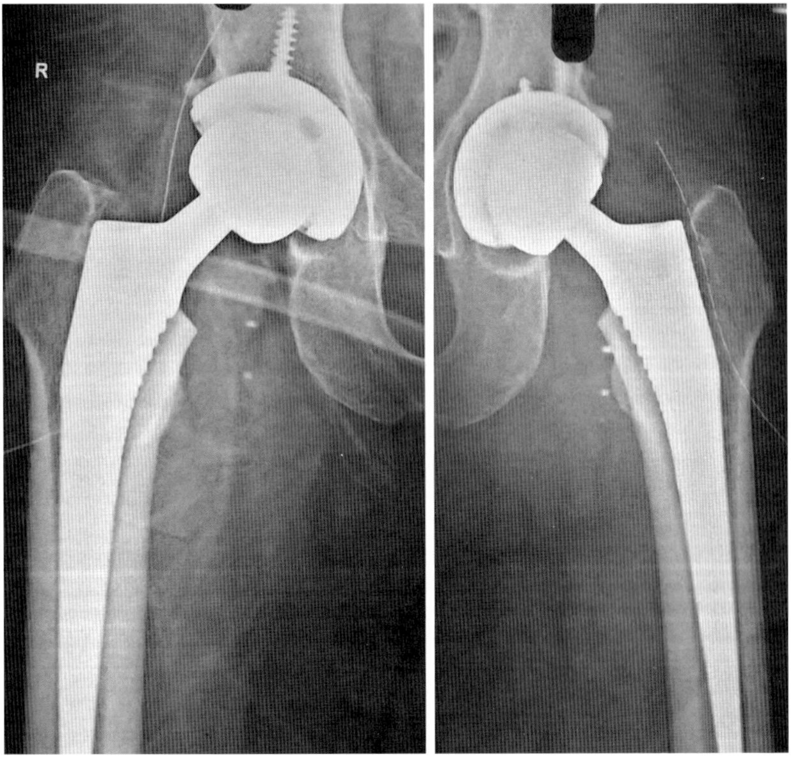

Treated with bilateral replacements, the components have been placed correctly.

Bibliography

1. Abrahams TG, Crothers OD. Radiographic analysis of an investigational hydroxyapatite-coated total hip replacement. Invest Radiol 1992;27: 779–784.

2. Agnelli G, Volpato R, Radicchia S, et al. Detection of asymptomatic deep vein thrombosis by real-time B-mode ultrasonography in hip surgery patients. Thromb Haemost1992;68:257–260.

3. Ahnfelt L, Herberts P, Malchau H, Anderson G. Prognosis of total hip replacement. Acta Orthop Scand (Suppl 238).

4. Ali Khan MA, Brakenbury PH, Reynolds IS. Dislocation following total hip replacement. J Bone Joint Surg Br.1981;63-B(2):214–218.

5. Altman DG. Better reporting of randomised controlled trials: the CONSORT statement. BMJ. 1996;313:570–571.

6. Amstutz HC, Yao J, Dorey FJ, Nugent JP. Survival analysis of T-28 hip arthroplasty with clinical implications. Orthop Clin North Am. 1988;19:491–503.

7. Anderson DR, O' Brien BJ, Levine MN, Roberts R, Wells PS, Hirsh J. Efficacy and cost of low-molecular-weight heparin compared with standard heparin for the prevention of deep vein thrombosis after total hip arthroplasty. Ann Intern Med 1993;119:1105–1112.

8. Arabmotlagh M, Rittmeister M, Hennigs T. Alendronate prevents femoral periprosthetic bone loss following total hip arthroplasty: prospective randomized double-blind study J Orthop Res 2006; 24: 1336–1341.

9. Atik M, Harkess JW, Wichman H. Prevention of fatal pulmonary embolism. *Surg Gynecol Obstet.* 1970 Mar;130(3):403–413.

10. Beckenbaugh RD, llstrup DM. Total hip arthroplasty. J Bone Joint Surg lAml 1978:60–A;306–313.

11. Belmont PJ Jr, Powers CC, Beykirch SE, Hopper RH Jr, Engh CA Jr, Engh CA. Results of the anatomic medullary locking total hip arthroplasty at a minimum of twenty years: A concise follow-up of previous reports. J Bone Joint Surg Am 2008;90:1524–1530.

12. Bergqvist D, Fredin H. Pulmonary embolism and mortality in patients with fractured hips—a prospective consecutive series. Eur J Surg 1991; 157:571–574.

13. Bergqvist D, Lindblad B, Matzsch T. Low molecular weight heparin for thromboprophylaxis and epidural/spinal anaesthesia—is there a risk? Acta Anaesthesiol Scand 1992;36:605–609.

14. Bergqvist D, Lindblad B. A 30-year survey of pulmonary embolism verified at autopsy: an analysis of 1274 surgical patients. Br J Surg 1985; 72:105–108.

15. Bergqvist D, Lindgren B, Mätzsch T. Cost-effectiveness of preventing postoperative deep vein thrombosis. In: Hull R, Pineo G, eds. Disorders of thrombosis. Philadelphia: W.B. Saunders, 1996:228–233.

16. Berry DJ, Harmsen WS, Cabanela ME, Morrey BF. Twenty-five-year survivorship of two thousand consecutive primary Charnley total hip replacements: factors affecting survivorship of acetabular and femoral components. J Bone Joint Surg Am. 2002;84A:171–177.

17. Bhandari M, Bajammal S, Guyatt GH, Griffith L, Busse JW, Schünemann H, et al. Effect of bisphosphonates on periprosthetic bone mineral density after total joint arthroplasty: a meta-analysis. J Bone Joint Surg Am 2005; 87:293–301.

18. Bjerkholt H, Hovik O, Reikeras O. Direct comparison of polyethylene wear in cemented and uncemented acetabular cups. J Orthop Traumatol. 2010;11:155–158. [PMC free article].

19. Bjorgul K, Novicoff WM, Andersen ST, et al. No differences in outcomes between cemented and uncemented acetabular components after 12–14 years: results from a randomized controlled trial comparing Duraloc with Charnley cups. J Orthop Traumatol.2010;11:37–45. [PMC free article].

20. Bordini B, Stea S, De Clerico M, et al. Factors affecting aseptic loosening of 4750 total hip arthroplasties: multivariate survival analysis. BMC Musculoskelet Disord. 2007;8:69. [PMC free article].

21. Borris LC, Lassen MR, Jensen HP, Andersen BS, Poulsen KS. Perioperative thrombosis prophylaxis with low molecular weight heparins in elective hip surgery: clinical and economic considerations. Int J Clin Pharmacol Ther 1994;32:262–268.

22. Bourne RB, Rorabeck CH, Laupacis A, et al. A randomized clinical trial comparing cemented to cementless total hip replacement in 250 osteoarthritic patients: the impact on health related quality of life and cost effectiveness. Iowa Orthop J.1994;14:108–114. [PMC free article] .

23. Bryant MJ, Kernohan WG, Nixon JR, Mollan RA. A statistical analysis of hip scores. *J Bone Joint Surg Br.* 1993 Sep;75(5):705–709.

24. Bugbee WD, Culpepper WJ 2nd, Engh CA Jr, Engh CA Sr. Longterm clinical consequences of stress-shielding after total hip arthroplasty without cement. J Bone Joint Surg Am 1997;79:1007–1012.

25. Campbell AC, Rorabeck CH, Bourne RB, Chess D, Nott L. Thigh pain after cementless hip arthroplasty. Annoyance or ill omen. *J Bone Joint Surg Br.* 1992 Jan;74(1):63–66.

26. Carlsson AS, Gentz CF. Radiographic versus clinical loosening of the acetabular component in noninfected total hip arthroplasty.Clin Orthop Relat Res. 1984:145–150.

27. Chambers B, St. Clair SF, Froimson MI. Hydroxyapatite-coated tapered cementless femoral components in total hip arthroplasty. J Arthroplasty 2007;22(suppl 1):71–74.

28. Chandran P, Azzabi M, Miles J, et al. Furlong hydroxyapatite-coated hip prosthesis vs the Charnley cemented hip prosthesis. J Arthroplasty. 2010;25:52–57.

29. Charnley J, Eftekhar N. Postoperative infection in total prosthetic replacement arthroplasty of the hip-joint. With special reference to the bacterial content of the air of the operating room. *Br J Surg.* 1969 Sep;56(9):641–649.

30. Charnley J, Kamangar A, Longfield MD. The optimum size of prosthetic heads in relation to the wear of plastic sockets in total replacement of the hip. *Med Biol Eng.* 1969 Jan;7(1):31–39.

31. Charnley J. Arthroplasty of the hip. A new operation. *Lancet.*1961 May 27;1(7187):1129–1132.

32. Charnley J. Surgery of the hip-joint: present and future developments. Br Med J. 1960;1:821–826. [PMC free article].

33. Charnley J. The long-term results of low-friction arthroplasty of the hip performed as a primary intervention. J Bone Joint Surg [Br] 1 972;54-B: 61–76.

34. Charnley J. Total hip replacement by low-friction arthroplasty. *Clin Orthop Relat Res.* 1970 Sep-Oct;72:7–21.

35. Clark CR. Cost containment: total joint implants. J Bone Joint Surg Am. 1994;76:799–800.

36. Clement ND, Biant LC, Breusch SJ. Total hip arthroplasty: to cement or not to cement the acetabular socket? A critical review of the literature. Arch Orthop Trauma Surg. 2012;132:411–27.

37. Cook SD, Thomas KA, Haddad RJ. Jr Histologic analysis of retrieved human porous-coated total joint components. Clin Orthop Relat Res. 1988:90–101.

38. Corten K, Bourne RB, Charron KD, et al. What works best, a cemented or cementless primary total hip arthroplasty?: minimum 17-year followup of a randomized controlled trial. Clin Orthop Relat Res. 2011;469:209–17. [PMC free article].

39. Coventry MB, Beckenbaugh RD, Nolan DR, Ustrup DM. 2, 01 2 total hip arthroplasties: a study of postoperative course and early complications.) Bone J#{252}iit Surg IAm] 1974;56-A:273–284.

40. Crowninshield RD, Brand RA, Johnston RC, Milroy JC. An analysis of femoral component stem design in total hip arthroplasty.J Bone Joint Surg Am. 1980;62:68–78.

41. Crowninshield RD, Brand RA , Pedersen DR. (1983) A stress analysis of acetabular reconstruction in protrusio acetabuli. J. Bone Joint Surg. 65-A, 495–499.

42. Crowther JD, Lachiewicz PF. Survival and polyethylene wear of porous-coated acetabular components in patients less than fifty years old: results at nine to fourteen years. J Bone Joint Surg Am 2002;84:729–735.

43. D'aubigne RM, Postel M. Functional results of hip arthroplasty with acrylic prosthesis. *J Bone Joint Surg Am.*1954 Jun;36-A(3):451–475.

44. Dahl OE, Andreassen G, Müller C, et al. The effect of prolonged thromboprophylaxis with dalteparin on the frequency of deep vein thrombosis (DVT) and pulmonary embolism (PE) 35 days after hip replacement surgery (HRS). Thromb Haemost 1995;73:1094–1094 abstract.

45. Dandy Di, Theodorou BC. The management of local complications of total hip replacement by the McKee-Farrar technique. J Bone Joint Surg [Br] 1975;57-B:30–35.

46. Devane PA, Robinson EJ, Bourne RB, et al. Measurement of polyethylene wear in acetabular components inserted with and without cement. A randomized trial. J Bone Joint Surg Am.1997;79:682–689.

47. Dorey F, Grigoris P, Amstutz H. Making do without randomised trials. J Bone Joint Surg Br. 1994;76:1–3.

48. Dorr LD, Wan Z, Song M, Ranawat A. Bilateral total hip arthroplasty comparing hydroxyapatite coating to porous-coated fixation. J Arthroplasty 1998;13:729–736.

49. Editorial. Quality control of implants. Acta Orthop Scand 48–55. 1990; 61: 1–33. 1987: 58: 477–478.

50. Eichler, J. (1973) Ein Vorschlag zur operativen Behandlung der F'rotrusio Acetabuli. Arch. Orthop. Unfall-Chir. 75, 76–80.

51. Engesaeter LB, Espehaug B, Lie SA, et al. Does cement increase the risk of infection in primary total hip arthroplasty? Revision rates in 56, 275 cemented and uncemented primary THAs followed for 0–16 years in the Norwegian Arthroplasty Register.Acta Orthop. 2006;77:351–358.

52. Engh CA Jr, Claus AM, Hopper RH Jr, Engh CA. Long-term results using the anatomic medullary locking hip prosthesis. Clin Orthop 2001; 393:137–146.

53. Engh CA, Bobyn JD, Glassman AH. Porous-coated hip replacement. The factors governing bone ingrowth, stress shielding, and clinical results. J Bone Joint Surg Br. 1987;69:45–55.

54. Engh CA, Hooten JP Jr, Zettl-Schaffer KF, Ghaffarpour M, McGovern TF, Macalino GE, et al. Porous-coated total hip replacement. Clin Orthop 1994;298:89–96.

55. Engh CA, Hopper RH Jr. The odyssey of porous-coated fixation. J Arthroplasty 2002;17(suppl 1):102–107.

56. Engh CA, Massin P, Suthers KE. Roentgenographic assessment of the biologic fixation of porous-surfaced femoral components. Clin Orthop 1990;257:107–128.

57. Engh CA, Massin P. Cementless total hip arthroplasty using the anatomic medullary locking stem: results using a survivorship analysis. Clin Orthop 1989;249:141–158.

58. Engh CA, Massin P. Cementless total hip replacement using the AML stem: 0–10 years results using a survivorship analysis. Nippon Seikeigeka Gakkai Zasshi 1989;63:653–666.

59. Eriksson BI, Zachrisson BE, Teger-Nilsson AC, Risberg B. Thrombosis prophylaxis with low molecular weight heparin in total hip replacement. Br J Surg 1988;75:1053–1057.

60. Eskelinen A, Remes V, Helenius I, et al. Total hip arthroplasty for primary osteoarthrosis in younger patients in the Finnish arthroplasty register. 4, 661 primary replacements followed for 0–22 years. Acta Orthop. 2005;76:28–41.

61. Etlenne A, Cupic Z, Charnley J. Postoperative dislocation after Charnley low-friction arthroplasty. Clin Orthop 1978;132:19–23.

62. Evarts CM, Feil EI. Thromboembolism after elective surgery of the hip. Detection, natural history, prophylaxis, and results with low molecular weight dextran. *Orthop Clin North Am.*1971 Mar;2(1):167–174.

63. Faro LMC, Huiskes R. Quality assurance of joint replacement. Acta Orthop Scand (Suppl 250) 1992; 63.

64. Fogelberg EV, Zitzmann EK, Stinchfield FE. Prophylactic penicillin in orthopaedic surgery. *J Bone Joint Surg Am.* 1970 Jan;52(1):95–98.

65. Fowler JL, Gie GA, Lee AJ, Ling RS. Experience with the Exeter total hip replacement since 1970. *Orthop Clin North Am.* 1988 Jul;19(3):477–489.

66. Furlong RJ, Osborn JF. Fixation of hip prostheses by hydroxyapatite ceramic coatings. *J Bone Joint Surg Br.* 1991 Sep;73(5):741–745.

67. Gaffey JL, Callaghan JJ, Pedersen DR, Goetz DD, Sullivan PM, Johnston RC. Cementless acetabular fixation at fifteen years: a comparison with the same surgeon's results following acetabular fixation with cement. *J Bone Joint Surg Am* 2004;86:257–261.

68. Garellick G, Malchau H, Herberts P. Survival of hip replacements. A comparison of a randomized trial and a registry.Clin Orthop Relat Res. 2000:157–67.

69. Ginsberg JS, Caco CC, Brill-Edwards PA, et al. Venous thrombosis in patients who have undergone major hip or knee surgery: detection with compression US and impedance plethysmography. Radiology 1991;181:651–654.

70. Godsiff SP, Emery RJ, Heywood-Waddington MB, Thomas TL. Cemented versus uncemented femoral components in the ring hip prosthesis. J Bone Joint Surg Br. 1992;74:822–824.

71. González Della Valle A, Ruzo PS, Li S, Pellicci P, Sculco TP, Salvati EA. Dislodgment of polyethylene liners in first and second-generation Harris-Galante acetabular components: a report of eighteen cases. J Bone Joint Surg Am 2001;83:553–559.

72. Grant P, Aamodt A, Falch J, Nordsletten L. Differences in stability and bone remodeling between a customized uncemented hydrox-yapatite coated and a standard cemented femoral stem. A randomized study with use of radiostereometry and bone densitometry. J Orthop Res. 2005;23:1280–1285.

73. Hailer NP, Garellick G, Karrholm J. Uncemented and cemented primary total hip arthroplasty in the Swedish Hip Arthroplasty Register. Acta Orthop. 2010;81:34–41. [PMC free article]

74. Hampson WGJ, Harris FC, Lucas HK, et al. Failure of low-dose heparin to prevent deep-vein thrombosis after hip-replacement arthroplasty. Lancet 1974;2:795–797.

75. Harada Y, Mitsuhashi S, Suzuki C, Yamashita K, Watanabe H, Akita T, et al. Anatomically designed prosthesis without cement for the treatment of osteoarthritis due to developmental dysplasia of the hip: 6-to 13-year follow-up study. J Orthop Sci 2007;12:127–133.

76. Harris WH, McGann WA. Loosening of the femoral component after use of the medullary-plug cementing technique. Follow-up note with a minimum five-year follow-up. J Bone Joint Surg Am.1986;68:1064–1066.

77. Harris WH. One step back; two steps forward. J Bone Joint Surg Am. 1993 Jul;75(7):959–960.

78. Harris WH, Jones WN. (1975) The use of wire mesh in total hip replacement. Clin. Orthop.106.

79. Hartofilakidis G, Georgiades G, Babis GC. A comparison of the outcome of cemented all-polyethylene and cementless metal-backed acetabular sockets in primary total hip arthroplasty. J Arthroplasty. 2009;24: 217–225.

80. Havelin LI, Engesaeter LB, Espehaug B, et al. The Norwegian Arthroplasty Register: 11 years and 73,000 arthroplasties. Acta Orthop Scand. 2000;71:337–353.

81. Hearn SL, Bicalho PS, Eng K, et al. Comparison of cemented and cementless total hip arthroplasty in patients with bilateral hip arthroplasties. J Arthroplasty. 1995;10:603–608.

82. Hendricks KJ, Harris WH. High placement of noncemented acetabular components in revision total hip arthroplasty: a concise follow-up, at a minimum of fifteen years, of a previous report. J Bone Joint Surg Am 2006;88:2231–2236.

83. Henrichsen E, Jansen K, Krough-Poulsen W. Experimental investigation of the tissue reaction to acrylic plastics. Acta Orthop Scand. 1952; 22(2):141–146.

84. Herberts P, Ahnfelt L, Malchau H, Stromberg C, Anderson G B J. Multi-centre clinical trials and their value in assessing total joint arthroplasty. Clin Orthop 1989; 249.

85. Heywood AWB. (1980) Arthroplasty with a solid bone graft for protrusio acetabuli. J. Bone Joint Surg. 62-B, 332–336.

86. Hooper GJ, Rothwell AG, Stringer M, Frampton C. Revision following cemented and uncemented primary total hip replacement: a seven-year analysis from the New Zealand Joint Registry. J Bone Joint Surg Br. 2009;91:451–458.

87. Hozack WJ, Rothman RH, Booth RE, Jr, et al. Survivorship analysis of 1, 041 Charnley total hip arthroplasties. J Arthroplasty.1990;5:41–47.

88. Huber O, Bounameaux H, Borst F, Rohner A. Postoperative pulmonary embolism after hospital discharge: an underestimated risk. Arch Surg 1992;127:310–313.

89. Huddleston HD. Femoral lysis after cemented hip arthroplasty. J Arthroplasty. 1988;3:285–97.

90. Huiskes R. (1979) Some fundamental aspects of human joint replacement. Analysis of stresses and heat conduction in bone prosthesis structures. Acta Orthop. Scand. Suppl. 185.

91. Jacob HAC, Huggler AH, Dietschi C. (1976) Mechanical function of subchondral bone as experimentally determined on the acetabulum of the human pelvis. J. Biomech. 9, 625–627. 117–121. Downloaded by [106.208.163.123] at 19:42 31 May 2016 596.

92. Jorgensen LN, Wille-Jorgensen P, Hauch O. Prophylaxis of postoperative thromboembolism with low molecular weight heparins. Br J Surg 1993;80:689–704.

93. Kaplan EL, Meier P. Nonparametric estimation from incomplete observation. Am Stat Ass Joum 1958: 457–481.

94. Karrholm J, Malchau H, Snorrason F, Herberts P. Micromotion of femoral stems in total hip arthroplasty. A randomized study of cemented, hydroxyapatite-coated, and porous-coated stems with roentgen stereo-photogrammetric analysis. J Bone Joint Surg Am.1994;76:1692–1705.

95. Kawamoto K, Hasegawa Y, Iwase T, Iwasada S, Kanamono T, Iwata H. Failed cementless total hip arthroplasty for osteoarthrosis due to hip dysplasia: a minimum five-year follow-up study. Bull Hosp Joint Dis 1998;57:130–135.

96. Kilgus DJ, Shimaoka EE, Tipton JS, Eberle RW. Dual-energy X-ray absorptiometry measurement of bone mineral density around porous-coated cementless femoral implants: methods and preliminary results. J Bone Joint Surg Br 1993;75:279–287.

97. Kim YH, Oh SH, Kim JS. Incidence and natural history of deep-vein thrombosis after total hip arthroplasty. A prospective and randomised clinical study. J Bone Joint Surg Br. 2003;85:661–665.

98. Kim YH, Suh JS. Low incidence of deep-vein thrombosis after cementless total hip replacement. J Bone Joint Surg Am.1988;70:878–882.

99. Kim YH. Bilateral cemented and cementless total hip arthroplasty. J Arthroplasty. 2002;17:434–440.

100. Kirk PG, Rorabeck CH, Bourne RB, Burkart B. Total hip arthroplasty in rheumatoid arthritis: comparison of cemented and uncemented implants. Can J Surg. 1993;36:229–32.

101. Kristiansen P, Bergentz SE, Bergqvist D, Nylander G. Thrombosis after elective phlebography as demonstrated with the 125I-fibrinogen test. Acta Radiol Diagn (Stockh)1981;22:577–580.

102. Laupacis A, Bourne R, Rorabeck C, et al. Comparison of total hip arthroplasty performed with and without cement: a randomized trial. J Bone Joint Surg Am. 2002; 84A:1823–1828.

103. Lazansky MG. Complications in total hip replacement with Charnley technic. C!in Orthop 1970;72:40–45.

104. Leizorovicz A, Haugh MC, Chapuis FR, Samama MM, Boissel JP. Low molecular weight heparin in prevention of perioperative thrombosis. BMJ 1992;305:913–920.

105. Lewinnek GE, Lewis JL, Tarr R, Compere CL, Zimmerman JR. Dislocations after total hip-replacement arthroplasties. J Bone Joint Surg [Am] 1 978;60-A:2 I 7.

106. Leyvraz PF, Bachmann F, Hoek J, et al. Prevention of deep vein thrombosis after hip replacement: randomised comparison between unfractionated heparin and low molecular weight heparin. BMJ 1991;303:543–548[Erratum, BMJ 1991;303:1243.].

107. Lidwell OM, Lowbury EJ, Whyte W, Blowers R, Stanley SJ, Lowe D. Effect of ultraclean air in operating rooms on deep sepsis in the joint after total hip or knee replacement: a randomised study. *Br Med J (Clin Res Ed)* 1982 Jul 3;285(6334):10–14. [PMC free article]

108. Lucht U. The Danish Hip Arthroplasty Register. Acta Orthop Scand. 2000;71:433–439.

109. Makela KT, Eskelinen A, Pulkkinen P, et al. Total hip arthroplasty for primary osteoarthritis in patients fifty-five years of age or older. An analysis of the Finnish arthroplasty registry. J Bone Joint Surg Am. 2008;90:2160–2170.

110. Malchau H, Herberts P, Eisler T, et al. The Swedish Total Hip. Replacement Register. J Bone Joint Surg Am. 2002;84A (Suppl 2): 2–20.

111. Malchau H, Herberts P, Eisler T, Garellick G, Söderman P. The Swedish Total Hip Replacement Register. J Bone Joint Surg Am 2002;84 (suppl 2): 2–20.

112. Maloney WJ. National joint replacement registries: has the time come? J Bone Joint Surg Am. 2001;83A:1582–1585.

113. Mannucci PM, Citterio LE, Panajotopoulos N. Low-dose heparin and deep-vein thrombosis after total hip replacement. Thromb Haemost 1976;36:157–164.

114. Marston RA, Cobb AG, Bentley G. Stanmore compared with Charnley total hip replacement. A prospective study of 413 arthroplasties. J Bone Joint Surg Br. 1996;78:178–184.

115. McCollum DE, Nunley JA, Harrelson JM. (1980) Bone grafting in total hip replacement for acetabular protrusion. J. Bone Joint Surg. 62 A, 1065–1073.

116. McCollum DE, Nunley JA. (1978) Bone grafting in acetabular protrusio. A biologic buttress. In: The Hip: Proceedings of the sixth open scientific meeting of the Hip Society, pp. 124–146. C. V. Mosby, St. Louis.

117. McCombe P, Williams SA. A comparison of polyethylene wear rates between cemented and cementless cups: a prospective, randomised trial. J Bone Joint Surg Br 2004;86:344–349.

118. McKee GK, Watson-Farrar J. Replacement of arthritic hips by the McKee-Farrar prosthesis. J Bone Joint Surg Br 1966;48:245–259.

119. McKee GK. Development of total prosthetic replacement of the hip. C!in Orthop 1970;72:85–l03.

120. McNally MA, Mollan RA. Venous thromboembolism and orthopaedic surgery. J Bone Joint Surg Br. 1993 Jul;75(4):517–519.

121. McNally MA, Mollan RAB. Total hip replacement, lower limb blood flow and venous thrombogenesis. J Bone Joint Surg Br 1993;75:640–644.

122. Moher D, Liberati A, Tetzlaff J, Altman DG. Preferred reporting items for systematic reviews and meta-analyses: the PRISMA statement. Int J Surg. 2010;8:336–341.

123. Mohr DN, Silverstein MD, Murtaugh PA, Harrison JM. Prophylactic agents for venous thrombosis in elective hip surgery: meta-analysis of studies using venographic assessment. Arch Intern Med 1993;153:2221–2228.

124. Möller G, Goldie I, Jonsson E. Hospital care versus home care for rehabilitation after hip replacement. Int J Technol Assess Health Care. 1992 Winter;8(1):93–101.

125. Morris J, Nicholson OR. A comparison between the Charnley low-friction hip arthroplasty and the McKee-Farrar all-metal hip joint. J Bone Joint Surg [Br] 1970;52-B:780–781.

126. Morshed S, Bozic KJ, Ries MD, et al. Comparison of cemented and uncemented fixation in total hip replacement: a meta-analysis. Acta Orthop. 2007;78:315–326.

127. Morshed S, Bozic KJ, Ries MD, Malchau H, Colford JM Jr. Comparison of cemented and uncemented fixation in total hip replacement: a meta-analysis. Acta Orthop 2007;78:315–326.

128. Mulliken B, Nayak N, Bourne R, et al. Early radiographic results comparing cemented and cementless total hip arthroplasty. J Arthroplasty. 1996;11:24–33.

129. Mulroy RD, Harris WH. The effect of improved cementing techniques on component loosening in total hip replacement. J Bone Joint Surg (Br) 1990; 72: 757–760.

130. National Joint Registry. The 2011 National Joint registry data for England and Wales. [Accessed: January 2013]; Available from:http://www.njrcentre.org.uk.

131. Nicolaides A, Arcelus J, Belcaro G, et al. Prevention of venous thromboembolism. Int Angiol 1992;11:151–159.

132. Nolan DR, Fitzgerald RH Jr, Beckenbaugh RD, Coventry MB. Complications of total hip arthroplasty treated by reoperation. J Bone Joint Surg [An] I 975 ;57-A:977–8 I.

133. Nurmohamed MT, Rosendaal FR, Buller HR, et al. Low molecular weight heparin versus standard heparin in general and orthopaedic surgery: a meta-analysis. Lancet1992;340:152–156.

134. Olsson SS, Jernberger A, Tryggö D. Clinical and radiological long-term results after Charnley-Müller total hip replacement: a 5 to 10 year follow-up study with special reference to aseptic loosening. Acta Orthop Scand 1981;52:531–542.

135. Onsten I, Carlsson AS. Cemented versus uncemented socket in hip arthroplasty. A radiostereometric study of 60 randomized hips followed for 2 years. Acta Orthop Scand. 1994;65:517–521.

136. Paiement GD, Schutzer SF, Wessinger SJ, Harris WH. Influence of prophylaxis on proximal venous thrombus formation after total hip arthroplasty. J Arthroplasty 1992;7:471–475.

137. Pakvis D, van Hellemondt G, de Visser E, et al. Is there evidence for a superior method of socket fixation in hip arthroplasty? A systematic review. Int Orthop. 2011;35:1109–1118.[PMC free article]

138. Parker SM, Hastings DC. (1974) Protrusio acetabuli in rheumatoid arthritis. J. Bone Joint Surg.

139. Paulsen A, Pedersen AB, Johnsen SP, Riis A, Lucht U, Overgaard S. Effect of hydroxyapatite coating on risk of revision after primary total hip arthroplasty in younger patients: findings from the Danish Hip Arthroplasty Registry. Acta Orthop 2007;78:622–628.

140. Pedersen DR, Crowninshield RD, Brand RA, Johnston RC. (1982) An axisymmetric model of acetabular components in total hip arthroplasty. J. Biomech. 15, 305–315.

141. Pekman WM 8c, Brown ThD. (1982) A finite element analysis of acetabular reconstruction following metastatic bone loss. In: Bio-mechanics Symposium, (Ed: Woo, S. L. Y.). A.M.D., Vol. 56, pp. 43–44. ASME. New York. 56-B, 587.

142. Peter B, Pioletti DP, Laïb S, Bujoli B, Pilet P, Janvier P, et al. Calcium phosphate drug delivery system: influence of local zoledronate release on bone implant osteointegration. Bone 2005;36:52–60.

143. Planes A, Vochelle N, Fagola M, et al. Persistence of the risk of deep venous thrombosis after hospital discharge in patients undergoing total hip replacement. Lancet (in press).

144. Planes A, Vochelle N, Fagola M. Total hip replacement and deep vein thrombosis: a venographic and necropsy study. J Bone Joint Surg Br 1990;72:9–13.

145. Planes A, Vochelle N, Mazas F, et al. Prevention of postoperative venous thrombosis: a randomized trial comparing unfractionated heparin with low molecular weight heparin in patients undergoing total hip replacement. Thromb Haemost 1988;60:407–410.

146. Pollard JP, Hughes SP, Scott JE, Evans MJ, Benson MK. Antibiotic prophylaxis in total hip replacement. Br Med J.1979 Mar 17;1(6165):707–709. [PMC free article].

147. Reigstad A, Rokkum M, Bye K, Brandt M. Femoral remodeling after arthroplasty of the hip. Prospective randomized 5-year comparison of 120 cemented/uncemented cases of arthrosis. Acta Orthop Scand. 1993;64:411–416.

148. Richards DJ. The results of Howse arthroplasty of the hip. J Bone Joint Surg [Br] 1978;60-B:137. Ring PA. Total replacement of the hip joint. J Bone Joint Surg [Br] 1974;56-B:44–58.

149. Ring PA. Complete replacement arthroplasty of the hip by the Ring prosthesis. J Bone Joint Surg Br 1968;50:720–731.

150. Roder C, Bach B, Berry DJ, et al. Obesity, age, sex, diagnosis, and fixation mode differently affect early cup failure in total hip arthroplasty: a matched case-control study of 4420 patients. J Bone Joint Surg Am. 2010; 92:1954–1963.

151. Roffman M, Silberman M, Mendes DG. (1982) Viability and osteogenicity of bone graft coated with methylmethacrylate cement. Acta Orthop. Scand. 53, 513–519.

152. Roffman M, Silberman M, Mendes DG. (1983) Incorporation of bone graft covered with methylmethacrylate onto acetabular wall. Acta Orthop. Scand. 54, 580–583.

153. Rorabeck CH, Bourne RB, Laupacis A, et al. A double-blind study of 250 cases comparing cemented with cementless total hip arthroplasty. Cost-effectiveness and its impact on health-related quality of life. Clin Orthop Relat Res. 1994:156–164.

154. Rorabeck CH, Bourne RB, Mulliken BD, et al. The Nicolas Andry award: comparative results of cemented and cementless total hip arthroplasty. Clin Orthop Relat Res. 1996:330–344.

155. Roth A, Winzer T, Sander K, Anders JO, Venbrocks RA. Press fit fixation of cementless cups: how much stability do we need indeed? Arch Orthop Trauma Surg 2006;126:77–81.

156. Rothman RH, Cohn JC. Cemented versus cementless total hip arthroplasty. A critical review. Clin Orthop Relat Res. 1990:153–169.

157. Russotti GM, Harris WH. Proximal placement of the acetabular component in total hip arthroplasty: a long-term follow-up study. J Bone Joint Surg Am 1991;73:587–592.

158. Salvati EA, Bullough P, Wilson PD Jr. (1975) Intrapelvic protrusion of the acetabular component following total hip replacement. Clin. Orth.

159. Santavirta S, Hoikka V, Eskola A, Konttinen YT, Paavilainen T, Tallroth K. Aggressive granulomatous lesions in cementless total hip arthroplasty. *J Bone Joint Surg Br.* 1990 Nov;72(6):980–984.

160. Schatzker J, Hastings DE, Broom RJ. (1979) Acetabular reinforcement in total hip replacement. Acta Orthop. Z'raumat. Surg. 94, 135–141.

161. Schmalzried TP, Brown IC, Amstutz HC, Engh CA, Harris WH. The role of acetabular component screw holes and/or screws in the development of pelvic osteolysis. Proc Inst Mech Eng [H] 1999;213: 147–153.

162. Schmalzried TP, Harris WH. The Harris-Galante porous-coated acetabular component with screw fixation. Radiographic analysis of eighty-three primary hip replacements at a minimum of five years. *J Bone Joint Surg Am.* 1992 Sep; 74(8):1130–1139.

163. Schneider, R. (1980) Die Armierung der Pfanne bei der Totalendoprothese der Hufte. Unfallheilk. 83, 482–488.

164. Schroder HM, Andreassen M. Autopsy-verified major pulmonary embolism after hip fracture. Clin Orthop 1993;293:196–203.

165. Sculco TP, Ranawat C. The use of spinal anesthesia for total hip-replacement arthroplasty. *J Bone Joint Surg Am.* 1975 Mar;57(2):173–177.

166. Scurr JH, Coleridge-Smith PD, Hasty JH. Deep venous thrombosis: a continuing problem.BMJ 1988;297:28.

167. Sevitt S, Gallagher N. Venous thrombosis and pulmonary embolism: a clinico-pathological study in injured and burned patients. Br J Surg 1961;48:475–489.

168. Shih CH, Lee PC, Chen JH, Tai CL, Chen LF, Wu JS, et al. Measurement of polyethylene wear in cementless total hip arthroplasty. J Bone Joint Surg Br 1997;79:361–365.

169. Sinha RK, Dungy DS, Yeon HB. Primary total hip arthroplasty with a proximally porous-coated femoral stem. J Bone Joint Surg Am. 2004;86A:1254–1261.

170. Sotelo-Garza A, Charnley J. (1978) The result of Charnley arthroplasty of the hip performed for protrusion acetabuli. Clin. Orthop. 132, 12–18.

171. Stamatakis JD, Kakkar VV, Sagar S, Lawrence D, Nairn D, Bentley PG. Femoral vein thrombosis and total hip replacement. BMJ 1977;2: 223–225.

172. Strom Hk, Kolstad K, Mallmin H, Sahlstedt B, Milbrink J. Comparison of the uncemented Cone and the cemented Bimetric hip prosthesis in

young patients with osteoarthritis: an RSA, clinical and radiographic study. Acta Orthop. 2006;77:71–78.

173. Sutherland CJ, Wilde AH, Borden LS, Marks KE. A ten-year follow-up of one hundred consecutive Müller curved-stem total hip-replacement arthroplasties. J Bone Joint Surg Am 1982;64:970–982.

174. T. J. J. H. Slooff et al. Marti RK, Besselaar PP. (1983) Bone grafts in primary and secondary total hip replacement. In: Progress in cemented total hip surgery and reuision. pp. 107–130. Excerpta Medica, Elsevier Science Publishers, Amsterdam.

175. Thanner J, Kärrholm J, Herberts P, Malchau H. Porous cups with and without hydroxylapatite-tricalcium phosphate coating: 23 matched pairs evaluated with radiostereometry. J Arthroplasty 1999;14:266–271.

176. Trowbridge A, Boese CK, Woodruff B, Brindley HH Sr, Lowry WE, Spiro TE. Incidence of posthospitalization proximal deep venous thrombosis after total hip arthroplasty: a pilot study. Clin Orthop 1994; 299:203–208.

177. Turpie AGG, Levine MN, Hirsh J, et al. A randomized controlled trial of a low-molecular-weight heparin (enoxaparin) to prevent deep-vein thrombosis in patients undergoing elective hip surgery. N Engl J Med 1986;315:925–929.

178. Unnanuntana A, Dimitroulias A, Bolognesi MP, et al. Cementless femoral prostheses cost more to implant than cemented femoral prostheses. Clin Orthop Relat Res. 2009;467:1546–1551.[PMC free article].

179. Vandermeulen EP, Van Aken H, Vermylen J. Anticoagulants and spinal-epidural anesthesia. Anesth Analg 1994;79:1165–1177.

180. Warwick D, Williams MH, Bannister GC. Death and thromboembolic disease after total hip replacement: a series of 1162 cases with no routine chemical prophylaxis. J Bone Joint Surg Br 1995;77:6–10.

181. Weiss RJ, Hailer NP, Stark A, Karrholm J. Survival of uncemented acetabular monoblock cups: evaluation of 210 hips in the Swedish Hip Arthroplasty Register. Acta Orthop. 2012;83:214–219. [PMC free article].

182. Wejkner B, Stenport J. Charnley total hip arthroplasty. A ten-to 14-year follow-up study. Clin Orthop Relat Res. 1988:113–119.

183. Wells PS, Lensing AW, Davidson BL, Prins MH, Hirsh J. Accuracy of ultrasound for the diagnosis of deep venous thrombosis in asymptomatic patients after orthopaedic surgery: a meta-analysis. Ann Intern Med 1995;122:47–53.

184. Willert HG, Ludwig J, Semlitsch M. (1974) Reaction of bone to methylmethacrylate after hip arthroplasty. J. Bone Joint Surg. 56-A, 1368–1382.

185. Wroblewski BM, Siney PD, Fleming PA. Charnley low-frictional torque arthroplasty in patients under the age of 51 years: followup to 33 years. J Bone Joint Surg Br 2002;84:540–543.

186. Wykman A, Olsson E, Axdorph G, Goldie I. Total hip arthroplasty. A comparison between cemented and press-fit noncemented fixation. J Arthroplasty. 1991;6:19–29.

187. Yoshihara Y, Henmi O, Kawaji Y, Date H, Morita M, Fujikawa K, et al. Quantitative analysis of femoral bone resorption after cementless total hip arthroplasty using AML-A stem. Nippon Jinko Kansetsu Gakkaishi 2003;33:159–160 (in Japanese).

188. Yoshihara Y, Hennmi O, Kawaji Y, Morita M, Date H, Fujikawa K, et al. Assessment of femoral bone resorption after cementless total hip arthroplasty using the AML stem. Hip Joint 2003;29:461–465 (in Japanese).

199. Yoshihara Y, Shiromoto Y, Kaneko M, Kono T, Ohashi K, Morita M, et al. Change of bone absorption of proximal femur after AML: a cementless total hip arthroplasty. Nippon Jinko Kansetsu Gakkaishi 2006;36:92–93 (in Japanese).

190. Zicat B, Engh CA, Gokcen E. Patterns of osteolysis around total hip components inserted with and without cement. J Bone Joint Surg Am. 1995;77:432–439.

191. Zweymuller K. A cementless titanium hip endoprosthesis system based on press-fit fixation: basic research and clinical results. Instr Course Lect. 1986;35:203–225.